REDUCING THE IMPACT OF
DEMENTIA IN AMERICA
A Decadal Survey of the Behavioral and Social Sciences

Committee on the Decadal Survey of Behavioral and
Social Science Research on Alzheimer's Disease and
Alzheimer's Disease-Related Dementias

Board on Behavioral, Cognitive, and Sensory Sciences
Division of Behavioral and Social Sciences and Education

A Consensus Study Report of

The National Academies of
SCIENCES · ENGINEERING · MEDICINE

THE NATIONAL ACADEMIES PRESS
Washington, DC
www.nap.edu

THE NATIONAL ACADEMIES PRESS   500 Fifth Street, NW   Washington, DC 20001

This activity was supported by contracts between the National Academy of Sciences and the AARP (Unnumbered), JPB Foundation (2019-1737), the National Institute on Aging (HHSN263201800029I/75N98020F00001), the National Institutes of Health (NNSN263201800029I/HHSN263000037), Office of the Assistant Secretary for Planning and Evaluation (HHSP233201400020B/75P00119F37098), and U.S. Department of Veterans Affairs (101D93004), with contributions to the project from the Alzheimer's Association, the American Psychological Association, and The John. A. Hartford Foundation. Support for the work of the Board on Behavioral, Cognitive, and Sensory Sciences is provided primarily by a grant from the National Science Foundation (Award No. BCS-1729167). Any opinions, findings, conclusions, or recommendations expressed in this publication do not necessarily reflect the views of any organization or agency that provided support for the project.

International Standard Book Number-13: 978-0-309-49503-5
International Standard Book Number-10: 0-309-49503-2
Digital Object Identifier: https://doi.org/10.17226/26175
Library of Congress Control Number: 2021946373

Additional copies of this publication are available from the National Academies Press, 500 Fifth Street, NW, Keck 360, Washington, DC 20001; (800) 624-6242 or (202) 334-3313; http://www.nap.edu.

Copyright 2021 by the National Academy of Sciences. All rights reserved.

Printed in the United States of America

Suggested citation: National Academies of Sciences, Engineering, and Medicine. (2021). *Reducing the Impact of Dementia in America: A Decadal Survey of the Behavioral and Social Sciences*. Washington, DC: The National Academies Press. https://doi.org/10.17226/26175.

The National Academies of
SCIENCES · ENGINEERING · MEDICINE

The **National Academy of Sciences** was established in 1863 by an Act of Congress, signed by President Lincoln, as a private, nongovernmental institution to advise the nation on issues related to science and technology. Members are elected by their peers for outstanding contributions to research. Dr. Marcia McNutt is president.

The **National Academy of Engineering** was established in 1964 under the charter of the National Academy of Sciences to bring the practices of engineering to advising the nation. Members are elected by their peers for extraordinary contributions to engineering. Dr. John L. Anderson is president

The **National Academy of Medicine** (formerly the Institute of Medicine) was established in 1970 under the charter of the National Academy of Sciences to advise the nation on medical and health issues. Members are elected by their peers for distinguished contributions to medicine and health. Dr. Victor J. Dzau is president.

The three Academies work together as the **National Academies of Sciences, Engineering, and Medicine** to provide independent, objective analysis and advice to the nation and conduct other activities to solve complex problems and inform public policy decisions. The National Academies also encourage education and research, recognize outstanding contributions to knowledge, and increase public understanding in matters of science, engineering, and medicine.

Learn more about the National Academies of Sciences, Engineering, and Medicine at www.nationalacademies.org.

The National Academies of
SCIENCES • ENGINEERING • MEDICINE

Consensus Study Reports published by the National Academies of Sciences, Engineering, and Medicine document the evidence-based consensus on the study's statement of task by an authoring committee of experts. Reports typically include findings, conclusions, and recommendations based on information gathered by the committee and the committee's deliberations. Each report has been subjected to a rigorous and independent peer-review process and it represents the position of the National Academies on the statement of task.

Proceedings published by the National Academies of Sciences, Engineering, and Medicine chronicle the presentations and discussions at a workshop, symposium, or other event convened by the National Academies. The statements and opinions contained in proceedings are those of the participants and are not endorsed by other participants, the planning committee, or the National Academies.

For information about other products and activities of the National Academies, please visit www.nationalacademies.org/about/whatwedo.

COMMITTEE ON THE DECADAL SURVEY OF BEHAVIORAL AND SOCIAL SCIENCE RESEARCH ON ALZHEIMER'S DISEASE AND ALZHEIMER'S DISEASE–RELATED DEMENTIAS

TIA POWELL (*Chair*), Montefiore Health System and Albert Einstein College of Medicine
KAREN S. COOK (*Vice Chair*) (NAS), Stanford University
MARGARITA ALEGRÍA (NAM), Massachusetts General Hospital and Harvard Medical School
DEBORAH BLACKER, Massachusetts General Hospital and Harvard University
M. MARIA GLYMOUR, University of California, San Francisco
ROEE GUTMAN, Brown University
MARK D. HAYWARD, University of Texas at Austin
RUTH KATZ, LeadingAge
SPERO M. MANSON (NAM), University of Colorado Anschutz Medical Campus
TERRIE E. MOFFITT (NAM), Duke University
VINCENT MOR (NAM), Brown University
DAVID B. REUBEN, University of California, Los Angeles
ROLAND J. THORPE JR., Johns Hopkins University
RACHEL M. WERNER (NAM), University of Pennsylvania
KRISTINE YAFFE (NAM), University of California, San Francisco
JULIE M. ZISSIMOPOULOS, University of Southern California

Advisory Panel

CYNTHIA HULING HUMMEL, living with dementia, Elmira, NY
MARIE MARTINEZ ISRAELITE, care partner/caregiver, Chevy Chase, MD
JOHN-RICHARD PAGAN, living with dementia, Woodbridge, VA
EDWARD PATTERSON, living with dementia, Clermont, FL
BRIAN VAN BUREN, living with dementia, Charlotte, NC
GERALDINE WOOLFOLK, care partner/caregiver, Oakland, CA

Study Staff

MOLLY CHECKSFIELD DORRIES, *Study Director*
ALEXANDRA BEATTY, *Senior Program Officer*
TINA M. WINTERS, *Associate Program Officer*
JACQUELINE L. COLE, *Senior Program Assistant*

BOARD ON BEHAVIORAL, COGNITIVE, AND SENSORY SCIENCES

TERRIE E. MOFFITT (*Chair*) (NAM), Duke University
RICHARD N. ASLIN (NAS), Yale University
JOHN BAUGH, Washington University in St. Louis
WILSON S. GEISLER (NAS), University of Texas at Austin
MICHELE GELFAND (NAS), University of Maryland, College Park
ULRICH MAYR, University of Oregon
KATHERINE L. MILKMAN, University of Pennsylvania
ELIZABETH A. PHELPS, Harvard University
DAVID E. POEPPEL, New York University
STACEY SINCLAIR, Princeton University
TIMOTHY J. STRAUMAN, Duke University

ADRIENNE STITH BUTLER, *Director*

About the Cover

Much of the American population has been directly affected by dementia; beyond the more than 6 million individuals in the United States currently living with dementia are millions more with close relatives, friends, or other loved ones who have received a dementia diagnosis. This reality is reflected on the cover, which includes a collage of images provided by members of the authoring committee for the report, the study staff, and the advisory panel for the study. Many of the committee members have had relatives who received a dementia diagnosis, as have all four members of the study staff, and the advisory panel for the study was composed of individuals living with a dementia diagnosis and individuals who have served as care partners to a person living with dementia; the collage reflects only a subset of those directly affected by dementia who contributed to the report. Each adult pictured on the cover received a dementia diagnosis (with one exception as noted in the captions below) and is either shown prior to their diagnosis or living life to the fullest postdiagnosis.

Elnora McCrimmon Edgerton, grandmother of Jacqueline Cole, National Academies' staff member.

Cynthia Huling Hummel, advisory panel member.

Patricia Hayden Powell, mother of Tia Powell, committee chair.

Lucille Martinez, mother of Maria Martinez Israelite, advisory panel member.

John-Richard Pagan, advisory panel member.

Dorothy Checksfield, with her granddaughter Molly Checksfield Dorries, study director.

Nordin and Donna Blacker, parents of Deborah Blacker, committee member. Her father was diagnosed with dementia, and her mother was his caregiver for the last 2 years of their marriage.

Terrie Montgomery, friend of Cynthia Huling Hummel, advisory panel member.

Florence Manson, Pambina Chippewa, grandmother of Spero Manson, committee member. Pictured with Quinn Manson, her 48th grandchild.

Mercedes Phelan Hayden, grandmother of Tia Powell, committee chair.

Brian Van Buren, advisory panel member.

Terry Moffitt, father of Terrie Moffitt, committee member.

Preface

There are few Americans who do not have a family member, friend, neighbor, or colleague living with Alzheimer's disease or another dementia. The members of this committee represent a broad range of academic expertise related to dementia, but many of us have also been touched by the disease in our own lives. We have seen first-hand its complexities and challenges.

There is no cure today for any of the dementias, and it is unclear when truly disease-modifying treatments will arrive. Even if medications soon emerge that can slow or prevent dementia, they are unlikely to provide relief for the more than 6 million Americans who have dementia today or for those whose brains have sufficiently changed that symptoms will likely follow in the next few years.

However, lack of a cure does not mean there is no hope for those with Alzheimer's disease and related dementias and those who care about them. Existing behavioral and social science research indicates promising directions for how it may be possible to slow the development of symptoms, support those who do have symptoms, and enhance the quality of life for both those living with dementia and their family caregivers.

This report offers a blueprint for the next decade of behavioral and social science research to reduce the negative impact of dementia for America's diverse population. It calls for research that addresses the causes and solutions for disparities in both developing dementia and receiving adequate treatment and support. It calls for research that sets goals meaningful not just for scientists but for people living with dementia and those who support them as well. It calls for significant improvements in research design to create interventions that will succeed in the real world, not only in the controlled context of research. The committee worked to devise a plan for research that will have a real impact for good for a broad range of people, including populations that are often bypassed by health care improvements. In this report, we call for research that will not only ameliorate symptoms but also enhance the quality of health care and quality of life.

For all of us, serving on this committee was a chance to work together to draft a plan that can deliver the full benefit of behavioral and social science research to a critically important common good: reducing the negative impacts of a debilitating and ultimately fatal disease. We are optimistic that the research agenda described here can advance that common good and so benefit the many among us living with the impact of dementia now or in the future.

This study would not have been possible without the contributions of many people. From its very first meeting and throughout the study, the committee benefitted tremendously from the efforts of a group of individuals who were living with a dementia diagnosis or had served as care partners to individuals with dementia and agreed to lend their time and energy to serve as an advisory panel to the study: Cynthia Huling Hummel (living with dementia), Marie Martinez Israelite (care partner), John-Richard Pagan (living with dementia), Ed Patterson (living with dementia), Brian Van Buren (living with dementia), and Geraldine Woolfolk (care partner). Members of the advisory panel gave presentations and served as discussants at our public workshops, participated in many in-person and virtual meetings, worked with staff to develop a call for commentaries from individuals with dementia and care partners, prepared a paper describing the experiences of individuals with dementia and care partners, and offered thoughtful comments on sections of the report. We are indebted for the grounding they provided in the experiences of those directly affected by dementia. In addition, Karen Love (Dementia Action Alliance) provided invaluable facilitation of the advisory panel's work and guidance to the study staff during the information gathering phase of the study, and we deeply appreciate her giving so generously of her time and wisdom.

We gained useful information and insights from several commissioned papers and thank the authors for their careful analyses and presentation of their work at public workshops: David A. Bennett (Rush University); Julie P.W. Bynum (University of Michigan) and Kenneth Langa (University of Michigan); Joseph E. Gaugler (University of Minnesota), Laura N. Gitlin (Drexel University), and Eric Jutkowitz (Brown University); Pei-Jung Lin (Tufts Medical Center); and Ana R. Quiñones (Oregon Health & Science University), Jeffrey Kaye (Oregon Health & Science University), Heather G. Allore (Yale University), Stephen Thielke (University of Washington), and Anda Botoseneanu (University of Michigan).

A number of other individuals lent their expertise to the study through presentations at public workshops: Scott Beach (University of Pittsburgh), Catherine A. Christian (New York County District Attorney's Office), Olivier Constant (Flanders Centre of Expertise on Dementia, Belgium), Leslie Chang Evertson (University of California, Los Angeles), Richard H. Fortinsky (UConn Health and UConn Center on Aging), Nathan Gray (Duke University), Jhamirah Howard (U.S. Department of Health and Human Services), Judith Kasper (University of Pittsburgh), Mika Kivimaki (University College London), Peter A. Lichtenberg (Wayne State University), Susan Mitchell (Hebrew SeniorLife), Mary Mittelman (New York University School of Medicine), Emily O'Brien (Duke University School of Medicine), Rani E. Snyder (The John A. Hartford Foundation), and David Stevenson (Vanderbilt University School of Medicine). We also thank Jim Butler (living with dementia), Michael Ellenbogen (living with dementia), Katie Jordan (care partner), and all those who responded to our call for white papers, participated in public comment sessions at workshops, and responded to the call for commentaries from individuals with dementia and care partners for their input to the study.

We express our appreciation for the staff team: study director Molly Checksfield Dorries, who worked tirelessly to keep the study organized and moving forward, along with Alix Beatty, Jacqueline Cole, and Tina Winters. We also thank Rebecca Krone for lending her graphic design talents, Kirsten Sampson Snyder for managing the report review process, Yvonne Wise for managing the report production process, and Rona Briere and Allison Boman for their skillful editing.

The committee is grateful to the AARP, the Alzheimer's Association, the American Psychological Association, The John. A. Hartford Foundation, the JPB Foundation, the National Institute on Aging, the National Institutes of Health, the Office of the Assistant Secretary for Planning and Evaluation within the U.S. Department of Health and Human Services, and the U.S. Department of Veterans Affairs.

This Consensus Study Report was reviewed in draft form by individuals chosen for their diverse perspectives and technical expertise. The purpose of this independent review is to provide candid and critical comments that will assist the National Academies of Sciences, Engineering, and Medicine in making each published report as sound as possible and to ensure that it meets the institutional standards for quality, objectivity, evidence, and responsiveness to the study charge. The review comments and draft manuscript remain confidential to protect the integrity of the deliberative process.

We thank the following individuals for their review of this report: Allison E. Aiello (Gillings School of Global Public Health at Chapel Hill, The University of North Carolina), Maria P. Aranda (Suzanne Dworak-Peck School of Social Work, Edward R. Roybal Institute on Aging, University of Southern California), Malaz Boustani (Center for Health Innovation and Implementation Science, Indiana University School of Medicine and Senior Care Innovation, Eskenazi Health), Christopher M. Callahan (Eskenazi Health and Indiana University School of Medicine and IU Center for Aging Research, Regenstrief Institute, Inc.), Maria M. Corrada (Institute for Memory Impairments and Neurological Disorders, University of California, Irvine), Kimberly Curyto (Center for Integrated Healthcare, VA Western New York Healthcare System), Gary Epstein-Lubow (Alpert Medical School and School of Public Health, Brown University), Karen I. Fredriksen Goldsen (Center for Aging and Health, Sexuality and Gender Research Center, University of Washington), J. Neil Henderson (Memory Keepers Medical Discovery Team–Health Equity and Department of Family Medicine & Biobehavioral Health, University of Minnesota Medical School), Kenneth M. Langa (School of Medicine, University of Michigan and VA Ann Arbor Healthcare System), Anne Montgomery (Center for Eldercare Improvement, Altarum, Washington, DC), Samuel H. Preston (Department of Sociology, University of Pennsylvania), Sally Sadoff (School of Management, University of California, San Diego), William M. Sage (School of Law and Dell Medical School, The University of Texas at Austin), Tetyana P. Shippee (School of Public Health and Center for Healthy Aging and Innovation, University of Minnesota), and Jennifer L. Wolff (Roger C. Lipitz Center for Integrated Health Care, Department of Health Policy and Management, Johns Hopkins Bloomberg School of Public Health).

Although the reviewers listed above provided many constructive comments and suggestions, they were not asked to endorse the conclusions or recommendations of this report, nor did they see the final draft before its release. The review of this report was overseen by Dan G. Blazer, Duke University Medical Center, and Eric B. Larson, Kaiser Foundation Health Plan, Inc. They were responsible for making certain that an independent examination of this report was carried out in accordance with the standards of the National Academies and that all review comments were carefully considered. Responsibility for the final content rests entirely with the authoring committee and the National Academies.

Tia Powell, *Chair*
Karen S. Cook, *Vice Chair*

Contents

Summary   1

1 Introduction   13
   About This Study, 16
     Study Charge, 17
     Purpose of a Decadal Survey, 18
     Applying the Social and Behavioral Sciences to the Study of Dementia, 19
   Context for Research on the Impacts of Dementia, 21
     A Large and Growing Problem, 22
     Disparities in Rates of Dementia and in Care and Resources, 22
     COVID-19 and Dementia, 24
   Study Approach and Scope, 25
     Study Scope, 26
     Information Gathering, 27
     Guiding Themes, 29
   Report Structure, 31
   References, 31

2 Prevention and Protective Factors   39
   Interpreting the Evidence, 41
   Influences on Cognitive Health in Individuals, 42
     Evidence About Risk and Protection for Cognitive Health, 43
       2017 National Academies Report, 44
       Lancet Commission Report, 46

        Potentially Important Risk Factors That Have Received
           Less Attention, 47
        Use of Emerging Evidence to Promote Public Health, 48
    Socioeconomic Risk, 50
        Socioeconomic Factors, 53
           Education, 54
           Occupation, 55
           Financial Resources, 56
        Racial/Ethnic Disparities in Dementia Risk, 56
    Research Directions, 60
    References, 65

3 Improving Outcomes for Individuals Living with Dementia   **73**
    Perspectives on Living with Dementia, 74
        Problems in Obtaining an Accurate and Timely
           Dementia Diagnosis, 74
        Problems in Obtaining Supports and Services, 75
        Challenges in Communicating with Doctors and
           Other Health Care Professionals, 76
        Fear and Loss, 77
    Research on Key Aspects of Living with Dementia, 77
        Diagnosing Dementia, 78
           Challenges in Arriving at a Diagnosis, 79
           Questions About Communicating a Dementia Diagnosis, 83
        Promoting Autonomy and Protecting from Harm, 83
           Financial Decisions and Potential for Abuse, 85
           Sexual Behavior, Risk, and Dementia, 88
           Resources for Assessing and Supporting Decisions, 89
        Interventions to Alleviate the Impact of Dementia, 91
           Goals for the Care of Persons Living with Dementia, 92
           Approaches for Addressing Key Dementia Symptoms, 95
    Research Directions, 98
    References, 101

4 Caregivers: Diversity in Demographics, Capacities, and Needs   **109**
    Reliance on Family Caregivers, 110
    Family Caregivers' Perspectives, 114
    Research on Family Caregiving, 116
        The Caregiving Experience, 116
        Caregiver Capacity and Screening, 119
    Supports for Family Caregivers, 121
        Intervention Research, 122

Focus on Three Key Issues: Care Transitions, Use of
  Assistive Technology, and Approaches for Addressing
  Behavioral and Psychological Symptoms, 124
  Care Transitions, 124
  Use of Technology to Support Caregiving, 126
  Approaches for Addressing Behavioral and Psychological
    Symptoms of Dementia, 128
Research Directions, 129
References, 132

5 **The Role of the Community** 137
   Disparities That Affect the Impact of Dementia, 138
     Links Between Community Characteristics and
       Cognitive Health, 141
     The Role of Race and Ethnicity, 144
   Looking Through a Community Lens, 145
   Opportunities to Support Communities, 147
     Types of Resources, 148
     A Patchwork of Resources and Supports, 150
     Building Community Responsiveness and Resilience, 153
     Housing for People Living with Dementia, 154
       Dementia Friendly Communities, 155
       Caregiver Support: Washington State, 157
       Aging in Place Challenge Program: Canada, 157
       The Village Movement: Beacon Hill, Boston,
         Massachusetts, 158
   Research Directions, 158
   References, 161

6 **Health Care, Long-Term Care, and End-of-Life Care** 171
   The Health Care System, 172
     Quality of Primary Care, 172
     Fragmentation of Care Delivery, 174
     Comprehensive Dementia Care, 174
     A Model of Comprehensive Care at the Population Level, 175
       Knowledge Gaps, 178
   Long-Term and End-of-Life Care, 179
     Assisted Living and Memory Units, 180
     Nursing Homes, 180
     Alternatives to Nursing Homes, 182
     Palliative and Hospice Care, 184
   Paying for Care: Medicare and Medicaid, 185
     Coverage, 186

The Federal Role in Innovation, 188
Managed Care, 189
    How Managed Care Works, 190
    Medicare Advantage and Dementia Care, 190
Research Directions, 194
References, 200

7   **Economic Costs of Dementia**   209
    Magnitude of Economic Costs, 210
    Drivers of Costs, 212
    The Economics of Innovation, 214
    Applying Behavioral Economics, 215
    A Word About the Costs of Aducanumab, 216
    Research Directions, 218
    References, 219

8   **Strengthening Data Collection and Research Methodology**   223
    Challenges of Quantitative Research on Dementia, 224
    Four Opportunities for Improvements in Methodology, 225
        Data Sources, 226
            Developing New Data Sources and Adding Items to Existing
                Sources, 227
            Linking Existing Data Sources in New Ways, 229
            Improving Recruitment, 232
        Measurement, 233
            Measuring Exposures, 234
            Identifying Valid Early Predictors of Cognitive Outcomes, 235
        Study Design, 237
            Broadening the Repertoire of Tools, 237
            Creating Opportunities for Quasi-Experimental Discovery,
                Including Leveraging Instrumental Variables Analyses, 239
            Enhancing Analyses of Randomized Controlled Trials, 239
            Moving from Evidence to Implementation, 240
            Conducting Pragmatic Clinical Trials Embedded in
                Health Systems, 242
            Evaluating Complex, Dynamic Interventions, 244
            Simulations, Microsimulations, Agent-Based Models,
                and Complex Systems Models, 245
            Formalizing Study Design Approaches, 245
        Evidence Integration, 247
            Methods for Assessing Heterogeneity and
                Generalizing Results, 248

　　　　　Tools for Systematically Combining Evidence, 248
　　　　　Tools for Quantifying Impacts of Policies, Interventions, or
　　　　　　Therapies, 249
　　　　Investment in Human Capital and Research Capacity, 252
　　　　Research Directions, 253
　　　　References, 256

9　**Ten-Year Research Priorities**　　　　　　　　　　　　　　263
　　　　Research Agenda, 267
　　　　Call to Action, 270

APPENDIXES
A　Biographical Sketches of Committee
　　and Advisory Panel Members　　　　　　　　　　　　　275
B　The Paid Health Care Workforce　　　　　　　　　　　　285
C　Synthesis of Reviews of Nonpharmacologic Interventions　293
D　Complete Research Agenda　　　　　　　　　　　　　　321

Summary

As the largest generation in U.S. history—the population born in the two decades immediately following World War II—enters the age of risk for cognitive impairment, growing numbers of people will experience dementia (including Alzheimer's disease and related dementias). By one estimate, nearly 14 million people in the United States will be living with dementia by 2060. Like other hardships, the experience of living with dementia can bring unexpected moments of intimacy, growth, and compassion, but these diseases also affect people's capacity to work and carry out other activities and alter their relationships with loved ones, friends, and coworkers. Those who live with and care for individuals experiencing these diseases face challenges that include physical and emotional stress, difficult changes and losses in their relationships with life partners, loss of income, and interrupted connections to other activities and friends. From a societal perspective, these diseases place substantial demands on communities and on the institutions and government entities that support people living with dementia and their families, including the health care system, the providers of direct care, and others. The economic cost of these diseases in the United States has been estimated at $305 billion for 2020 and is projected to rise to $1,500 trillion by 2050.

Dementia will be a fact of life for the foreseeable future. Although a medication that effectively slows or even prevents dementia may someday be discovered and approved, dementia will not be eradicated by one or even several medications, including the recently approved drug aducanumab. Multiple diseases and causes lead to dementia, and researchers seeking pharmacological remedies are focused on the earliest stages of disease.

Those who already have dementia or will develop it in the next 10 years have lived for multiple decades and been exposed to risk and protective factors, and likely would not benefit materially from a pharmacological breakthrough.

Nevertheless, research in the social and behavioral sciences points to possibilities for preventing or slowing the development of dementia and for substantially reducing its social and economic impacts. Accordingly, the National Institute on Aging of the U.S. Department of Health and Human Services requested that the National Academies of Sciences, Engineering, and Medicine conduct a consensus study to produce a decadal survey of research in the social and behavioral sciences with the potential to mitigate the negative impacts of Alzheimer's disease and related dementias and identify a research agenda for the coming decade.[1] To carry out this study, the National Academies convened the Committee on the Decadal Survey of Behavioral and Social Science Research on Alzheimer's Disease and Alzheimer's Disease–Related Dementias, whose members have expertise in sociology, epidemiology, biostatistics, public health, psychology, geriatric medicine, psychiatry and neurology, bioethics, and public policy. The committee's charge is shown in Box S-1.

The study charge focuses on research that can improve the experience of living with dementia. Therefore, this report is concerned primarily with the impacts of dementia on those for whom symptoms have become salient and their caregivers.

To carry out this study, the committee followed the approach established in previous decadal surveys by (1) assessing the needs of the communities the study was intended to benefit, and (2) surveying the landscape of potentially relevant research for ideas with the greatest promise for advancing the objective of mitigating the impacts of dementias on all of the constituencies they affect. We examined evidence on the impacts of dementia from multiple perspectives and identified research directions for each.

RISK AND PREVENTIVE FACTORS FOR DEMENTIA AND HOW THEY RELATE TO THE SOCIAL AND ECONOMIC CONDITIONS THAT AFFECT HEALTH CARE AND HEALTH OUTCOMES

A large proportion of dementia could be prevented, but rigorous causal evidence with enough precision to guide evidence translation and the development of interventions is limited for nearly every domain of prevention,

---

[1] A decadal survey is a method for engaging members of a scholarly community to identify lines of research with the greatest potential to be of use over a 10-year period in pursuit of a particular goal. The National Academies developed this type of survey to support the planning of future research for government agencies and other entities.

SUMMARY 3

> **BOX S-1**
> **Committee Charge**
>
> The committee will conduct a decadal survey focusing on developing a research agenda for the next decade in the behavioral and social sciences as it relates to Alzheimer's disease (AD) and Alzheimer's disease-related dementias (ADRD). Drawing on extensive input from the scientific community and other stakeholders, the committee will assess the role of the social and behavioral sciences (including data sources and other resources) in reducing the burden[a] of AD/ADRD.
> The following areas will be reviewed:
>
> 1. research using the methods of behavioral and social sciences on the burden of AD/ADRD on individuals, families, medical and long-term care systems;
> 2. challenges associated with AD/ADRD care;
> 3. intervention development for persons with dementia and their caregivers at different stages of illness;
> 4. cognitive and AD/ADRD epidemiology;
> 5. AD/ADRD prevention, leveraging basic and translational research on behavioral and social pathways to AD/ADRD and cognitive decline;
> 6. detection of AD/ADRD-related change;
> 7. the causes and consequences of AD/ADRD health disparities; and
> 8. AD/ADRD data infrastructure needs.
>
> A final report will include recommendations for an agenda for social and behavioral science research on AD/ADRD during the next decade (2020–2030).
>
> ---
>
> [a]The committee notes that although our charge refers to the "burden" of Alzheimer's and related diseases, we instead use such words as "impact" and "effect" to avoid the implication that people living with dementia themselves pose a burden.

including behavioral changes, socioeconomic conditions, and structural and interpersonal racism and discrimination. For example, robust evidence suggests that people who take such common-sense measures as eating a healthy diet, exercising regularly, maintaining a healthy weight, and reducing cardiovascular risk have a lower risk of dementia. Similarly, clear evidence shows that disparities in socioeconomic resources, negative social interactions (e.g., overt racism and discrimination), systemic racism, and other socioeconomic factors contribute to stark disparities in dementia risk across population groups. Research is needed to follow up on these findings so that interventions can be designed for the benefit of individuals and at the population level, and rigorously evaluated for effectiveness. High-priority research in this area would address

- the causal effects of social factors on the incidence and rate of progression of dementia;
- the effects of health-related behaviors and their management over the life course;
- modifiable drivers of racial/ethnic inequality in dementia incidence, as well as other dimensions of inequality (e.g., geography);
- the mechanisms through which socioeconomic factors influence brain health, including physiologic changes, behavioral mechanisms, and medical care pathways;
- understanding of identified risk factors that is needed to support more precise recommendations to individuals about and the development of population-level policies; and
- effective means of communicating the magnitude and degree of potential risk and protective factors to support informed decision making.

THE PERSONAL EXPERIENCE OF LIVING WITH DEMENTIA AND ISSUES ASSOCIATED WITH DIAGNOSIS, CARE, AND TREATMENT

Much of the research on interventions for people living with dementia is primarily observational or conducted using conventional rather than pragmatic trials. The committee identified the need for both qualitative and quantitative research related to the needs of people at all stages of dementia that is interdisciplinary, involving ethicists and legal experts as well as clinicians and researchers. Related is the need for improved measures that can be used in assessing outcomes relevant to persons living with dementia and their caregivers throughout the course of the disease. High-priority research in this area would address

- improved screening and diagnosis to identify persons living with dementia, including guidance for clinicians that also addresses issues related to disclosure;
- the development of guidance to support ethical and responsible decision making by and for people living with dementia;
- the development and validation of outcome measures that reflect the perspectives of people living with dementia, their family caregivers,[2] and communities; and

---

[2] The committee uses the terms "family caregivers" and "caregivers" to refer to those who provide any level of care, usually unpaid, to a person with dementia primarily because of their prior personal relationship with that person. The term here encompasses both care partners, who support people living with dementia during the early stages of disease, and those who provide more intensive direct care during later stages.

- improved design and evaluation of nonpharmacologic interventions to slow or prevent cognitive and functional decline, reduce or ameliorate behavioral and psychological symptoms, improve comfort and well-being, and adequately and equitably serve diverse populations.

THE EXPERIENCES OF FAMILY CAREGIVERS AND RESOURCES AVAILABLE TO THEM

There is evidence that many interventions to support family caregivers can provide benefit, but as in the other areas discussed above, there are also significant gaps in the existing research. Many existing studies lack the methodological rigor needed to support wide dissemination. Moreover, important aspects of the caregiving experience and its effects on both caregivers and people living with dementia have not yet been documented and studied. High-priority research in this area would address

- identification of the highest-priority needs for resources and support for family caregivers, particularly assessment of how caregivers' needs vary across race and ethnicity, and community;
- means of identifying the assets that family caregivers bring to this role, as well as their needs for supplemental skills and training and other resources to enhance their capacity to provide care while maintaining the safety and well-being of both care recipients and caregivers;
- continued development and evaluation of interventions to support and enhance family caregiving and address the practical and logistical challenges; and
- continued progress in data collection and research methods.

HOW COMMUNITY CHARACTERISTICS AFFECT DEMENTIA RISK AND QUALITY OF LIFE FOR PEOPLE LIVING WITH DEMENTIA AND THEIR FAMILIES

There is strong evidence that community factors shape the exposures and behaviors that influence dementia risk, the way people interpret the meaning of the experience of living with the disease, their expectations for social interactions, and the availability of needed resources. Researchers have not yet fully documented the impacts on dementia of interventions to circumvent negative influences on cognitive health at the community level. At the same time, community supports are known to be key resources, and community is an important lens for understanding ways to reduce the negative impacts of dementia. Innovative approaches to the design of communities in which people living with dementia can thrive do indeed show promise, although their application to diverse contexts and populations has yet to be systematically demonstrated. High-priority research in this area would address

- systematic analysis of the characteristics of communities that influence the risk of developing dementia and the experience of living with the disease, with particular attention to the sources of disparities in dementia incidence and disease trajectory;
- the collection of data to document the opportunities and resources available in communities both historically and currently and evaluation of their impact, with particular attention to disparities in population groups' access to resources and including development of the infrastructure needed for data collection;
- analysis of the community characteristics needed to foster dementia friendly environments, including assessment of alternative community models that foster dementia friendly environments in communities that have different constellations of resources and serve diverse populations; and
- evaluation of innovative approaches to adapting housing, services, and supports so that persons with dementia can remain in the community and out of institutional care.

THE HEALTH CARE SYSTEM AND THE INSTITUTIONS THAT PROVIDE RESIDENTIAL LONG-TERM CARE AND HOSPICE AND PALLIATIVE CARE

People living with dementia interact with many different institutions that provide health care and social support as their dementia symptoms become more severe and they lose their ability to function independently. Many spend time living in long-term care facilities and ultimately receive such care as hospice resources at the end of life. These experiences involve relationships with numerous professionals and institutions—often a great many, over time—including neurologists, psychiatrists, geriatricians, and nurse practitioners who specialize in dementia care; social workers; and public and private entities that provide residential and end-of-life care. Each interaction may be comforting and beneficial, or may fall short of that ideal.

Highest-priority research on how persons living with dementia and their caregivers interact with and are served by the health care and social service systems would address

- how to strengthen the quality and structure of the health care provided to people living with dementia, including

- documentation of the diagnosis and care management received by persons living with dementia,
    - clarification of disease trajectories,
    - identification of effective methods for providing comprehensive dementia-related services,
    - development and evaluation of standardized systems of coordinated care for comprehensively managing multiple comorbidities for persons with dementia, and
    - identification of effective approaches for integrating care services across health care delivery and community-based organizations;
- how to strengthen the quality and structure of long-term and end-of-life care provided to people living with dementia, including
    - identification of future long-term and end-of-life needs and available care,
    - description and monitoring of factors that contribute to problems with nursing home quality,
    - development and evaluation of alternatives to traditional nursing home facilities including home care options and innovative facility designs, and
    - improved understanding of how and when persons living with dementia use palliative and hospice care options and of variations in the end-of-life care available across regions and populations; and
- how to strengthen the arrangements through which most dementia care is funded (traditional Medicare, Medicare Advantage, alternative payment models, Medicaid), including
    - comparison of the effects of different financing structures on the quality of care and clinical outcomes,
    - examination of ways to modify incentives in reimbursement models to optimize care and reduce unnecessary hospitalizations and other negative outcomes, and
    - development and testing of approaches to integrated financing of medical and social services.

The health care and long-term care systems employ millions of individuals who care for people living with dementia and possess a wide range of experience and skills. Issues that affect the workforces in these two sectors—including shortages of qualified workers, limitations of available training and education, and national-level policies and economic trends—undoubtedly have important impacts for those affected by dementia. It was beyond the scope of this study to conduct a review of the state of the research in each of the relevant areas that would be detailed enough to support specific conclusions about the research directions that should be given highest priority. Nevertheless, the committee regards emerging knowledge about workforce issues as a vital complement to the research directions described here.

THE ECONOMIC COSTS OF DEMENTIA TO INDIVIDUALS AND SOCIETY

Understanding the full extent of the economic impacts of dementia and how they can be reduced will be key to mitigating the overall impact of the disease on individuals and society. Both reducing unnecessary costs and increasing value—that is, achieving significant improvements in health, quality of life, and other outcomes that justify the associated costs—will bring economic benefit. High-priority research to improve understanding of the economic impact of dementia and identify ways to reduce costs without reducing quality of care would include

- assessment and quantification of the total economic impact of dementia for individuals and families, including current and future national costs;
- improved understanding of drivers of dementia-related costs; and
- estimation of the value to individuals, families, and society of innovations in prevention, diagnostics, and treatment, including pharmacologic treatments.

STRENGTHENING DATA COLLECTION AND RESEARCH METHODOLOGY

Advances in data collection and research methodology are needed to support progress in virtually every domain of dementia research. Progress toward four key methodological objectives will support a research agenda to reduce the negative impacts of dementia:

1. Expansion of data infrastructure.
2. Improved measurement of exposure and outcomes.
3. Support for the adoption of more rigorous study designs, particularly in the realm of implementation science, so that research findings can be successfully integrated into clinical and community practices.
4. Development of systematic approaches for integrating evidence from disparate studies.

Advances in these areas will be relevant to and strengthen research in every other area discussed in this report. Social and behavioral scientists from numerous specific disciplines are the natural leaders in meeting these methodological challenges.

TEN-YEAR RESEARCH PRIORITIES

Collectively, the priority research outlined above constitutes a substantial body of work that will provide the basis for powerful benefits to people living with dementia, their families and communities, and society. Recognizing that resources are finite, however, the committee identified the highest priorities from that set of research challenges to help ensure that the research undertaken in the next 10 years will contribute more than the sum of its parts. These priorities emerge from themes that can be traced across the report, and can be used to structure funding for a research agenda that addresses the full range of negative impacts of dementia and to guide decisions about the research likely to have the greatest impact in the coming decade.

> CONCLUSION 9-1:[3] A 10-year research agenda for the behavioral and social sciences will have maximal impact in reducing the negative impacts of dementia and improving quality of life if it distributes attention and resources across five priorities:
> 1. Improvements in the lives of people affected by dementia, including those who develop it and their families and caregivers, as well as in the social and clinical networks that surround them, through research on factors that affect the development of disease and its outcomes, promising innovative practices and new models of care, and policies that can facilitate the dissemination of interventions found to be effective.
> 2. Rectifying of disparities across groups and geographic regions that affect who develops dementia, how the disease progresses, outcomes and quality of life, and access to health care and supportive services.
> 3. Development of innovations with the potential to improve the quality of care and social supports for individuals and communities and to support improved quality of life (e.g., reducing financial abuse and stressors, finding relevant affordable housing and care facilities, gaining access to important services).

---

[3] The conclusions and recommendation are listed here with the numbers they are assigned within Chapter 9.

4. Easing of the financial and economic costs of dementia to individuals, families, and society and balancing of long-term costs with long-term outcomes across the life span.
5. Pursuit of advances in research capability, including study design, measurement, analysis, and evidence integration, as well as the development of data infrastructure needed to study key dementia-related topics.

In addition to these broad priorities, the committee offers guidelines for the design of an effective portfolio of research.

CONCLUSION 9-2: A 10-year research agenda will be optimally effective if it
- is coordinated to ensure that the various research topics identified in this report are addressed sufficiently without redundancy and competing initiatives;
- consistently takes into account fundamental socioeconomic factors that influence who develops dementia, access to high-quality care, and outcomes;
- includes pragmatic, implementation, and dissemination research needed to ensure that findings can be implemented effectively in clinical and community settings; and
- addresses potential policy implications that are articulated beginning in the planning stages and assessed during the course of the investigations.

CALL TO ACTION

A 10-year research agenda that meets the above objectives will require sustained leadership; integration of effort across multiple, sometimes competing domains; and the capacity to deliver research findings to individuals, communities, and health systems to change the lives of people with dementia and caregivers for the better. This research agenda defines goals and priorities for the vital task of supporting better lives for people with dementia and caregivers, but its existence alone will not be sufficient: action is needed to ensure that the United States benefits from the potential in this body of research. The committee therefore makes the following recommendation:

RECOMMENDATION 9-1: Funders of dementia-related research, including federal agencies, such as the National Institutes of Health and the Agency for Healthcare Research and Quality, along with relevant philanthropic and other organizations, such as the Patient-Centered

Outcomes Research Institute, should use guidelines for the awarding of research grants to establish incentives for
- coordination of research objectives with the research agenda priorities identified in this report to ensure that key areas are funded without undue overlap and to foster links across research efforts;
- interdisciplinary research and inclusion of stakeholders in research partnerships;
- attention to topics that have not typically been part of standard medical research but are important to those living with dementia, including isolation, financial security, and housing options;
- rigorous evaluation and implementation research needed to translate findings into programs with impact on a broad scale; and
- dissemination of research findings to policy makers.

This report documents the multifold challenges dementia is expected to bring in the coming decades, and it was written as the COVID-19 pandemic was exposing and seriously exacerbating long-standing deficiencies in the support systems for people living with dementia. The report lays out a broad research roadmap for the behavioral and social sciences over the next decade. It notes promising intervention programs that require additional confirmatory evidence. And it describes social and behavioral research that can provide the foundation for the development of programs and policies, as well as ethical safeguards that would serve the needs of all Americans affected by dementia. The committee notes that funding for the research agenda proposed in this report may require difficult choices within the federal agencies to which our recommendations are directed.

The committee's objective was to set priorities for research aimed at reducing the negative impacts of dementia, taking into account broad societal and community-level impacts on risk and prevention and on access to care and resources, as well as developments that can improve the quality and delivery of care and improve the lives of persons with dementia and their caregivers. Scrupulous reliance on evidence is the foundation on which society can protect and improve the public health of the nation. It is our hope that by identifying these priorities for social and behavioral science research and recommending ways in which they can be pursued in a coordinated fashion, this report will help produce research that improves the lives of all those affected by dementia. By 2030, an estimated 8.5 million Americans will have Alzheimer's disease and many more will have other forms of dementia. If the nation is to ensure that the lives of these individuals are better than those of people living with dementia in 2021, the time to act is now.

1

Introduction

More than 6 million people in the United States are currently living with Alzheimer's disease, a number that will rise to nearly 14 million by 2060 if current demographic trends continue (Rajan et al., 2021; Matthews et al., 2019; Bynum and Langa, 2020; Zissimopoulos et al., 2014, 2018).[1] It is estimated that approximately one-third of older Americans have Alzheimer's or another dementia at death (Weuve et al., 2014). The economic cost of dementia in the United States has been estimated at $305 billion in 2020, and is projected to rise to $1.5 trillion by 2050 (Zissimopoulos et al., 2014; Alzheimer's Association, 2021).[2] The financial and emotional costs to patients and families are enormous and impossible to fully measure.

Dementia is a syndrome that can result from several different, often co-occurring, diseases, of which Alzheimer's is the most common; see Box 1-1 for an explanation of the terminology used to refer to these diseases in this report, as well as other key terms used throughout the report (terms that have more specific application are defined as they appear). Most forms of dementia develop gradually, and changes in an individual's functioning vary widely in pace and nature; moreover, each person living with dementia does so in a unique context. Regardless of the underlying causes, these diseases begin to affect people's capacity to work and carry out other activities,

---

[1] These figures are likely to be underestimates because they include only persons living with Alzheimer's disease, not other forms of dementia.

[2] Worldwide, the cost of dementia as of 2015 has been estimated to be $818 billion (Wimo et al., 2017).

as well as their relationships with loved ones, friends, and coworkers. Those who live with and care for individuals experiencing these diseases face challenges that include physical and emotional stress, difficult changes and losses in their relationships with life partners, loss of income, and interrupted connections to other activities and friends.

From a societal perspective, dementia places substantial demands on communities and on the institutions and government entities that support people living with dementia and their families—strains that are likely to

---

BOX 1-1
Key Terminology Used in This Report

In general, the committee attempted to avoid language that could be offensive or demeaning to those living with dementia or their caregivers, and to respect the terminology used in different contexts by researchers and others. We particularly took note of the recommendations from members of the advisory panel for this study (see the description of the study approach later in this chapter), such as that the word "demented" never be used to describe people living with the disease. The advisory panel encouraged us to recognize the importance of focusing on what a person living with dementia can do and highlighting positive aspects of living with dementia, rather than focusing solely on negative outcomes. The advisory panel emphasized that language plays an important role in the stigma that can be associated with dementia. Accordingly, we have tried to avoid using jargon and acronyms that can dehumanize individuals and the important issues that affect them.

Alzheimer's disease and Alzheimer's-related dementias: This report examines issues related to Alzheimer's disease and related dementias—progressive cognitive disorders of midlife and especially late life—of which Alzheimer's is the most common. All are forms of dementia—an acquired loss of cognitive function severe enough to interfere with independence, irrespective of cause—although the 5th edition of the Diagnostic and Statistical Manual of Mental Disorders (DSM-5) replaced the term dementia with the term "neurocognitive disorder," which may by mild or major (American Psychiatric Association, 2013; Crisis Prevention Institute, 2021; McKhann et al., 2011). Other common types or causes of dementia include cerebrovascular disease, Lewy body dementia, and frontotemporal lobar degeneration. Although there are important differences among types of dementia, they share many symptoms and outcomes and have similar impacts; in this report, the term "dementia" is used to refer to this set of diseases, with specific diseases identified when relevant to the discussion. In referring to people living with dementia, we mean those who manifest symptoms of these diseases. Where other issues, such as biomarkers or risk factors in people who are not showing symptoms, arise, we discuss them explicitly. Chapter 3 describes the various types of dementia and their diagnosis.

INTRODUCTION 15

grow as the number of persons living with dementia rises. By 2034, people over age 65 will outnumber children under 18 in the United States, and by 2060, they will make up 23 percent of the U.S. population (Vespa, 2018). Thus, there will be fewer adult children to provide care, as well as a shortage in the supply of paid care providers (those who provide medical care and direct care).

Research in the biomedical sciences has made important contributions to understanding of the pathophysiology of Alzheimer's disease and related

---

(Family) caregiver: An important decision was which term to use for those individuals who provide care for people living with dementia. There is no single, universally accepted term for these individuals. For the purposes of this report, family caregivers (or simply caregivers) are defined as those who provide any level of care, usually unpaid, to a person with dementia primarily because of their prior personal relationship with that person.[a] Many persons with dementia live alone or with paid caregivers, and family caregivers may or may not live with the person receiving care. Indeed, this category of caregiver includes people who may not be formal family members by blood or marriage, such as neighbors, members of shared faith congregations, coworkers, and friends, who provide regular uncompensated help to a person living with dementia. We distinguish this group from paid caregivers, although there is overlap between the two categories.

Note that there are many other names for the group we are calling caregivers. They are sometimes referred to as "informal" caregivers, although this term diminishes the enormous importance and scale of the care they deliver. They are sometimes referred to as "care partners," a term that may be apt for those who provide care in the early phases of dementia but does not capture the relationship and activities that are needed toward the end of a life. In this report, these individuals are encompassed by the term "(family) caregivers." We acknowledge the value of alternative terms, but are guided by the fact that several large national organizations, including the Family Caregiver Alliance, the National Family Caregivers Association, and the Caregiver Action Network, use "caregiver" as part of their naming convention. We are also following the convention of much of the relevant research literature in using the term "family caregiver."

Burden/impact/effect: Although the committee's charge refers to the "burden of Alzheimer's and related diseases," we instead use such words as "impact" and effect." We wish both to avoid the implication that people living with dementia themselves pose a burden and to highlight possibilities for improving conditions and quality of life for all affected by the disease.

[a] This definition is used in *Families Caring for an Aging America* (National Academies of Sciences, Engineering, and Medicine [NASEM], 2016a, Ch. 1). See also Gitlin and colleagues (2020) for further discussion of the implications of definitions and terms used in research and policy contexts.

conditions, but this work has yet to be translated into effective preventive therapies or pharmaceuticals that can halt the progression of the disease or mitigate its impacts. Until recently, no new medications targeting dementia symptoms had been approved in the United States since 2005, and currently available medications offer modest benefits at best (Cummings et al., 2014). It is hoped that aducanumab, a drug that was recently approved by the U.S. Food and Drug Administration despite the objections of its advisory panel, may slow or temporarily arrest some symptoms of Alzheimer's disease, but research has not yet demonstrated that it will have that benefit (issues surrounding the approval of aducanumab are discussed in Chapters 7 and 9). A wide array of social and behavioral influences has been associated with the risk of developing dementia, its trajectory, and the nature of the experience of living with the disease, as discussed in Chapter 2, but growing understanding of these influences has not yet led to the development of broadly effective interventions.

Thus dementia, with its profound impacts on individuals, families, and society, will be a fact of life for the foreseeable future. However, research in the social and behavioral sciences points to possibilities for preventing or slowing the development of dementia and for substantially reducing its negative impacts. This research can shed light on social, behavioral, economic, environmental, cultural, and other contextual factors that influence the development of the disease; its course; and its effects on individuals, families, caregivers, communities, and the health care system. Such research can be the foundation for strategies to address the challenges dementia brings and improve the lives of those affected by it.

ABOUT THIS STUDY

In this context, the National Institute on Aging within the National Institutes of Health (NIH) of the U.S. Department of Health and Human Services requested that the National Academies of Sciences, Engineering, and Medicine conduct a consensus study to produce a decadal survey[3] assessing the contributions of research in the social and behavioral sciences to mitigation of the negative impacts of Alzheimer's disease and related dementias and identifying a research agenda for the coming decade. This effort complements an array of initiatives occurring as part of the National Plan to Address Alzheimer's, a project of the U.S. Department of Health and Human Services.[4]

---

[3] A decadal survey is a method for engaging members of a scholarly community to identify lines of research with the greatest potential to be of use over a 10-year period in pursuit of a particular goal. The National Academies developed this type of survey to support the planning of future research for government agencies and other entities.

[4] https://aspe.hhs.gov/national-plan-address-alzheimers-disease

Study Charge

The study charge, shown in Box 1-2, focuses on research that can improve the experience of living with dementia, so this report is concerned primarily with the impacts of dementia on those for whom symptoms have become salient and their caregivers (see Chapter 3). Issues related to diagnosis and recognition of early symptoms, people who are at risk for developing dementia, and those with conditions that can lead to dementia who are not showing symptoms are also important, and we touch on those as well.

To carry out this study, the National Academies convened the Committee on the Decadal Survey of Behavioral and Social Science Research on Alzheimer's Disease and Alzheimer's Disease-Related Dementias, whose members have expertise in sociology, epidemiology, biostatistics, public health, psychology, anthropology, geriatric medicine, psychiatry and neurology, bioethics, and public policy (see Appendix A for biosketches of the committee members). The project was supported by the AARP, the

---

BOX 1-2
Committee Charge

The committee will conduct a decadal survey focusing on developing a research agenda for the next decade in the behavioral and social sciences as it relates to Alzheimer's disease (AD) and Alzheimer's disease-related dementias (ADRD). Drawing on extensive input from the scientific community and other stakeholders, the committee will assess the role of the social and behavioral sciences (including data sources and other resources) in reducing the burden of AD/ADRD.

The following areas will be reviewed:

- research using the methods of behavioral and social sciences on the burden of AD/ADRD on individuals, families, medical and long-term care systems;
- challenges associated with AD/ADRD care;
- intervention development for persons with dementia and their caregivers at different stages of illness;
- cognitive and AD/ADRD epidemiology;
- AD/ADRD prevention, leveraging basic and translational research on behavioral and social pathways to AD/ADRD and cognitive decline;
- detection of AD/ADRD-related change;
- the causes and consequences of AD/ADRD health disparities; and
- AD/ADRD data infrastructure needs.

A final report will include recommendations for an agenda for social and behavioral science research on AD/ADRD during the next decade (2020–2030).

Alzheimer's Association, the American Psychological Association, The John. A. Hartford Foundation, the JPB Foundation, the National Institute on Aging, the National Institutes of Health, the Office of the Assistant Secretary for Planning and Evaluation within the U.S. Department of Health and Human Services, and the U.S. Department of Veterans Affairs. This report presents the committee's conclusions and the evidence that supports them, which collectively provide the basis for a 10-year research agenda that can ultimately yield powerful benefits to people living with dementia, their caregivers and communities, and society.

Purpose of a Decadal Survey

As noted earlier, a decadal survey is a method for engaging members of a scholarly community to identify lines of research with the greatest potential impact over a 10-year period in pursuit of a particular goal. The National Academies developed this type of survey to support the planning of future research for a range of government entities with missions in the earth and space sciences, including the National Aeronautics and Space Administration, the National Science Foundation, the U.S. Department of Energy, the National Oceanic and Atmospheric Administration, and the U.S. Geological Survey. More recently, the decadal method was applied for the first time to research in the social and behavioral sciences in a study of research to strengthen intelligence analysis and enhance national security, which includes a detailed discussion of the National Academies' decadal process (NASEM, 2019a; see also NASEM, 2015). Regardless of the field of study, decadal surveys are a powerful tool for identifying research whose relevance to policy priorities may have been overlooked, as well as for identifying key questions to answer in the coming decade.

The decadal process was developed to meet urgent public policy needs, and there are compelling reasons for viewing dementia in this light and launching the first decadal survey of research related to the lived experience of dementia. As noted above, the numbers of persons affected by dementia are large and growing rapidly, and the impact of these diseases on individuals and their families and on society is substantial. There is also strong evidence that members of some racial/ethnic groups, as well as economically disadvantaged populations, are at greater risk for dementia, and that the availability, quality, and financing of care may be more limited for these populations (Quiñones et al., 2020a, 2020b; Favreault et al., 2015). Attention to the rapidly growing challenges of dementia has increased. Congress sent a powerful message when it tripled research spending on dementia at the National Institute on Aging over the 3-year period 2015–2018. The only precedents for this level of increase at NIH were the war on cancer, initiated in 1971, and the dramatic expansion of AIDS funding in the late

1980s (Kaiser, 2018). However, this spending has targeted primarily biomedical research rather than research in the social and behavioral sciences.

Applying the Social and Behavioral Sciences to the Study of Dementia

The committee looked across the landscape of the social and behavioral sciences for research that could help to ameliorate what we understand to be the "burden" of Alzheimer's disease and related dementias: their negative impacts on individuals, families, and communities, and the social and economic costs of ensuring that professional care and resources are available to people at all stages of disease. Researchers in social and behavioral fields are making a critical contribution to the overall landscape of dementia-related research by offering key pieces to the puzzle that biological and pharmaceutical research cannot provide. The past few decades have produced a vast amount of research on the biological mechanisms that lead to dementia, as well as potential pharmacologic interventions that can ameliorate that pathology. As noted above, however, no disease-altering medications—ones that can prevent, delay, or cure dementia—have been approved. The drugs that are available may mitigate symptoms of the disease but do not address its underlying causes. There is enormous interest in finding a drug for a common and fatal disease that causes so much suffering, but research outcomes to date have been disappointing. Although aducanumab may ultimately provide more benefit than many observers expect—or another new medication that effectively slows or prevents dementia may be discovered and approved in the next few years—dementia will not be eradicated by one or even several medications, for a number of reasons.

First, evidence suggests that many types of dementia are multifactorial. While the pathology of Alzheimer's disease is common, it often occurs in conjunction with vascular and other pathologies. It is unlikely that a single medication will effectively eradicate all neuropathology, and indeed those medications under study are not designed to do so. Most medical advances—for instance, those related to cancer or HIV—occur when several interventions can be combined to address different aspects of a disease. Thus, multiple different successful discoveries may be needed to have a meaningful impact on dementia at the individual and population levels.

Second, the development of a drug that slows the progression of dementia may mean that *more*, not *fewer*, people will be experiencing the disease's early phases at a given time. That is, people living with dementia may live longer and spend more years affected by the disease. Although such a delay would benefit those who maintained a higher level of function longer, it would also create the need for more support for larger numbers of people whose dementia was progressing more slowly than is currently typical.

Third, the committee is aware of no funded research that is exploring ways to cure or reverse dementia beyond the earliest phases. Brain pathology that is severe is understood to be permanent and irreversible, and brain pathology related to dementia is believed to precede symptoms by at least several years—perhaps more. There is not consensus among researchers that the elimination of senile plaques, as aducanumab is designed to do, will have a significant effect on the symptoms of Alzheimer's disease. Thus, those millions of Americans who currently have moderate to severe dementia, as well as those who develop dementia in the next decade, are unlikely to benefit from medications aimed at prevention that emerge during that period.

Finally, any approved drug for dementia will be costly (Garde and Feuerstein, 2020). The expected costs for aducanumab are not clear but estimates just for the drug itself (to be marketed as Aduhelm) could be as high as $112 billion per year, not including necessary associated costs (see Chapter 7 for a detailed discussion of the cost estimates).[5] Millions of aging Americans will wish to receive aducanumab or any other new drug. At the population level, the cost of such a drug would represent a substantial addition to Medicare and other insurance programs. Moreover, the growing population of older people would still require medical and social support for other conditions apart from dementia, and would not benefit if funding for those needs were reduced.

These realities highlight the continuing need for dementia-related research in the social and behavioral sciences. The disciplines that fall into this broad category make use of diverse methods and types of data, but they all share a focus on understanding human and social behavior, responses, and motivations, as well as institutional, social, cultural, and contextual factors that constrain or shape behavior, relationships, access to resources, and exposure to advantage or disadvantage from before conception through late life. Important domains relevant to dementia risk and living with dementia include the study of disparities in access to medical care, the socioeconomic factors that affect cognitive health, psychological study of emotional responses to disease, policies governing health care reimbursement, and many others.

Research in social and behavioral fields also is instrumental to such public health efforts as effectively disseminating information and education, supporting the adoption of innovations in care and treatment, identifying and monitoring trends, and suggesting policy remedies for disparities and health inequities. It also plays a key part in such methodological issues as

---

[5]This estimate is based on the manufacturer's estimate that as many as 2 million people may be currently eligible for the medication, which is expected to be priced at $56,000 per year; see Chapter 7.

interpretation of observational evidence, measurement of important exposures (e.g., racism) and outcomes (e.g., costs, quality of life), the design of clinical trials, and integration of evidence from disparate sources. Social and behavioral research can illuminate the factors that exacerbate or ameliorate dementia, and support better lives for those living with dementia and their caregivers.

Finally, dementia is a progressive and ultimately fatal illness with potentially profound impacts on the lives of all who experience it and their families. As discussed below, however, the risk of developing dementia and its impacts vary across subgroups of the population. Social and behavioral research is vital precisely because this variation is not an accident. The experiences of individuals and families are affected by factors as personal as their own financial resources, physical and emotional health, and relationships, but also by broader systemic and societal factors, including the functioning of medical and long-term care systems, the role of policy and law, the allocation of public resources, and socioeconomic factors that shape health and health care in the United States. The impacts of dementia strain all of the institutions involved, and those strains in turn increase the pressure on individuals and families. Research on the social determinants of health and related issues offers insights relevant to the disparities in both the incidence of dementia and the care and resources available.

While researchers often target average effects in populations, the impacts on individuals are just as important, and these vary markedly. One individual may have numerous advantages that both slow the development of disease and mitigate aspects of the experience, including the resources to support a healthy lifestyle, a stable family, and the financial resources to afford expert care. For another, early-life disadvantages, physically demanding work, subpar health care, a stressed family, and economic hardship may bring a very different experience. From diagnosis to the end of life, individuals with dementia and their caregivers have a wide range of experiences and outcomes. The committee sought to understand the reasons for these discrepancies and what it would take to promote wellness, well-being, and opportunities for life satisfaction for all individuals who develop dementia and their families.

CONTEXT FOR RESEARCH ON THE IMPACTS OF DEMENTIA

The committee began its work with a broad look at the possible impacts of dementia in the United States, including data on the scope of this significant problem and evidence of disparities and inequality. The COVID-19 pandemic emerged after the project began, and we sought evidence of its impact as well.

A Large and Growing Problem

Dementia is primarily a disease of older age. Its prevalence (defined as the percentage of individuals in the population who have a condition) increases steeply after age 60. Incidence (defined as the rate of new cases in the population) also increases steeply with age, according to recent large studies (Lucca et al., 2020; Gilsanz et al., 2019; Corrada et al., 2010). The lifetime risk of developing dementia is approximately twice as great for women as for men, in part because women live longer (Langa et al., 2017; Wolters et al., 2020; Chene et al., 2015). Black and Hispanic people are significantly more likely to develop the disease than are White people (Chen and Zissimopoulos, 2018; Plassman et al., 2007). For an important but small number of people (e.g., persons with Down syndrome), dementia can occur in midlife—in rare cases as early as the 30s but more commonly during the 40s or 50s (National Down Syndrome Society, 2021).

Dementia is expected to become more common as life expectancy increases and the largest generation in history enters the age of risk. Evidence that age-specific rates of dementia have declined in recent decades—in high-income countries—has provided a ray of hope, but the magnitude of these declining rates is modest overall, estimated at about 13 percent per decade over the past 25 years (Wolters et al., 2020). There also is no reason to assume that observed declines in age-specific incidence will continue, since one driver of the declines—rising education levels—has leveled off, and the full range of contributing causes has not been established. Moreover, the impact of any such declines will likely be more than offset by the rapidly growing numbers of people reaching the age of risk (Langa, 2015; Wolters et al., 2020). And as the U.S. population lives longer, the number of years an average person will likely live with dementia is growing (Mayeda et al., 2017b; Zissimopoulos et al., 2014; Langa, 2018).

Disparities in Rates of Dementia and in Care and Resources

Emerging evidence indicates that dementia does not affect all population groups in the United States equally, for complex reasons addressed throughout this report. For example, Table 1-1 shows differences by race and ethnicity reflecting 2000 census data (analyses based on the 2020 census were not yet available). These data include person-years[6] affected by the disease (to account for both the different sizes of the groups themselves and differences in survival rates after onset), as well as age-adjusted incidence

---

[6]Person-years is a measure used to calculate both the number of people in a group and the amount of time each was affected by the circumstance being studied.

rates by group. However, these data do not capture differences among subgroups in these populations, such as the many different subgroups counted as Hispanic for purposes of census data collection.

Estimates using other data also identify sharp disparities across racial/ethnic groups. For example, a population study of the epidemiology of Alzheimer's disease indicated even starker differences, showing that both prevalence and incidence were approximately double for African American people in the study compared with those of European ancestry, although the authors note the challenges of arriving at precise estimates (Rajan et al., 2019). Research also has found that the prevalence of dementia is greatest in low-income neighborhoods and rural areas (Powell et al., 2020a; Wing et al., 2020). Research focused on locations with the highest prevalence has shown further that all groups in lower-income areas have higher rates of disease. In those areas, incidence rates are higher among Black and some Latino populations than among White people of the same age. The rates are lower among Asian American people than among their White counterparts, but there is substantial heterogeneity among Asian American groups (Dilworth-Anderson et al., 2008; Mayeda et al., 2016, 2017a; Mudrazija et al., 2020; Mehta and Yeo, 2017).

These disparities may largely reflect the legacy of systematic inequality, although contemporary conditions also influence both dementia risk and quality of life and well-being for individuals living with dementia. What have been termed the social determinants of health—such factors as education, financial stability, housing, food security, work and work conditions, social isolation, experiences of discrimination and racism, and unhealthy environments—have profound impacts on health and on experiences with the health care system (NASEM, 2016b, 2020; Plough and Christopher, 2020; Yaffe et al., 2013). These issues shaped every section of this report.

TABLE 1-1 Disparities in the Incidence and Impact of Dementia

Racial/Ethnic Group	Total Person-Years	Age-Adjusted Incidence Rate, per 1,000 People
African American	157,118	26.60
American Indian/Alaska Native	41,182	22.18
Latino	195,686	19.59
Pacific Islander	3,246	19.63
White	1,750,252	19.35
Asian American	224,120	15.24

SOURCE: Adapted from Mayeda et al. (2016).

COVID-19 and Dementia

After the committee began its work, COVID-19 began to spread in the United States, and it quickly became apparent that older adults, particularly those living in residential settings, were among the hardest hit (Powell et al., 2020b). The infection spread at lightning speed through many nursing homes and assisted living facilities. By August 2020, it was estimated that 35 to 40 percent of all those who had died from COVID-19 in the United States were residents of nursing homes (Severns, 2020; Chidabaram, 2020; Chidabaram and Garfield, 2021; Chidabaram et al., 2020a; Bernstein, 2020; Soucheray, 2020; Powell et al., 2020b). People living with dementia constitute almost one-half of nursing home residents (Harris-Kojetin et al., 2019). Because of the shocking rate of illness and death in nursing homes, they became the focus of numerous interventions, including heightened testing of both staff and residents, drastic restrictions on visiting, and early access to vaccines when they became available. Significant reductions in the rate of morbidity and mortality followed. The most recent estimate available for this report was that more than 130,000 fatalities, among nearly 600,000 total U.S. fatalities, were nursing home residents (Centers for Medicare & Medicaid Services, 2021).

Policy makers and the operators of care facilities were slow to recognize and act on the threat to vulnerable residents and especially those living with dementia; for example, many facilities did not immediately effectively isolate COVID patients (Jewett, 2020). Facilities and their staffs were also coping with many challenges: stress and illness among staff members; lack of access to COVID testing; staffing shortages; hospitals sending COVID-positive patients to nursing homes to make room for new admissions; the challenge and expense of instituting virus protection measures, especially dire shortages of personal protective equipment and egregious cost increases; and the difficulties of caring safely for residents who contracted the virus. Facilities serving traditionally disadvantaged populations, including low-income residents and members of racial/ethnic subgroups, were particularly hard hit (Chidabaram et al., 2020b). The rate of COVID in any residential setting generally reflected the rate of COVID in the surrounding community, but at least one study suggests that mortality rates were highest in facilities serving the largest percentages of non-White residents (Altman, 2020; Gorges and Konetzka, 2020, 2021).

In addition to the risk of serious illness and death, the virus posed challenges for persons living with dementia, regardless of whether they resided in care facilities, including social isolation and loss of access to vital resources, overcrowded and intergenerational households, shortages of care options, and risks to their care partners, to name but a few. Many communities that had active adult day programs, arts activities, multigenerational community gardens, and other opportunities for social engagement closed these programs until they could be operated safely. Guidance for protecting residents unfortunately increased isolation. For example, a nationwide survey of nursing home residents conducted in summer 2020 found that only 13 percent of residents were eating meals in the dining room, compared with 69 percent before COVID restrictions began (Montgomery et al., 2020).

While researchers are just beginning to explore these issues, it is clear that for a person living with dementia, the loss of regular community or church activities; the inability to see health care providers in person; the demands of using technologies such as Zoom to communicate with providers, caregivers, or family and friends; and the disorienting nature of communication with people whose faces are covered by masks can be devastating. COVID produced exceptional stress for family caregivers as well. Not being able to visit loved ones in nursing homes, especially as rates of disease and death rose across the country, was extraordinarily painful. One distressed daughter described the isolation of a nursing home without visitors as "a slow killer" (Healy et al., 2020). Many families withdrew loved ones from nursing homes or declined admission, choosing instead to provide advanced care at home, hoping to decrease the risk of exposure to COVID (Lin, 2021).

These problems were compounded by the disparate impact of the virus. Although rates varied over time and across regions, Black, Hispanic, American Indian, and Asian people in the United States had disproportionately high rates of infection, hospitalization, and death compared with White people (Rubin-Miller et al., 2020; Manson and Buchwald, 2021). Social and economic inequities in the rates of infection were exacerbated by disparities in access to care (Grabowski and Mor, 2020).

In short, the pandemic exposed profound deficiencies in the care and support available in the United States for people living with dementia and their caregivers. Nevertheless, the pandemic also presented an opportunity to systematically examine an infrastructure that is not only vulnerable to disaster but also inadequate in ordinary times. This report, which outlines a 10-year research agenda for reducing adverse impacts of Alzheimer's disease and other dementias and promoting the well-being of people living with dementia, was conceived long before the pandemic began. As the report goes to press, while the ultimate impact of COVID-19 is not yet known, the pandemic clearly has only heightened the urgency of the report's purpose.

STUDY APPROACH AND SCOPE

To carry out this decadal study of the impact of Alzheimer's disease and related dementias, the committee followed the approach established in previous decadal studies by (1) assessing the needs of the communities the study was intended to benefit, and (2) surveying the landscape of potentially relevant research for ideas with the greatest promise for advancing the objective of mitigating the impact of dementias on all of the constituencies they affect.

Study Scope

As with other decadal studies, the committee was aware that systematically uncovering every potentially valuable research direction would be impossible. Our criteria for identifying candidate research directions were straightforward. We looked for

- problems that are both common and serious for people living with dementia and their caregivers and can be addressed through research in the social and behavioral sciences;
- gaps in the existing research that signal opportunities for meaningful developments in interventions, policies, dementia prevention, or promotion of the well-being of people with dementia and their loved ones; and
- reason to believe those gaps could be filled within a decade using data and methods that are currently or could become available.

A decadal study of necessity reviews a wide landscape, but even within the above parameters, we could not address every relevant topic. Throughout the report we note specific areas we were unable to examine in sufficient depth to support clear research directions, but one key area deserves mention here. The health care system and the entities that provide direct care to people living with dementia (both in their homes and in residential facilities) employ millions of people, including employees ranging from highly trained medical specialists and other clinicians to the individuals who provide assistance with bathing and toileting. The United States is facing moderate to severe shortages of most categories of workers needed to care for people living with dementia, and these shortages are growing. While we recognized the critical importance of a sufficiently supplied and adequately prepared workforce in reducing the impact of dementia, we also appreciated the complexity of the issues involved. Valuable research directions would be based on understanding such issues as the nuances of workforce recruitment, training, and retention related to dementia care; broad societal factors that affect labor supply and demand; benefit structures; and immigration policies. Although a responsible examination of these issues was beyond the scope of this study, we wish to underscore their importance. Appendix B provides a brief review of these issues and the related research recommendations of the 2017 National Research Summit on Dementia Care.

Information Gathering

The committee members brought to this study a significant body of expertise, as well as in many cases personal experiences with family members and friends who either had dementia or cared for loved ones who did. We were determined to learn all we could about the experiences of people living with dementia and those who care for people at all stages of these diseases. An advisory panel made up of individuals living with dementia and having experience as caregivers was appointed to assist in this effort; they are listed in Box 1-3 (biographical sketches of the members appear in Appendix A). Members of the advisory panel spent countless hours with us, contributing to our meetings, participating in conference calls, and assisting us in an effort to solicit perspectives from a much broader population.

The advisory panel also prepared a paper summarizing the ideas they thought were most important for the committee to understand, titled "A Summary of Commentaries Submitted by Those Living with Dementia and Care Partners" (Huling Hummel et al., 2020). This paper includes insights gained from a public call for comments from people living with dementia and caregivers about their experiences and the challenges they face, as well as the panel members' own insights. These perspectives were very valuable as the committee developed this report, particularly Chapters 3, 4, and 5. We have included perspectives shared by advisory panel members and others throughout the report to highlight the impact of the issues discussed on families' lives. We are indebted to the entire advisory panel for all of their contributions.

The public call for commentaries yielded 17 written responses from persons living with dementia and caregivers, as well as three responses delivered orally. We also sought input through committee members' participation in town halls and professional meetings at which they described the project and solicited input, and through a call for white papers that was issued in fall 2019. We received 12 white papers in total and reviewed

---

BOX 1-3
Members of the Advisory Panel to the Committee

Cynthia Huling Hummel
Marie Israelite
John-Richard (JR) Pagan
Ed Patterson
Brian Van Buren
Geraldine Woolfolk

each carefully. We also invited public comment through the project website and a series of e-blasts. Four public workshops held in conjunction with committee meetings allowed us to hear presentations both from persons who have lived with dementia and from traditional academic experts, and to engage in discussions with them and other participants. These workshops addressed

1. Quality of Life for Individuals with Dementia: Preventing Elder Abuse and Fostering Living Well After a Dementia Diagnosis;[7]
2. Nursing Home, Hospice, and Palliative Care for Individuals with Later-Stage Dementia: Making Health Systems More Responsive to Dementia;[8]
3. Challenging Questions About Epidemiology, Care, and Caregiving for People with Alzheimer's Disease and Related Dementias and Their Families;[9] and
4. ADRD Experience and Caregiving, Epidemiology, and Models of Care.[10]

Finally, the committee commissioned six papers to delve more deeply into key topics:[11]

1. Bennett, D. (2020). Commissioned Paper on Defining Different Types of Dementia;
2. Bynum, J.P.W, and Langa, K. (2020). Prevalence Measurement for Alzheimer's Disease and Dementia: Current Status and Future Prospects;
3. Gaugler, J., Jutkowitz, E., and Gitlin, L.N. (2020). Non-Pharmacological Interventions for Persons Living with Alzheimer's Disease: Decadal Review and Recommendations;

---

[7] https://www.nationalacademies.org/event/07-07-2020/meeting-3-decadal-survey-of-behavioral-and-social-science-research-on-alzheimers-disease-and-alzheimers-disease-related-dementias-and-workshop-3

[8] https://www.nationalacademies.org/event/07-08-2020/meeting-3-decadal-survey-of-behavioral-and-social-science-research-on-alzheimers-disease-and-alzheimers-disease-related-dementias-and-workshop-4

[9] https://www.nationalacademies.org/event/10-17-2019/meeting-2-decadal-survey-of-behavioral-and-social-science-research-on-alzheimers-disease-and-alzheimers-disease-related-dementias

[10] https://www.nationalacademies.org/event/08-14-2019/workshop-on-adrd-experience-and-caregiving-epidemiology-and-models-of-care

[11] All commissioned papers are available on the study website at https://www.nationalacademies.org/event/10-17-2019/meeting-2-decadal-survey-of-behavioral-and-social-science-research-on-alzheimers-disease-and-alzheimers-disease-related-dementias.

4. Gitlin, L.N., Jutkowitz, E., and Gaugler, J.E. (2020). Dementia Caregiver Intervention Research Now and into the Future: Review and Recommendations;
5. Lin, P.J. (2020). Commissioned Paper on AD/ADRD Health Economics and Public Policy; and
6. Quiñones, A.R., Kaye, J., Allore, H.G., Thielke, S., and Botoseneanu, A. (2020). Sociocultural Aspects and Determinants of Care for Alzheimer's Disease and Related Dementias (ADRD) Among Minority Ethnic Populations.

We also reviewed research literature related to each of the domains we identified as key to the lived experience of dementia. Several other National Academies' committees have addressed related topics, and we relied on their conclusions where they were relevant; see Box 1-4.

Guiding Themes

Several themes from social and behavioral research shaped the committee's work and run through this report. These include the critical importance of context and development across the life course; the intertwined impacts of dementia on those who have the disease and their caregivers; and ethical issues, such as the balance between safety and autonomy.

Context, from the immediate influences that shape the life of an individual to the larger societal influences that affect health and well-being at a population level, is increasingly recognized as essential to understanding many phenomena. It was particularly important for understanding the stark disparities in both the incidence of dementia and access to high-quality care discussed above. The importance of context to human development was notably articulated in the 1970s by psychologist Urie Bronfenbrenner, who proposed an ecological perspective for understanding the interactions among biological and social influences (Bronfenbrenner, 1977, 1994; for a detailed discussion of research on the influences of environment and context, see, e.g., NASEM, 2019b, 2019c). Researchers in numerous disciplines have built on this idea, particularly in the area of fetal and early-childhood development. They have identified linkages between characteristics of the individual's environment and neurodevelopment, and even the expression of genes later in life. Researchers have also traced the negative impacts of numerous environmental influences on development in the most vulnerable and disadvantaged populations of children, and have pointed to cross-generational effects that serve to perpetuate disadvantage (NASEM, 2019b).

Similarly, in studying dementia and its impacts, it is critical to recognize that every individual affected by dementia is embedded in the context of home, family, community, and society. Factors ranging from characteristics

> **BOX 1-4**
> **National Academies' Reports on Related Topics**
>
> - *Retooling for an Aging America: Building the Health Care Workforce* (2008)
> - *Redesigning Continuing Education in the Health Professions* (2010)
> - *Cognitive Aging: Progress in Understanding and Opportunities for Action* (2015)
> - *Dying in America: Improving Quality and Honoring Individual Preferences Near the End of Life* (2015)
> - *Improving Diagnosis in Health Care* (2015)
> - *A Framework for Educating Health Professionals to Address the Social Determinants of Health* (2016)
> - *Families Caring for an Aging America* (2016)
> - *Communities in Action: Pathways to Health Equity* (2017)
> - *Effective Care for High Need Patients: Opportunities for Improving Outcomes, Value, and Health* (2017)
> - *Preventing Cognitive Decline and Dementia: A Way Forward* (2017)
> - *Integrating Social Care into the Delivery of Health Care: Moving Upstream to Improve the Nation's Health* (2019)
> - *Social Isolation and Loneliness in Older Adults: Opportunities for the Health Care System* (2020)
> - *Leading Health Indicators 2030: Advancing Health, Equity, and Well-Being* (2020)
> - *Meeting the Challenge of Caring for Persons Living with Dementia and Their Care Partners and Caregivers: A Way Forward* (2021)

of neighborhoods, to the legacy of racial discrimination in local housing policies, to the long-standing lingering effects of residential segregation, to federal policies regarding Medicare or the clean-up of toxic pollutants are relevant to dementia risk and progression. These factors interact in ways that can amplify both positive and negative effects on the health and well-being of families and individuals.

Like many contemporary researchers, we also considered a life-course approach in examining cognitive function and dementia in late life (Alwin et al., 2016; Glymour and Manly, 2008; Livingston et al., 2020; Richards and Deary, 2005; Whalley et al., 2006; Zhang et al., 2016). The life-course framework—a way of examining change across the life span—is related to the ecological approach and has also been applied in many contexts (Alwin, 2012).[12] Taking a life-course perspective led the committee to look not only

---

[12] These contexts include the study of chronic disease, physical functioning, and mortality (see, e.g., Ben-Shlomo and Kuh, 2002; Haas, 2008; Hayward and Gorman, 2004; Kuh, 2007; Kuh et al., 2002).

at the experiences that begin when symptoms appear or when medical care is required, but also at the factors that may eliminate, ameliorate, or exacerbate risk beginning long before the onset of disease.

REPORT STRUCTURE

With the above ideas in mind, the committee looked across the potential impacts of dementia and identified those areas in which we saw the greatest potential leverage for improving outcomes. Accordingly, the report is structured around these primary areas:

- Risk and preventive factors for dementia and how they relate to the social determinants of health—the social and economic conditions that affect health care and health outcomes (Chapter 2).
- The personal experience of living with dementia and the issues associated with diagnosis, care, and treatment (Chapter 3).
- The experiences of family caregivers and resources available to them (Chapter 4).
- How characteristics of communities affect dementia risk and quality of life for people living with dementia and their families, and the broad social forces that shape communities (Chapter 5).
- The health care system and the institutions that provide residential long-term care and hospice and palliative care (Chapter 6).
- The economic costs of dementia to individuals and to society (Chapter 7).

Each of these chapters offers directions for research in the coming decade. Chapter 8 reviews methodological issues that affect research across these areas and suggests pathways for strengthening the evidence base to support progress in reducing the negative impacts of dementia. Chapter 9 summarizes the committee's recommended research agenda.

REFERENCES

Altman, D. (2020, July 21). *Hotspot States See More COVID Cases in Nursing Homes*. https://www.axios.com/coronavirus-cases-infections-nursing-homes-b5260d20-47f2-4a56-9574-e63e9dafd012.html

Alwin, D. (2012). Integrating varieties of life course concepts. *Journals of Gerontology, Series B, 67*(2), 206–220. https://doi.org/10.1093/geronb/gbr146

Alwin, D.F., Thomas, J.R., and Wray, L.A. (2016). Cognitive development and the life course: Growth, stability and decline. In M. Shanahan, J. Mortimer, and M.K. Johnson (Eds.), *Handbook of the Life Course* (vol. 2, pp. 451–488). Cham: Springer International Publishing. https://doi.org/10.1007/978-3-319-20880-0_21

Alzheimer's Association. (2021). *2021 Alzheimer's Disease Facts and Figures*. https://www.alz.org/media/Documents/alzheimers-facts-and-figures.pdf

American Psychiatric Association. (2013). *Diagnostic and Statistical Manual of Mental Disorders* (5th ed.). Washington, DC: Author.

Bennett, D. (2020). *Commissioned Paper on Defining Different Types of Dementia*. Paper prepared for the National Academies of Sciences, Engineering, and Medicine, Decadal Survey of Behavioral and Social Science Research on Alzheimer's Disease and Alzheimer's Disease-Related Dementias. https://www.nationalacademies.org/event/10-17-2019/meeting-2-decadal-survey-of-behavioral-and-social-science-research-on-alzheimers-disease-and-alzheimers-disease-related-dementias

Ben-Shlomo, Y., and Kuh, D. (2002). A life course approach to chronic disease epidemiology: Conceptual models, empirical challenges and interdisciplinary perspectives. *International Journal of Epidemiology*, 31(2), 285–293.

Bernstein, L. (2020, August 13). Covid-19 surges back into nursing homes in coronavirus hot spots. *Washington Post*. https://www.washingtonpost.com/health/covid-19-surges-back-into-nursing-homes-in-coronavirus-hot-spots/2020/08/13/edbff5fe-dd75-11ea-b205-ff838e15a9a6_story.html

Bronfenbrenner, U. (1977). Toward an experimental ecology of human development. *American Psychologist*, 32(7), 513–531.

———. (1994). Ecological models of human development. In *International Encyclopedia of Education* (2nd ed., vol. 3). Oxford: Elsevier.

Bynum, J.P.W., and Langa, K. (2020). *Prevalence Measurement for Alzheimer's Disease and Dementia: Current Status and Future Prospects*. Paper prepared for the National Academies of Sciences, Engineering, and Medicine, Decadal Survey of Behavioral and Social Science Research on Alzheimer's Disease and Alzheimer's Disease-Related Dementias. https://www.nationalacademies.org/event/10-17-2019/meeting-2-decadal-survey-of-behavioral-and-social-science-research-on-alzheimers-disease-and-alzheimers-disease-related-dementias

Centers for Medicare & Medicaid Services. (2021). *COVID-19 Nursing Home Data*. https://data.cms.gov/stories/s/COVID-19-Nursing-Home-Data/bkwz-xpvg

Chen, C., and Zissimopoulos, J. (2018). Racial and ethnic disparities in dementia prevalence and risk factors from 2000 to 2012 in the United States. *Alzheimer's and Dementia Translational Research*, 4(1), 510–520. https://doi.org/10.1016/j.trci.2018.08.009

Chene, G., Beiser, A., Au, R., Preis, S., Wolf, P., Dufouil, C., and Seshadri, S. (2015). Gender and incidence of dementia in the Framingham Heart Study from mid-adult life. *Alzheimer's & Dementia*, 11(3), 310–320. https://doi.org/10.1016/j.jalz.2013.10.005

Chidabaram, P. (2020, July 21). *Rising Cases in Long-Term Care Facilities Are Cause for Concern*. Kaiser Family Foundation. https://www.kff.org/coronavirus-covid-19/issue-brief/rising-cases-in-long-term-care-facilities-are-cause-for-concern

Chidabaram, P., and Garfield, R. (2021, January 14). *Patterns in COVID-19 Cases and Deaths in Long-Term Care Facilities in 2020*. Kaiser Family Foundation. https://www.kff.org/coronavirus-covid-19/issue-brief/patterns-in-covid-19-cases-and-deaths-in-long-term-care-facilities-in-2020

Chidabaram, P., Garfield, R., and Neuman, T. (2020a, November 25). *COVID-19 Has Claimed the Lives of 100,000 Long-Term Care Residents and Staff*. Kaiser Family Foundation. https://www.kff.org/policy-watch/covid-19-has-claimed-the-lives-of-100000-long-term-care-residents-and-staff

Chidabaram, P., Neuman, T., and Garfield, R. (2020b, October 27). *Racial and Ethnic Disparities in COVID-19 Cases and Deaths in Nursing Homes*. Kaiser Family Foundation. https://www.kff.org/coronavirus-covid-19/issue-brief/racial-and-ethnic-disparities-in-covid-19-cases-and-deaths-in-nursing-homes

Corrada, M., Brookmeyer, R., Paganini-Hill, A., Berlau, D., and Kawas, C. (2010). Dementia incidence continues to increase with age in the oldest old: The 90+ study. *Annals of Neurology, 67*(1), 114–121. https://doi.org/10.1002/ana.21915

Crisis Prevention Institute. (2021). Major neurocognitive disorder: The DSM-5's new term for dementia. Blog post. https://www.crisisprevention.com/Blog/Major-Neurocognitive-Disorder-Dementia

Cummings, J., Morstorf, T., and Zhong, K. (2014). Alzheimer's disease drug development pipeline: Few candidates, frequent failure. *Alzheimer's Research and Therapy, 6*(37). https://doi.org/10.1186/alzrt269

Dilworth-Anderson, P., Hendrie, H.C., Manly, J.J., Khachaturian, A.S., and Fazio, S. (2008). Diagnosis and assessment of Alzheimer's disease in diverse populations. *Alzheimer's & Dementia, 4*(4), 305–309. https://doi.org/10.1016/j.jalz.2008.03.001

Favreault, M.M., Gleckman, H., and Johnson, R.W. (2015). Financing long-term services and supports: Options reflect trade-offs for older Americans and federal spending. *Health Affairs, 30*(12), 2181–2191. https://doi.org/10.1377/hlthaff.2015.1226

Garde, D., and Feuerstein, A. (2020, November 4). FDA scientists appear to offer major endorsement of Biogen's controversial Alzheimer's treatment. *STAT.* https://www.statnews.com/2020/11/04/fda-scientists-appear-to-offer-major-endorsement-of-biogens-controversial-alzheimers-treatment

Gaugler, J., Jutkowitz, E., and Gitlin, L. (2020). *Non-pharmacological Interventions for Persons Living with Alzheimer's Disease: Decadal Review and Recommendations.* Paper prepared for the National Academies of Sciences, Engineering, and Medicine, Decadal Survey of Behavioral and Social Science Research on Alzheimer's Disease and Alzheimer's Disease-Related Dementias. https://www.nationalacademies.org/event/10-17-2019/meeting-2-decadal-survey-of-behavioral-and-social-science-research-on-alzheimers-disease-and-alzheimers-disease-related-dementias

Gilsanz, P., Corrada, M., Kawas, C., Mayeda, E., Glymour, M., Quesenberry, C., Lee, C., and Whitmer, R. (2019). Incidence of dementia after age 90 in a multiracial cohort. *Alzheimer's & Dementia, 15*(4), 497–505. https://doi.org/10.1016/j.jalz.2018.12.006

Gitlin, L., Jutkowitz, E., and Gaugler, J. (2020). *Dementia Caregiver Intervention Research Now and into the Future: Review and Recommendations.* Paper prepared for the National Academies of Sciences, Engineering, and Medicine, Decadal Survey of Behavioral and Social Science Research on Alzheimer's Disease and Alzheimer's Disease-Related Dementias. https://www.nationalacademies.org/event/10-17-2019/meeting-2-decadal-survey-of-behavioral-and-social-science-research-on-alzheimers-disease-and-alzheimers-disease-related-dementias

Glymour, M.M., and Manly, J.J. (2008). Lifecourse social conditions and racial and ethnic patterns of cognitive aging. *Neuropsychology Review, 18*(3), 223–254. https://doi.org/10.1007/s11065-008-9064-z

Gorges, R.J., and Konetzka, R.T. (2020). Staffing levels and COVID-19 cases and outbreaks in U.S. nursing homes. *Journal of the American Geriatrics Society, 68*(11), 2462–2466. https://doi.org/10.1111/jgs.16787

———. (2021). Factors associated with racial differences in deaths among nursing home residents with COVID-19 infection in the U.S. *JAMA Network Open, 4*(2), e2037431. https://doi.org/10.1001/jamanetworkopen.2020.37431

Grabowski, D.C., and Mor, V. (2020, May 22). Nursing home care in crisis in the wake of COVID-19. *JAMA Network Open.* https://jamanetwork.com/journals/jama/fullarticle/2766599

Haas, S. (2008). Trajectories of functional health: The "long arm" of childhood health and socioeconomic factors. *Social Science & Medicine, 66*(4), 849–861. https://doi.org/10.1016/j.socscimed.2007.11.004

Harris-Kojetin, L., Sengupta, M., Lendon, J.P., Rome, V., Valverde, R., and Caffrey, C. (2019). Long-term care providers and services users in the United States, 2015–2016. *National Center for Health Statistics: Vital and Health Statistics*, *3*(43). https://www.cdc.gov/nchs/data/series/sr_03/sr03_43-508.pdf

Hayward, M.D., and Gorman, B.K. (2004). The long arm of childhood: The influence of early-life social conditions on men's mortality. *Demography*, *41*(1), 87–107. https://doi.org/10.1353/dem.2004.0005

Healy, J., Ivory, D., and Kovaleski, S.F. (2020, October 30). "A slow killer": Nursing home residents wither in isolation forced by the virus. *New York Times*. https://www.nytimes.com/2020/10/30/us/nursing-homes-isolation-virus.html

Huling Hummel, C., Pagan, J.R., Israelite, M., Patterson, E., Van Buren, B., and Woolcock, G. (2020). *A Summary of Commentaries Submitted by Those Living with Dementia and Care Partners*. Paper prepared for the National Academies of Sciences, Engineering, and Medicine, Decadal Survey of Behavioral and Social Science Research on Alzheimer's Disease and Alzheimer's Disease-Related Dementias. https://www.nationalacademies.org/our-work/decadal-survey-of-behavioral-and-social-science-research-on-alzheimers-and-alzheimers-disease-related-dementias

Jewett, C. (2020, September 10). Hospitals, nursing homes fail to separate COVID patients, putting others at risk. *Kaiser Health News*. https://khn.org/news/hospitals-nursing-homes-fail-to-separate-covid-patients-putting-others-at-risk

Kaiser, J. (2018). The Alzheimer's gamble. *Science*, *31*(361), 838–841. https://doi.org/10.1126/science.361.6405.838

Kuh, D. (2007). A life course approach to healthy aging, frailty, and capability. *Journals of Gerontology: Series A*, *62*(7), 717–721. https://doi.org/10.1093/gerona/62.7.717

Kuh, D., Hardy, R., Langenberg, C., Richards, M., and Wadsworth, M.E.J. (2002). Mortality in adults aged 26-54 years related to socioeconomic conditions in childhood and adulthood: Post war birth cohort study. *British Medical Journal*, *325*(7372), 1076–1080. https://doi.org/10.1136/bmj.325.7372.1076

Langa, K.M. (2015). Is the risk of Alzheimer's disease and dementia declining? *Alzheimer's Research & Therapy*, *7*(1), 34. https://doi.org/10.1186/s13195-015-0118-1

———. (2018). Cognitive aging, dementia, and the future of an aging population. In *Future Directions for the Demography of Aging: Proceedings of a Workshop*. Washington, DC: The National Academies Press. https://www.nap.edu/read/25064/chapter/15

Langa, K.M., Larson, E.B., Crimmins, E.M., Faul, J.D, Levine, D.A., Kabeto, M.A., and Weir, D.R. (2017). A comparison of the prevalence of dementia in the United States in 2000 and 2012. *JAMA Internal Medicine*, *177*(1), 51–58. https://doi.org/10.1001/jamainternmed.2016.6807

Lin, P. (2020). *Commissioned Paper on AD/ADRD Health Economics and Public Policy*. Paper prepared for the National Academies of Sciences, Engineering, and Medicine, Decadal Survey of Behavioral and Social Science Research on Alzheimer's Disease and Alzheimer's Disease-Related Dementias. https://www.nationalacademies.org/event/10-17-2019/meeting-2-decadal-survey-of-behavioral-and-social-science-research-on-alzheimers-disease-and-alzheimers-disease-related-dementias

Lin, K. (2021, January 1). Because of you guys I'm stuck in my room. *New York Times*. https://www.nytimes.com/2021/01/01/opinion/nursing-home-senior-living-coronavirus.html

Livingston, G., Huntley, J., Sommerlad, A., Ames, D., Ballard, C., Banerjee, S., Brayne, C., Burns, A., Cohen-Mansfield, J., Cooper, C., Costafreda, S.G., Dias, A., Fox, N., Gitlin, L.N., Howard, R., Kales, H.C., Kivimäki, M., Larson, E.B., Ogunniyi, A., Orgeta, V., Ritchie, K., Rockwood, K., Sampson, E.L., Samus, Q., Schneider, L.S., Selbæk, G., Teri, L., and Mukadam, N. (2020). Dementia prevention, intervention, and care: 2020 report of the Lancet Commission. *Lancet*, *396*(10248), P413–P446. https://doi.org/10.1016/S0140-6736(20)30367-6

Lucca, U., Tettamanti, M., Tiraboschi, P., Logroscino, G., Landi, C., Sacco, L., Garri, M., Ammesso, S., Biotti, A., Gargantini, E., Piedicorcia, A., Mandelli, S., Riva. E., Galbussera, A., and Recchia, A. (2020). Incidence of dementia in the oldest-old and its relationship with age: The Monzino 80-plus population-based study. *Alzheimer's & Dementia*, 16(3), 472–481. https://doi.org/10.1016/j.jalz.2019.09.083

Manson, S.M., and Buchwald, D.S. (2021). Bringing light to the darkness: COVID-19 and survivance of American Indians and Alaska Natives. *Health Equity*, 5(1). https://doi.org/10.1089/heq.2020.0123

Matthews, K.A., Xu, W., Gaglioti, A.H., Holt, J.B., Croft, J.B., Mack, D., and McGuire, L.C. (2019). Racial and ethnic estimates of Alzheimer's disease and related dementias in the United States (2015-2060) in adults aged ≥65 years. *Alzheimer's & Dementia*, 15(1), 17–24. https://doi.org/10.1016/j.jalz.2018.06.3063

Mayeda, E.R., Glymour, M.M., Quesenberry, C.P., and Whitmer, R.A. (2016). Inequalities in dementia incidence between six racial and ethnic groups over 14 years. *Alzheimer's & Dementia*, 12(3), 216–224. https://doi.org/10.1016/j.jalz.2015.12.007

Mayeda, E.R., Glymour, M.M., Quesenberry, C.P., and Whitmer, R.A. (2017a). Heterogeneity in 14-year dementia incidence between Asian American subgroups. *Alzheimer Disease & Associated Disorders*, 31(3), 181–186. https://doi.org/10.1097/WAD.0000000000000189

Mayeda, E.R., Glymour, M.M., Quesenberry, C.P., Johnson, J.K., Pérez-Stable, E.J., and Whitmer, R.A. (2017b). Survival after dementia diagnosis in five racial/ethnic groups. *Alzheimer's & Dementia*, 13(7), 761–769. https://doi.org/10.1016/j.jalz.2016.12.008

McKhann, G.M., Knopman, D.S., Chertkow, H., Hyman, B.T., Jack, Jr., C.R., Kawas, C.H., Klunk, W.E., Koroshetz, W.J., Manly, J.J., Mayeux, R., Mohs, R.C., Morris, J.C., Rossor, M.N., Scheltens, P., Carrillo, M.C., Thies, B., Weintraub, S., and Phelps, C.H. (2011). The diagnosis of dementia due to Alzheimer's disease: Recommendations from the National Institute on Aging-Alzheimer's Association workgroups on diagnostic guidelines for Alzheimer's disease. *Alzheimer's & Dementia*, 7(3), 263–269. https://doi.org/10.1016/j.jalz.2011.03.005

Mehta, K.M., and Yeo, G.W. (2017). Systematic review of dementia prevalence and incidence in United States race/ethnic populations. *Alzheimer's & Dementia*, 13(1), 72–83. https://doi.org/10.1016/j.jalz.2016.06.2360

Montgomery, A., Slocum, S., and Stanik, K. (2020). *Experiences of Nursing Home Residents during the Pandemic: What We Learned from Residents About Life Under Covid-19 Restrictions and What We Can Do About It*. Altarum. https://altarum.org/sites/default/files/uploaded-publication-files/Nursing-Home-Resident-Survey_Altarum-Special-Report_FINAL.pdf

Mudrazija, S., Vega, W., Resendez, J., and Monroe, S. (2020). *Place & Brain Health Equity: Understanding the County-Level Impacts of Alzheimer's*. UsAgainstAlzheimer's and Urban Institute. https://www.usagainstalzheimers.org/sites/default/files/2020-11/Urban_UsA2%20Brain%20Health%20Equity%20Report_11-15-20_FINAL.pdf

NASEM (National Academies of Sciences, Engineering, and Medicine). (2015). *The Space Science Decadal Surveys: Lessons Learned and Best Practices*. Washington, DC: The National Academies Press.

———. (2016a). *Families Caring for an Aging America*. Washington, DC: The National Academies Press. https://doi.org/10.17226/23606

———. (2016b). *A Framework for Educating Health Professionals to Address the Social Determinants of Health*. Washington, DC: The National Academies Press.

———. (2019a). *A Decadal Survey of the Social and Behavioral Sciences: A Research Agenda for Advancing Intelligence Analysis*. Washington, DC: The National Academies Press.

———. (2019b). *Fostering Healthy Mental, Emotional, and Behavioral Development in Children and Youth*. Washington, DC: The National Academies Press. https://doi.org/10.17226/25201

———. (2019c). *How People Learn II*. Washington, DC: The National Academies Press.
———. (2020). *Leading Health Indicators 2030: Advancing Health, Equity, and Well-Being*. Washington, DC: The National Academies Press. https://doi.org/10.17226/25682
National Down Syndrome Society. (2021). *Alzheimer's Disease and Down Syndrome*. https://www.ndss.org/resources/alzheimers
Plassman, B.L., Langa, K.M., Fisher, G.G., Heeringa, S.G., Weir, D.R., Ofstedal, M.B., Burke, J.R., Hurd, M.D., Potter, G.G., Rodgers, W.L., Steffens, D.C., Willis, R.J., and Wallace, R.B. (2007). Prevalence of dementia in the United States: The aging, demographics, and memory study. *Neuroepidemiology*, 29(1–2), 125–132. https://doi.org/10.1159/000109998
Plough, A., and Christopher, G. (2020). The role of racial justice in building a culture of health. *Health Affairs Blog*. https://www.healthaffairs.org/do/10.1377/hblog20200914.537608/full
Powell, W.R., Buckingman, W.R., Larson, J.L., Yu, M., Salamat, M.S., Bendlin, B.B., Rissman, R.A., and Kind, A.J.H. (2020a). Association of neighborhood level disadvantage with Alzheimer disease neuropathology. *JAMA Network Open*, 3(6), e207559. https://doi.org/10.1001/jamanetworkopen.2020.7559
Powell, T., Bellin, E., and Ehrlich, A.R. (2020b). Older adults and COVID-19: The most vulnerable are the hardest hit. *Hastings Center Report*, 50(3), 61–63. https://doi.org/10.1002/hast.1136
Quiñones, A.R, Kaye, J., Allore, H.G., Thielke, S., and Botoseneanu, A. (2020a). *Sociocultural Aspects and Determinants of Care for Alzheimer's Disease and Related Dementias (ADRD) among Minority Ethnic Populations*. Paper prepared for the National Academies of Sciences, Engineering, and Medicine, Decadal Survey of Behavioral and Social Science Research on Alzheimer's Disease and Alzheimer's Disease-Related Dementias. https://www.nationalacademies.org/event/10-17-2019/meeting-2-decadal-survey-of-behavioral-and-social-science-research-on-alzheimers-disease-and-alzheimers-disease-related-dementias
Quiñones, A.R., Kaye, J., Allore, H.G., Botoseneanu, A., and Thielke, S.M. (2020b). An agenda for addressing multimorbidity and racial and ethnic disparities in Alzheimer's disease and related dementia. *American Journal of Alzheimer's Disease & Other Dementias*, 35, 1–7. https://doi.org/10.1177/1533317520960874
Rajan, K., Weuve, J., Barnes, L., Wilson, R., and Evans, D. (2019). Prevalence and incidence of clinically diagnosed Alzheimer's disease dementia from 1994 to 2012 in a population study. *Alzheimer's & Dementia*, 15(1), 1–7. https://doi.org/10.1016/j.jalz.2018.07.216
Rajan, K., Weuve, J., Barnes, L., McAninch, E., Wilson, R., and Evans, D. (2021). Population estimate of people with clinical AD and mild cognitive impairment in the United States (2020-2060). *Alzheimer's & Dementia*, 15(1), 1–7. https://doi.org/10.1016/j.jalz.2018.07.216
Richards, M., and Deary, I.J. (2005). A life course approach to cognitive reserve: A model for cognitive aging and development? *Annals of Neurology*, 58(4), 617–622. https://doi.org/10.1002/ana.20637
Rubin-Miller, L. Alban, C., Artiga, S., and Sullivan, S. (2020, September 16). *COVID-19 Racial Disparities in Testing, Infection, Hospitalization, and Death: Analysis of Epic Patient Data*. Kaiser Family Foundation. https://www.kff.org/coronavirus-covid-19/issue-brief/covid-19-racial-disparities-testing-infection-hospitalization-death-analysis-epic-patient-data
Severns, M. (2020, August 10). Could massive numbers of nursing home deaths have been prevented? *Politico*. https://www.politico.com/states/florida/story/2020/08/10/could-massive-numbers-of-nursing-home-deaths-have-been-prevented-1307016

Soucheray, S. (2020, June 16). Nursing homes might account for 40% of U.S. COVID-19 deaths. *Center for Infectious Disease Research and Policy News*. https://www.cidrap.umn.edu/news-perspective/2020/06/nursing-homes-might-account-40-us-covid-19-deaths

Vespa, J. (2018, March 13). *The Graying of America: More Adults than Kids by 2035*. U.S. Census Bureau. https://www.census.gov/library/stories/2018/03/graying-america.html

Weuve, J., Hebert, L., Scherr, P., and Evans, D. (2014). Deaths in the United States among persons with Alzheimer's disease (2010-2050). *Alzheimer's & Dementia, 10*(2), E40–E46. https://doi.org/10.1016/j.jalz.2014.01.004

Whalley, L.J., Dick, F.D., and McNeill, G. (2006) A life-course approach to the aetiology of late-onset dementias. *Lancet Neurology, 5*(1), 87–96. https://doi.org/10.1016/S1474-4422(05)70286-6

Wimo, A., Guerchet, M., Ali, G.-C., Wu, Y.-T., Prina, A.M., Winblad, B., Jönsson, L., Liu, Z., and Prince, M. (2017). The worldwide costs of dementia 2015 and comparisons with 2010. *Alzheimer's & Dementia, 13*(1), 1–7. https://doi.org/10.1016/j.jalz.2016.07.150

Wing, J., Levine, D., Ramamurthy, A., and Reider, C. (2020). Alzheimer's disease and related disorders prevalence differs by Appalachian residence in Ohio. *Journal of Alzheimer's Disease, 76*(4), 1309–1316. https://pubmed.ncbi.nlm.nih.gov/32597814

Wolters, F.J., Chibnik, L.B., Waziry, R., Anderson, R., Berr, C., Beiser, A., Bis, J.C., Blacker, D., Bos, D., Brayne, C., Dartigues, J.-F., Darweesh, S.K.L., Davis-Plourde, K.L., De Wolf, F., Debette, S., Dufouil, C., Fornage, M., Goudsmit, J., Grasset, L., Gudnason, V., Hadjichrysanthou, C., Helmer, C., Ikram, M.A., Ikram, M.K., Joas, E., Kern, S., Kuller, L.H., Launer, L., Lopez, O.L., Matthews, F.E., McRae-McKee, K., Meirelles, O., Mosley, T.H., Pase, M.P., Psaty, B.M., Satizabal, C.L., Seshadri, S., Skoog, I., Stephan, B.C.M., Wetterberg, H., Wong, M.M., Zettergren, A., and Hofman, A. (2020). Twenty-seven-year time trends in dementia incidence in Europe and the United States. *Neurology, 95*(5), e519–e531. https://doi.org/10.1212/WNL.0000000000010022

Yaffe, K., Falvey, C., Harris, T., Newman, A., Satterfield, S., Koster, A., Ayonayon, H., and Simonsick, E. (2013). Effect of socioeconomic disparities on incidence of dementia among biracial older adults: Prospective study. *British Medical Journal, 347*, f7051. https://doi.org/10.1136/bmj.f7051

Zhang, Z., Hayward, M.D., and Yu, Y.-L. (2016). Life course pathways to racial disparities in cognitive impairment among older Americans. *Journal of Health and Social Behavior, 57*(2), 184–199. https://doi.org/10.1177/0022146516645925

Zissimopoulos, J.M., Crimmins, E.M., and St. Clair, P.A. (2014). The value of delaying Alzheimer's disease onset. *Forum for Health Economics and Policy, 18*(1), 25–39. https://doi.org/10.1515/fhep-2014-0013

Zissimopoulos, J.M., Tysinger, B.C., St. Clair, P.A., and Crimmins, E.M. (2018). The impact of changes in population health and mortality on future prevalence of Alzheimer's disease and other dementias in the United States. *Journals of Gerontology: Series B, 73*(Suppl_1), S38–S47. https://doi.org/10.1093/geronb/gbx147

2

Prevention and Protective Factors

Multiple lines of evidence suggest that a large proportion of all dementia could be prevented, delayed, or slowed by social or behavioral changes. Researchers have not yet established, however, which specific risk factors are most important or how interventions to modify behaviors and conditions could have the greatest impact on dementia. Many aspects of an individual's life—socioeconomic resources; education level; health-relevant behaviors, including diet and exercise patterns; trauma; medical and psychiatric conditions; and characteristics of the physical and social environment—play a role in dementia and intersect with genetic risks. Yet while social and behavioral factors may influence the risk of developing dementia or the progression of disease, their impacts are not inevitable. Modifications, either at the individual level (through changes in behaviors or exposures) or at the population level (through changes to local, state, or federal policies or reorganization of institutional regulations, programs, and practices) may affect outcomes.

Although clear causal relationships are challenging to establish definitively, some researchers have suggested that as much as 40 percent of dementia may be attributable at least in part to modifiable risk factors (Barnes and Yaffe, 2011; Norton et al., 2014; Livingston et al., 2020).[1] Identifying a firm percentage would be challenging, however, because dementia risk is associated with many factors beginning very early in life,

---

[1] Modifiable risk factors account for an additional portion of the overall impact of dementia that is not explained by either identified genetic or identified environmental factors (Livingston et al., 2020).

which vary significantly across population groups. Although some genetic factors are important, healthier social and behavioral patterns predict lower dementia risk, virtually regardless of genetic background (Lourida et al., 2019).[2] Overall, these estimates are approximate at best and fail to account for the joint impact of multiple correlated risk factors or changes in the pattern of risk factors over time, as discussed below. What is important to note is that prevention efforts can alter the risk of dementia in any population, at any time of life.

Several public health initiatives to modify harmful influences on health—including reductions in the prevalence of smoking (leading to extraordinary declines in cardiovascular disease), reductions in motor vehicle crash fatalities per mile traveled, and reductions in exposure to lead—have been quite successful (Ruiz-Hernandez et al., 2017). Although these initiatives are by no means completed and often were slow to initiate, they have yielded tremendous public health gains and offer insight into how to approach complex public health problems (Gielen and Green, 2015). These successful campaigns highlight the importance of targeting multiple levels of influence, as was done, for example, in the campaign to reduce smoking, which targeted both individual behavior (e.g., smoking cessation classes) and factors at the population or systems level (e.g., cigarette taxes and bans on smoking in public spaces).[3]

Successes in combating cardiometabolic conditions are especially relevant because many types of dementia are influenced by mechanisms or processes that contribute to other diseases (e.g., vascular changes, metabolic dysregulation, inflammation). A substantial proportion of cases of late-onset dementia (defined as dementia symptoms starting at age 65 and older [McMurtray et al., 2006]) reflect the combined effects of mixed pathologies, such as amyloid and tau deposition and vascular changes. Improved understanding of the relationships among these factors and how to exploit them to slow disease progression, reduce the severity of disease, or prevent or delay disease in some people could be an important means of reducing the incidence and severity of dementia (Schneider et al., 2009; Barnes et al., 2015; Kawas et al., 2015). Likewise, such population trends as the obesity epidemic and associated increasing prevalence of diabetes are relevant for anticipating future increases in the risk of dementia.

This chapter examines the state of the research on prevention and risk factors for dementia, beginning with an overview of the nature of the

---

[2] This statement does not apply to rare autosomal-dominant dementias that occur early in life.

[3] See Frieden (2010) for discussion of the tension between interventions that require increasing individual effort (e.g., counseling, education, or clinical interventions) and interventions that are likely to have large population impact (e.g., socioeconomic factors or systems changes to make healthy choices the default).

available evidence. The chapter then looks in detail at two primary lenses for thinking about prevention. First, it explores evidence about how various factors affect cognitive health and disease in individuals, including evidence about preventive strategies and policies that have been pursued in targeting chronic diseases that are medically linked to dementia, such as cardiovascular disease and diabetes. The chapter then turns to the evidence about broader social and environmental factors and policies that play a role in increasing or diminishing risk over the life span.

INTERPRETING THE EVIDENCE

In assessing the evidence about risk and protective factors for dementia, the committee was able to rely on systematic reviews, meta-analyses, and the work of previous National Academies of Sciences, Engineering, and Medicine committees that have synthesized relevant research. In general, these syntheses make clear that the body of evidence provided by randomized controlled trials (RCTs) is limited. RCTs are regarded as providing the highest-quality evidence for establishing a causal link between an exposure and an outcome in at least some people. But very few RCTs targeting behavior change and including follow-up for dementia or related outcomes have been carried out. Moreover, existing RCTs in this area are often underpowered, involving modest sample sizes, relatively brief interventions, and short follow-up periods. The findings they yield are sometimes inconsistent across trials and between outcomes within the same trial. And even when RCTs are available, they often do not reflect the demographic characteristics or health status of the broader population, and so must be augmented with evidence on heterogeneity of effects and generalizability to other populations. There are also many situations in which conducting RCTs can be considered unethical, such as when the intervention is known to be beneficial for another outcome and it is not offered to one group. And in other settings, RCTs are infeasible because the time periods over which risk factors are thought to operate are so long.

A significantly larger body of observational (non-RCT) data implicates several factors associated with subsequent dementia risk. However, many of these observational studies are vulnerable to at least one of two sources of bias. One is "confounding," the term used when an association is ascribed to one factor, the putative cause, but is driven by another factor that is associated with both the putative cause and the outcome. For example, cognitive activity appears to reduce the risk of dementia, but it is possible that some or all of the apparent effect may result from the association of cognitive activity with other protective factors, such as education. Researchers address this problem by using analytic adjustment for such confounding factors, but residual or unmeasured confounders are always a concern in observational studies. A second potential source of bias is reverse causation—when early symptoms of the disease outcome lead to changes in the apparent risk factor rather than the other way around. For example, mild cognitive changes could make cognitive activities less enjoyable and thus decrease participation, leading to a spurious impression that lower cognitive activity increases the risk of dementia (Floud et al., 2021; Sajeev et al., 2016). Similarly, while social isolation may be a risk factor for dementia, incipient dementia may also lead to social isolation.

In addition to these two forms of bias, other challenges need to be considered when evaluating observational studies, including

- difficulties measuring cognition, especially subtle cognitive changes or change in those with very high or low levels of education, and while this is true in all dementia research, in observational studies it can interact with the hypothesis or a key covariate and lead to bias;
- selective survival, or differences in the characteristics of populations that survive to older ages that can lead to spurious statistical associations;
- a lack of diversity in the samples or nonrepresentative samples of the population;
- short follow-up periods in many studies, particularly given that many risk factors are thought to contribute to risk over long periods of time;
- selective recruitment into and retention in research studies, leading to both uncertainty (because of small sample sizes) and spurious associations (caused by selection bias); and
- testing of multiple hypotheses without correction for the multiplicity of tests.

These concerns are well known, but biases can be minimized, quantified, or possibly avoided with appropriate study designs and analytical tools, and ancillary evidence may aid in the interpretation of results from observational studies. Nevertheless, biases and the other challenges outlined above remain a significant concern if observational findings are to be translated into preventive interventions. These issues are discussed further in Chapter 8.

INFLUENCES ON COGNITIVE HEALTH IN INDIVIDUALS

Researchers have explored factors that may affect the risk of dementia directly, influences on cardiovascular health that in turn have implications for cognitive health, and other possible culprits. This section explores the evidence and reviews the implications for individuals and public health experts.

Evidence About Risk and Protection for Cognitive Health

Interest in preventing or minimizing the impact of dementia has stimulated a wealth of research, as well as the development of many hypotheses and recommendations to the public. Expert advice is neither unanimous nor conclusive, however. Different experts who have assessed the available work have reached somewhat different conclusions as a result of decisions about which type of evidence to focus on or how to weigh the evidence. Two National Academies' committees and a group writing for the medical journal *The Lancet* have reviewed the available research and summarized their conclusions about preventive factors. These summaries offer a clear picture of the current state of the research.

As a backdrop, a 2015 National Academies' report titled *Cognitive Aging: Progress in Understanding and Opportunities for Action* focuses not on preventing such diseases as dementia but on optimal cognitive aging overall. The report summarizes ways to support cognitive health and functioning as people experience the "process of gradual, ongoing, yet highly variable changes in cognitive functions that occur as people get older" (Institute of Medicine, 2015, p. 2). The authors offer broad recommendations about steps individuals can take to support their cognitive health (p. 7):

- Be physically active.
- Reduce and manage cardiovascular disease risk factors (including hypertension, diabetes, and smoking).
- Regularly discuss and review health conditions and medications that might influence cognitive health with a health care professional.

The report also endorses some actions more cautiously, indicating that they "may" promote cognitive health:

- Be socially and intellectually engaged and engaged in lifelong learning.
- Get adequate sleep and receive treatment for sleep disorders if needed.
- Take steps to avoid the risk of cognitive changes due to delirium if hospitalized.

The authors suggest careful evaluation of products advertised to consumers for improving cognitive health, such as medications, nutritional supplements, and cognitive training.

The willingness of these authors to recommend these actions likely was based on the observation that they have other potential benefits (e.g., prevention of cardiovascular disease) and are certainly unlikely to harm anyone, rather than on the strength of evidence that they ameliorate cognitive aging per se. The authors also reviewed evidence about other factors, such as exposure to pollution, tobacco smoke, and stress; diet; and such conditions as hearing loss and depression, but found it difficult to draw conclusions about this evidence because of variation in the available studies and the paucity of studies for some topics. In general, the quality of evidence was such that it was difficult to support recommendations for anything one might not already recommend for other reasons.

2017 National Academies' Report

The 2017 National Academies of Sciences, Engineering, and Medicine report *Preventing Cognitive Decline and Dementia: A Way Forward* summarizes the evidence about interventions that may be effective in preventing dementia and other types of cognitive decline (National Academies of Sciences, Engineering, and Medicine [NASEM], 2017). The report examines evidence that changes in the brain associated with dementia and other forms of cognitive impairment may begin many years before they are expressed as symptoms. This evidence provides reason to think that interventions implemented long before a person is impaired could have significant impact and that making changes decades before the typical age of onset may even be essential. This possibility is supported by the data showing declines in both the incidence and prevalence of dementia in high-income countries (see Chapter 1), suggesting that shifts in risk factors have influenced dementia risk.

The authors of the 2017 report coordinated their work with a systematic review commissioned by the Agency for Healthcare Research and Quality (AHRQ), which focused on evidence from RCTs. However, they note the difficulty of conducting this type of investigation on interventions targeting conditions that develop later in life and often in conjunction with other medical conditions. For example, they observe that the National Institute on Aging, the primary funder of research related to dementia, generally funds only research on older adults, which would not encompass risk factors that occur in earlier phases of the life course. Because of these challenges, the report's authors found very few randomized studies that could support public health recommendations. They supplemented their work with a review of observational data, studies of risk factors, and assessments of the possible effects of interventions on the body, but also note the limitations of these studies.

The authors found that three types of interventions are "supported by encouraging although inconclusive evidence" (NASEM, 2017, p. 7):

- cognitive training—a broad set of interventions, such as those aimed at enhancing reasoning, memory, and speed of processing—to delay or slow age-related cognitive decline;

- blood pressure management for people with hypertension to prevent, delay, or slow clinical Alzheimer's-type dementia; and
- increased physical activity to delay or slow age-related cognitive decline.

The report notes that methods of *cognitive training*—including structured exercises designed to improve reasoning or problem solving, boost memory, and increase processing speed, as well as cognitively stimulating activities, such as learning a new language or playing challenging games—can improve performance on the task involved, at least in the short term. But the authors found only limited or mixed evidence about whether such benefits would translate to improved capacity on other cognitive tasks, to general cognitive functioning over time, or to decreased risk of dementia.

With respect to *hypertension*, the authors cite research that has established multiple connections between dementia and the health of the brain's vascular system. Atherosclerosis in blood vessels in the brain, microbleeds, and silent strokes, for example, have been identified as contributors to dementia. It is possible that vascular risk factors increase dementia risk by other mechanisms as well (e.g., decreased blood flow in the brain may lessen the body's capacity to clear Alzheimer's disease proteins or increase their production). In any event, reducing the risk of stroke or other cerebrovascular disease could plausibly reduce the risk of dementia. Since the publication of this 2017 National Academies' report, results reported from the SPRINT-MIND RCT have demonstrated that more aggressive systolic blood pressure management led to a lower risk of dementia and mild cognitive impairment (SPRINT-MIND Investigators et al., 2019).

Physical activity, including aerobic activities, resistance or weight training, and stretching, is generally recognized as important for healthy aging, sustaining physical functioning and reducing the risk of cardiovascular disease. While there is substantial observational evidence to support the hypothesis that physical activity may reduce the risk of cognitive decline or dementia, the 2017 report's authors (drawing on a previous systematic review from AHRQ) found that the data from intervention studies designed to confirm this effect remained sparse. Most studies the authors identified were not of sufficient duration or size to detect plausible effect sizes. Other study designs (e.g., isolating different types of physical activity) might have identified truly heterogeneous effects.

The caution that characterizes the conclusions of the 2017 report reflects the authors' strict filters for the types of evidence on which they would rely, particularly the decision to accord the greatest weight to evidence from RCTs. The authors also highlight the need for further research and methodological improvements to build understanding of the differences among populations and other issues.

Lancet Commission Report

A 2020 Lancet Commission report also summarizes the evidence on dementia prevention and possible interventions, offering a more expansive view of the possibilities for prevention (Livingston et al., 2020). The authors interpreted a wide array of expert opinion in building on findings from their own 2017 report on the subject, which identified nine potentially modifiable risk factors for dementia that could account for approximately 35 percent of dementia cases (Livingston et al., 2017). By 2020, Livingston and colleagues had found the evidence to be stronger and identified three additional factors for which they found recent evidence to be compelling. The resulting set of 12 factors is

1. lower education levels,
2. hypertension,
3. hearing impairment,
4. smoking,
5. obesity,
6. depression,
7. physical inactivity,
8. diabetes,
9. low social contact,
10. excessive alcohol consumption,
11. traumatic brain injury, and
12. air pollution.

These lifestyle behaviors are linked to the development of other diseases, particularly cardiovascular disease, and may also be linked to dementia risk. For example, cigarette smokers have been found to be at higher risk for developing dementia relative to those who do not smoke. Thus, targeting these lifestyle risk behaviors has the dual benefit of reducing the risk of common chronic diseases while likely reducing the risk of dementia as well.

The authors found that these 12 factors collectively "account for around 40 percent of worldwide dementias," meaning that that proportion of dementias could be "prevented or delayed" with intervention (Livingston et al., 2020, p. 413). This estimate should be interpreted with caution, however, because it depends on the current distribution of risk factors in a population and overall population risk, which differ across current demographic and other population features and are expected to change over time. In addition, these calculations do not take into account the simultaneous impact of multiple risk factors, many of which are highly correlated. In any event, the authors suggest that the potential benefits are likely to be highest in low-income countries.

The report advocates for broad prevention efforts, such as providing all children with primary and secondary education and reducing exposure to air pollution. It also makes very specific recommendations, such as maintaining a systolic blood pressure of 130 mm Hg or less from age 40. The recommendation regarding blood pressure likely reflects the influence of the above-mentioned clinical trial data from the SPRINT-MIND study, in which tighter blood pressure control was associated with better outcomes. However, it should be noted that data specific to older individuals, for whom lower blood pressures may not be as well tolerated, were limited (Yaffe, 2019; SPRINT-MIND Investigators et al., 2019).

The authors of this 2020 Lancet Commission report based their conclusions on observational studies and expert opinion, with limited evidence from experimental or even quasi-experimental studies. As noted above, these observational studies are vulnerable to two important sources of bias—confounding and reverse causation—as well as measurement errors and selection bias. Because some recommendations based on observational evidence appear to be innocuous and may have ancillary benefits, the assumptions under which that evidence would support causal inferences may be evaluated less rigorously.

Potentially Important Risk Factors That Have Received Less Attention

The role of medications and polypharmacy receives little attention in the reports discussed above but may be important. An estimated 85 percent of adults ages 65 and older live with at least one chronic condition, and nearly 60 percent have two or more such conditions. The conditions associated with dementia risk (e.g., diabetes, hyperlipidemia, depression) are among the most prevalent, and most older Americans use drug therapies to treat them. There are questions about whether some drug therapies themselves may be associated with that risk, even though they offer the benefits of treating a condition that increases dementia risk. Some drugs may also interact with dementia-related pathophysiological pathways by way of mechanisms unrelated to their original therapeutic indication. For example, such drugs as benzodiazepines (used for anxiety), antispasmodics (for overactive bladder), and anticholinergics (used for a variety of conditions and also present in over-the-counter sleep medications) have been associated with increased risk of dementia (Barthold et al., 2020; Chatterjee et al., 2020; see Thunell et al., 2021, for an overview of research on the relationship between pharmaceuticals and dementia risk).[4] However, the caveats

---

[4]In the case of benzodiazepines for anxiety, the association may be driven by reverse causality, as anxiety can be a prodromal symptom of dementia.

noted above regarding confounding, reverse causation, measurement error, and selection bias should be noted regarding some of these findings.

The physical environment also likely influences dementia risk. While the effects of specific environmental factors on dementia risk are generally not well understood, there is compelling evidence that a wide variety of toxic exposures are influential (Finch and Kulminski, 2019; Mortamais et al., 2021). For example, female participants in the Women's Health Initiative Memory Study who were exposed to air pollution above the risk standard identified by the Environmental Protection Agency in 2012 had nearly twice the risk of dementia compared with their counterparts who did not have that exposure (Cacciottolo et al., 2017). Similarly, exposure to lead is associated with dementia risk. As climate change increases temperature extremes and volatility and such adverse events as wildfires, these effects are likely to influence the risk of incident dementia and the well-being of people living with dementia (Wei et al., 2019; Milton and White, 2020). Because environmental risk factors are unequally distributed in terms of geographic location, socioeconomic conditions, and other social factors, research on this topic needs to be linked with the research on disparities discussed below.

Significant research and funding have also been devoted to identifying modifiable risk factors that may help prevent cancer, hypertension, and other diseases. As noted above, cardiovascular diseases themselves may increase the risk of dementia; moreover, many of the risk factors that have been studied appear to affect the risk of multiple diseases, including dementia. Thus, the reduction of risk factors for these other diseases can contribute to reducing the risk for dementia. Successful efforts to reduce risk for these diseases can also offer insights for public health activities targeting dementia directly. Cardiovascular disease in particular may contribute to dementia risk, and relationships among major chronic conditions, including hypertension, heart disease, and stroke, and dementia heighten the importance of attention to modifiable factors that affect risk.[5]

Use of Emerging Evidence to Promote Public Health

The major challenge related to findings such as those reported above has been identifying ways to act on the evidence and change long-term behaviors, which may involve addictive substances or strong social norms and are constrained by built and social environments, as well as socioeconomic resources. There is little evidence to suggest that telling individuals to change their behavior will bring about enduring behavior change in most

---

[5] https://www.ninds.nih.gov/Disorders/Patient-Caregiver-Education/Preventing-Stroke research

of the population. However, a look at the campaign to reduce tobacco use illustrates the possibilities for altering harmful individual behaviors. Smoking declined by 58 percent among adults between the 1960s and the early 2000s, and this campaign has been identified as one of the most successful public health efforts of the 20th century (Institute of Medicine, 2007) and a major driver of declines in lung cancer and cardiovascular disease (Lu et al., 2019). As noted earlier, the campaign to reduce smoking, which is still ongoing, demonstrates the importance of targeting multiple levels of influence for prevention, including individual behavior change and population- or systems-level factors. Other major public health achievements, such as reductions in motor vehicle crashes and lead exposure, were also achieved through multiple levels of intervention. Another successful example is a clinical trial testing the effectiveness of lifestyle interventions for preventing diabetes—the Diabetes Prevention Program[6]—and the program's successful dissemination in a wide variety of settings and populations (Jiang et al., 2013; Ackermann et al., 2015).

The campaign to reduce tobacco use was a massive effort based on strong evidence for the causal relationship between smoking and serious adverse health outcomes. In general, sound decisions about devoting resources to such interventions rest on solid evidence that

- the change being promoted has the capacity to reduce risk,
- changing the behavior or environment to a degree likely to have a significant effect is feasible and sustainable, and
- there is a tested means of effecting the change that could work in the intended setting or circumstances.

There is evidence that interventions can improve or maintain cognitive function in older individuals (see, e.g., Ngandu et al., 2015). But in the context of health-related behaviors with possible implications for dementia risk, it is important to weigh a variety of competing considerations. The causal role of some risk factors that have been linked with dementia remains uncertain, and the estimated impact of any one individual risk factor may be small. In other words, the fraction of dementia cases that could potentially be prevented if it were possible to convince everyone to adopt a particular behavior might be small. Researchers also have not yet been able to establish whether combined risk factors have multiplicative effects. Thus, it would be reasonable to prioritize efforts to modify behaviors by considering the feasibility of changing those risk factors, the opportunity cost of such changes (given that most would have impact if achieved in

---

[6]https://coveragetoolkit.org/about-national-dpp/evidence

middle age or earlier), and the potential population impact of such changes on the overall incidence of or disparities in dementia.

Conveying the above uncertainties clearly so that individuals can make informed decisions about behavioral changes will be key to the usefulness of behavioral interventions. The greatest success may be achieved with interventions that are collaborative rather than prescriptive and help people decide what they believe is worth doing and how to do it if they are interested. A holistic perspective that considers the potential impact of a behavior change on overall health and quality of life may be key to helping individuals navigate these types of decisions.[7] Interventions that target systems or structures to make healthy behaviors the default (e.g., active transportation options, policies that subsidize or increase access to healthy dietary patterns or tax or decrease access to unhealthy ones) are likely to be especially valuable.

The impact of such behavior changes on common risk factors could be substantial for a population, even if individual-level benefits were small. However, the population-level effects of behavior changes that reduce the risk of cardiovascular and other health conditions associated with dementia could also bring corresponding changes in population mortality risk. If reduced risk in associated health conditions resulted in longer lives, there could be a corresponding increased cumulative lifetime risk of dementia as more people reached older and older ages (Zissimopoulos et al., 2018). Thus, from a population perspective, it would make sense to base action on improved understanding of the point in the life course at which interventions would both improve population health and longevity and reduce the cumulative lifetime risk of dementia.

SOCIOECONOMIC RISK

The advances in understanding of how individual behaviors may influence the development of dementia and related diseases discussed in the first part of this chapter offer valuable benefits, but researchers have also looked more broadly at influences on risk. Work that has emerged in the past few decades from economics, epidemiology, and neuropsychology, among other disciplines, has substantially broadened understanding of how social, environmental, and economic factors contribute to risk, as well as how racism and racial discrimination have interacted with those factors to amplify risk for certain groups.

A full understanding of these influences starts with a look at the entire life course, as noted in Chapter 1. Beginning in infancy and early childhood,

---

[7]For an example of this type of communication, see https://siteman.wustl.edu/prevention/ydr.

such factors as health and nutrition, material well-being, social ties, stressful experiences, and education affect how an individual develops physically, cognitively, and emotionally in ways that, decades later, can have substantial impacts on cognitive health (see, e.g., Zhang et al., 2010; Lövdén et al., 2020; Sharp and Gatz, 2011; Jirout et al., 2019). As the individual ages, health behaviors, leisure activities, and factors associated with an array of social advantages and disadvantages continue to shape later cognitive health outcomes (see, e.g., Bowling et al., 2016; Nelson et al., 2020; Arpino et al., 2018). And, as discussed above, the development of such adult disease conditions as diabetes and stroke, many of which are themselves associated with these social factors, is associated with risk of dementia.

It is increasingly clear that factors operating at multiple geographic levels (neighborhood, city, state) and through such social institutions as school, workplaces, and houses of worship have the potential to modify the associations between risk factors and both the incidence and progression of dementia. It is also important to examine who lives in a particular environment and why (e.g., racial segregation), and the characteristics of an area (e.g., levels of crime, availability of such resources as health care providers and support networks, exposures to such toxins as air pollution) that may also be influential.

Taking a life-course approach sensitizes researchers to the importance of historical factors (e.g., technological developments, policies, and such cultural forces as racism). For example, the so-called Jim Crow laws that enforced segregation in the South were not ended until the Civil Rights Act passed in 1965. Thus, many Black Americans alive today were born into a racialized caste system that substantially affected their lives: they attended primary schools legally segregated by race, which were systematically underresourced, and experienced higher rates of childhood adversity compared to White populations (Zhang et al., 2016). Indeed, de facto segregation persists in many American localities, and despite minor advances toward racial equity, the United States can still be described as a racialized caste system (Wilkerson, 2020). The effects of these experiences will likely continue to contribute to racial disparities in dementia risk for years to come (see, e.g., Zuelsdorff et al., 2020; Coogan et al., 2020; Caunca et al., 2020). For instance, analyses of the results of the Health and Retirement Study between 1998 and 2010 found that higher rates of childhood adversity among Black populations put Black adults at significantly greater risk of cognitive impairment in later life (Zhang et al., 2016).

Figure 2-1 illustrates the life-course approach to the development of dementia. The figure highlights two major phases of the human life course—the developmental phase and the aging phase. The developmental phase corresponds roughly to childhood, when a substantial amount of cognitive and brain development occurs. During the aging phase, general declines in functioning occur in healthy individuals; neurodegeneration and pathology can lead to dementia when a threshold is crossed in terms of the individual's comparative cognitive functioning.

The figure roughly illustrates how the effects of experience and environmental exposures compound over a lifetime, pushing in both positive and negative directions. The blue curve represents possible trajectories in the course of a lifetime and shows that the individuals who are most affected by risks across the life span may have significantly poorer cognitive health after decades of such exposures and experiences, relative to their counterparts who experience fewer risks and much greater protections. In other words, outcomes diverge significantly as people age because their cumulative experiences may combine either to support cognitive health or to make dementia more likely.

The figure significantly oversimplifies these processes. An individual's trajectory is not likely to follow a smooth arc, and it is difficult to portray the interplay of influences and effects that occur across the life course, such as exposures or learning occurring later in life. What is too complex to represent in a figure is what lies behind the differences in exposures: the social, environmental, and economic factors that multiply the risks for certain groups and afford cushions of protection for others. Nevertheless, it highlights the critical influence of environment and experience on cognitive health.

The precise biological, behavioral, and psychosocial mechanisms through which such life-course risk factors influence dementia and the timing of greatest influence are not clearly established. Researchers have posited numerous possible pathways, including cellular (e.g., neuroplasticity), behavioral (e.g., physical activity), material (e.g., lead exposure), and medical (e.g., hypertension control) mechanisms. For example, children who grow up in poverty may experience nutritional deprivation, which may harm brain development. Growing up in poverty may also limit an

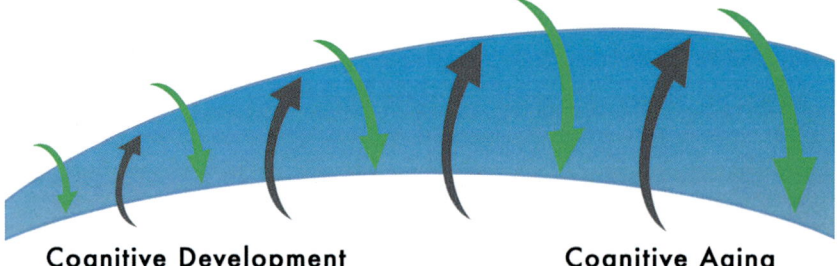

FIGURE 2-1 Cumulative impact of risks and protective factors on cognitive health.
NOTE: The upward arrows represent experiences and exposures that protect cognitive health; the downward arrows represent risk factors that may impair it.

individual's employment opportunities in adulthood and therefore also limit access to high-quality medical care that would manage hypertension—increasing the risk of dementia. And both pathways contribute to risk. Such hypotheses are plausible, but establishing their relative impact is not easy.

Pinpointing such connections is challenging in part because ways of measuring mediators (factors that explain the links among variables) in this context are not well developed (see Chapter 8). For example: What mediates the association between years of education in early life and dementia in late life? Does education have a direct effect on brain development, or does its impact come through its effects on income, access to health care, health behaviors, or other factors, or some combination of these and other factors? Many questions about how factors combine over the life course to influence the risk of dementia have not been answered. For example, few of the existing studies of associations among these factors were designed to address questions about the accumulation of risk from childhood through adulthood. Emerging data sources along with improved statistical methods will support progress in understanding these mechanisms in the coming decade, as discussed in Chapter 8.

Although much more work is needed to understand these issues, there is a growing body of work on three socioeconomic factors that influence dementia risk: education, occupation, and financial resources. There is also a growing literature on the role of race and ethnicity in disparities in dementia prevalence and incidence. These factors are discussed in turn below.

Socioeconomic Factors

Policies to alter socioeconomic conditions, including employment, education, and financial security, hold the potential to bring substantial benefits to the cognitive health of future cohorts of people as they age. Because policy remedies are expensive, however, clear evidence that they could have meaningful impact on dementia would be important. Improving understanding of the effects of socioeconomic factors on dementia will also contribute to understanding of the effects of other modifiable risk factors because nearly every behavior (physical activity, diet, alcohol use, smoking) is influenced by socioeconomic conditions. Yet few studies of these issues have included measures of socioeconomic conditions that would make it possible to disentangle such related factors, and there is limited systematic information on the magnitude of bias potentially introduced by this omission. A detailed exploration of these areas was beyond the scope of this study, but the issues related to education, occupation, and financial resources are briefly discussed below.

Education

The contribution of educational inequities in early life to disparities in the incidence of dementia in later life is perhaps the best studied of the socioeconomic factors (Walsemann and Ailshire, 2020). The causal evidence linking education and dementia risk includes both observational and quasi-experimental findings in many settings. For example, a systematic review of studies of the effects of lower education on risk for dementia showed a significant relationship (Sharp and Gatz, 2011). A study that explored the effects of changes in rules about compulsory schooling showed that individuals who completed more years of school had better cognitive outcomes and lower dementia risk decades later (Nguyen et al., 2016). And a meta-analysis of dose-response and dementia suggests that higher education significantly reduces dementia risk (Xu et al., 2016). Similar results from another longitudinal study indicated that these associations were robust when models controlled for indicators of childhood IQ (Wolters et al., 2020).

This finding points to a promising area for further study. Cohorts now reaching old age benefited from dramatic increases in educational opportunity and attainment since the mid-20th century—increases in K–12 enrollment, high school graduation, and college enrollment and graduation, for example (National Center for Education Statistics, 1993)—and recently documented declines in age-specific dementia incidence have been linked to educational improvements (Hayward et al., 2021).

Education may offer protection from dementia in several ways. It may strengthen cognitive reserve, the brain's ability to optimize or maximize performance by recruiting different brain networks and tapping alternative cognitive strategies (Stern, 2009). It may also prevent the progressive pathophysiologic processes that lead to dementia (e.g., cerebrovascular disease or amyloid deposition) or offer protection in other ways. Research on the protection that may be afforded by education has explored links between cognitive decline and educational attainment in varied settings and at varied stages of the life cycle (see, e.g., Crimmins et al., 2018; Seblova et al., 2019; Lövdén et al., 2020; Weden et al., 2018).

However, there is some inconsistency across studies, which may be the result of chance or sampling or measurement issues, or may reflect limits on the power of education to protect an individual from other negative forces. For example, despite significant improvements in the quality of and access to education in the United States in the 1960s and 1970s, race-based discrimination often prevented Black men from obtaining jobs appropriate to their education levels, thus denying them many of the social benefits of education (Hayward et al., 2021). Some evidence suggests that although education may strengthen an individual's cognitive level, later-life influences, such as level of income or wealth, have greater impacts on the rate of cognitive change (Glymour and Manly, 2008; Marden et al., 2017). Finding a factor that is theoretically modifiable throughout life, such as income level, affects cognitive health would be useful, as it would point to opportunities for intervention.

Although education may seem a simple concept to measure, it is a multifaceted construct, and each of those facets is challenging to measure. Nearly all evidence on the effects of education is based on easily quantifiable measures, such as test scores, number of years completed, or major credentials (see, e.g., Zahodne et al., 2015). However, more difficult-to-measure aspects of educational quality are likely as important for cognitive development and health. At the same time, there is strong evidence that some educational assets—such as high-quality preschool—have multiple benefits, such as for social and emotional development, academic attainment, and earnings, that are observable even decades later (see, e.g., Child Trends, 2018). On the other hand, there is surprisingly little evidence on the benefits of educational experiences people have later in life, although such experiences are quite common. These same ambiguities apply to nearly every other social determinant of health, such as work and retirement, financial resources, and social networks and support.

Occupation

Employment and occupation merit special consideration because of the multiple mechanisms through which they may influence dementia risk. Researchers have examined the effects of types of occupation, occupational autonomy, stress, and unemployment. For example, a study of work during midlife and later dementia risk found that mentally stimulating or complex work is associated with lower risk of dementia and may even compensate for the risks that come with lower educational attainment (Karp et al., 2009).

There is growing evidence that retirement is associated with cognitive deterioration, increasing the risk of dementia (Karp et al., 2009; Rohwedder and Willis, 2010; Celidoni et al., 2017). However, individuals' responses to retirement vary significantly, by number of years in retirement, occupation, and postretirement environment (Denier et al., 2017). Assessing the role of retirement is also challenging because of the possibility of reverse causality (early cognitive decline may cause someone to retire early), as well as selection bias (those with physically demanding jobs may be more likely to retire early). Because retirement age reflects both personal preferences and policy interventions, evidence on how retirement influences dementia risk and what aspects of postretirement life may reduce the risk would be valuable. The link between education and cognition is sometimes interpreted as support for the "use it or lose it" hypothesis of cognitive aging, that is, the idea that cognitive demands are important for maintaining cognitive health (Denier et al., 2017). If so, enhancing retirement from the paid labor force with alternative cognitively engaging activities may provide opportunities for reducing cognitive decline.

Financial Resources

A factor related to many others that have possible effects on cognitive health is inequality in wealth and income. Establishing direct links between cognitive health and poverty, economic hardship, and financial security would open intriguing possibilities for population-level interventions. The pernicious effects of poverty on human health and well-being have been documented, but policy responses are still emerging (see, e.g., NASEM, 2019a, 2019b).

Racial/Ethnic Disparities in Dementia Risk

As noted in Chapter 1, significant disparities across racial/ethnic groups in dementia prevalence and incidence persist in the United States, although the magnitude of these disparities has shifted over time (Matthews et al., 2019; Mayeda et al., 2016). Box 2-1 summarizes some key recent evidence documenting these disparities in dementia outcomes.

The magnitude of racial/ethnic disparities in dementia risk and the heterogeneity of these disparities across subpopulations point to the potential impact of social and interpersonal experiences on people's risk for dementia. Multiple explanations for the disparities in dementia risk have been posited, many of which emphasize structural racism (Zhang et al., 2016; Plassman et al., 2007). For example, researchers studying racial/ethnic differences in dementia risk found that environmental factors and social determinants of health could be responsible for inequities in dementia risk (Plassman et al., 2007; Yaffe et al., 2013). Structural racism that has been embedded in policies and laws as well in the delivery of medical care has contributed to disparities across health outcomes (Bailey et al., 2021; Park and Chen, 2020). Disparities in access to care, quality of care, and health outcomes of care for communities of color in the United States all likely contribute to disparities in dementia risk and outcomes (Chen and Zissimopoulos, 2018; Lines et al., 2014; Werner, 2019). In a 2021 survey, 36 percent of Black Americans, 18 percent of Hispanic Americans, and 19 percent of Asian Americans reported that discrimination is a barrier to receiving dementia care and that they expected to be treated differently because of their race, color, or ethnicity (Alzheimer's Association, 2021).

> **BOX 2-1**
> **Disparities in the Incidence and Risk of Dementia**
>
> There is accumulating evidence that the risk of dementia varies by race and ethnicity. For example, a nationally representative longitudinal survey of Americans aged 65 and above showed that, even after controlling for measured risk factors, Black and Hispanic individuals had 2.0 and 1.5 times the odds of developing dementia, respectively, compared with non-Latinx White individuals (Chen and Zissimopoulos, 2018). Evidence from a large study of members of a single health care system involving individuals from five different racial/ethnic groups showed that the Asian American elderly had a lower incidence of dementia relative to any other group and that elderly African Americans had an approximately 65 percent higher incidence than their Asian American counterparts. In this sample, based in California, where more granular disaggregation was possible, Mexican American and White elderly people had a similar incidence of dementia (Mayeda et al., 2017a, 2017b). Yet in a systematic review, African American and Caribbean Latinx populations had the highest annual incidence of dementia compared with Mexican Americans, Japanese Americans, and non-Latinx White populations (Mehta and Yeo, 2017).
>
> There are also significant disparities across populations in the length of time people live with cognitive impairment and dementia. The contrast in the mean years living with cognitive impairment or dementia after age 50 is stark: 3.9 years for Black women, 4.7 years for U.S.-born Latina women, and 6.0 years for foreign-born Latina women, compared with White women (1.6 years). For men, the pattern is comparable: 3.1 years for Black men, 3.0 years for U.S.-born Latino men, and 3.2 years for foreign-born Latino men, compared with 1.1 years for White men (Farina et al., 2020; Mayeda et al., 2017b).

Respondents also reported that it is more difficult for them to get excellent dementia care, and caregivers also reported that they had witnessed racial discrimination in their recipient's health care settings.

Researchers have focused on effects of the interlocking processes that maintain race-based power inequalities in the United States, which

- expose people of color to interpersonal racism;
- reduce their socioeconomic opportunities, such as educational attainment;
- impose intense psychosocial stressors, such as threats of violence and incarceration; and
- create barriers to quality medical care (Glymour and Manly, 2008).

These processes operate across the life course and across generations. They tend to be cumulative, and it is therefore difficult to isolate single factors contributing to the observed disparities. Nevertheless, as researchers have sought to identify modifiable targets for which change is likely to have large impacts, their attention has increasingly turned to the interplay among the effects of race and ethnicity, risk factors for dementia, and the role of public policy. A detailed analysis of how domestic policies in the United States have contributed to current disparities is beyond the scope of this study, but several examples can illustrate the importance of these issues.

An example is education. As discussed above, there is reason to believe that having limited educational experiences (including both attainment and quality of schooling) plays a role in the development of dementia. At the same time, minority and immigrant populations that are disproportionately affected by dementia are also more likely than other groups to have experienced limited educational opportunities (Garcia et al., 2018). An extensive body of work in education has documented inequities by race and ethnicity as well as income in educational opportunity (see, e.g., Duncan and Murnane, 2011). Looking specifically at dementia risk, researchers have explored differences across groups. For example, one study showed that although foreign-born Latina women and Black males are more likely to experience cognitive impairment and dementia relative to their White counterparts, these differences are attenuated after adjusting for years of education (Garcia et al., 2018).[8] Yet the benefits of education in terms of healthy cognitive life expectancy appear greatest for Black men and women and U.S.-born Latina women with some college education (Garcia et al., 2021). As evidence of the importance of education in explaining disparities in healthy cognitive life expectancy grows, it will underscore the urgency of addressing educational disparities and the role of local, state, and federal policy in ameliorating them (Montez et al., 2019; see especially Farina et al., 2020).

Policy makers also influence economic well-being, which, as discussed above, has an influence on dementia risk. A few examples illustrate the connections between economic policies and health. Increasing state minimum wages and expanding earned income tax credits has been associated with decreasing the risk of disability, such as being deaf or blind or being unable to perform activities of daily living (Montez et al., 2017). Similarly, expanding Medicaid to cover working-age adults with incomes up to 138 percent of the federal poverty level can significantly narrow the insurance gap between Black and Latinx households and White households (Buchmueller et al., 2016; Griffith et al., 2017). Increasing opportunities for health care coverage would contribute to opportunities for early diagnosis of many health conditions, including hypertension and diabetes, both

---

[8] The disparities persist for U.S.-born Latinx and Black older adults.

of which increase the risk for dementia. Insurance policies that reduce financial obstacles in health care can contribute to improved access to and quality of care and health outcomes (Sommers et al., 2015; Simon et al., 2017; Guth et al., 2020). Also of note, an estimated 65 percent of Medicaid enrollees lose their Medicaid coverage when they transition to traditional Medicare at age 65, which means they begin to bear substantially higher costs for services just at the stage of life when they may have increased need for care, such as provision of hearing aids and blood pressure control, that may contribute to dementia prevention (Kaiser Family Foundation, 2020).

Limited access to high-quality health care may also have significant effects on cognitive health, as evidence on American Indian populations illustrates. Both limitations of the Indian Health Service (a division of the U.S. Department of Health and Human Services) and very low rates of health insurance among many Native American groups have been documented (Artiga and Orgera, 2019). American Indian and Alaska Native adults are more likely than their White counterparts to have been unable to see a doctor in the past year because of cost (19% vs. 13%) and to have delayed care for other reasons (36% vs. 19%). Lost opportunities for preventive care (e.g., having blood pressure under control or obtaining hearing aids) and for connections with community resources (i.e., avoiding isolation) likely have significant effects on health, including cognitive outcomes, although researchers have not effectively disentangled the effects of race from the effects of disadvantaged socioeconomic status (Zahodne et al., 2017). Furthermore, access to health care, including such services as cognitive impairment screening (discussed further in Chapter 3), is critical to the early detection of dementia, which in turn can positively influence decision making and promote better health outcomes (Patnode et al., 2020).

Evidence for other population groups supports the importance of insurance and health care access. For example, a study of social correlates of likely dementia for the oldest old Mexican origin populations in Mexico and the United States showed that most of these individuals depend on their extended family for care (Mejia-Arango et al., 2020). Lack of medical, rehabilitative, and preventive services for this group, and others, can translate to significant economic challenges for families (e.g., paying for costly hearing aids that are important to many outcomes for the elderly [Brewster et al., 2020]). Inadequate nutrition, financial hardship, environmental stressors, and reduced opportunities for physical and social activity in their neighborhoods also play a key role in cognitive outcomes, and the groups they hit hardest are both members of minority populations and those who are economically disadvantaged.

The strong relationship between the race and ethnicity of a population and places where its members reside and the benefits they can access is discussed in greater detail in Chapter 5, but here we note that the United States spends significantly less on social services for the elderly compared with 11 other high-income countries (Osborn et al., 2017). The resulting financial strains affect the racial/ethnic subgroups that are also disproportionally poor. The conditions in homes and neighborhoods experiencing these strains are associated with an increased risk of premature mortality that is comparable to the risks posed by obesity, smoking, and a sedentary lifestyle (Fulmer et al., 2021). In other words, it is the intersection of many risk factors at the policy, community, and individual levels that either increases risk for or offers protection against dementia for racial/ethnic minorities.

Many researchers who study these issues use the concept of structural racism to capture the intersection of the multiple processes that drive differential outcomes in dementia risk (as well as many other health outcomes).[9] Much more research is needed to identify and document the effects of inequitable policies and systems in health care, education, housing, and social services; to identify specific discriminatory practices; and to document unequal distribution of resources that has adverse impacts on the health of populations of color. Also needed is evaluation of initiatives that have begun to address such sources of inequality—such as Seattle's Race and Social Justice Initiative, an effort to eliminate racial disparities and foster racial equity.[10] Needed as well is study of the interactive, embedded, and reciprocal dynamics that operate in the relationships among patient, provider, community, service systems, and policy to identify additional pathways for mitigating the impact of institutional racism on cognitive health.

RESEARCH DIRECTIONS

A look across the landscape of preventive and protective factors suggests that a large proportion of dementia could be prevented or delayed, but there is limited rigorous causal evidence with enough precision to guide evidence translation and the development of interventions. The uncertainties relate to nearly every domain of prevention, including behavioral changes, socioeconomic conditions, and structural and interpersonal racism and

---

[9] Structural racism has been defined as the "totality of ways in which societies foster racial discrimination through mutually reinforcing systems of housing, education, employment, earnings, benefits, credit, media, health care, and criminal justice" (Zinzi et al., 2017, p. 1453).

[10] http://www.seattle.gov/rsji

discrimination. This chapter has noted as well important potential impacts of risk factors that have received less attention, including polypharmacy and environmental conditions. For all these factors, there is an urgent need for better evidence on how to translate their well-documented correlations with the prevalence, incidence, and course of dementia into effective policies, system changes, or interventions.

For example, although there is robust evidence that people who take such common-sense measures as eating a healthy diet, exercising regularly, maintaining a healthy weight, and reducing cardiovascular risk have a lower risk of dementia, it remains unclear whether interventions on these factors would reduce dementia risk. The specifics of how to design such interventions are even less clear: Must healthy behavior be sustained throughout life, or can older adults who have recently modified their behavior derive benefits? What duration and intensity of exercise are necessary, and does it matter whether the exercise is primarily aerobic or strength training? Are there some groups of people who would benefit more or less from particular behavioral interventions? For individuals seeking to reduce their risk of dementia, the research provides little firm evidence but rather suggests a set of behaviors that might be helpful for brain health, are almost certainly not harmful, and probably have ancillary benefits for other health domains.

There are similar gaps regarding the causal effects of structural racism, socioeconomic disadvantage, and negative social interactions (e.g., perceived overt racism and discrimination), with the exception of relatively strong evidence that education improves cognitive reserve. To understand how to design interventions for any of these factors may require better understanding of mechanisms and mediators. To the extent that socioeconomic resources, such as education, do reduce dementia risk, these factors may well operate through behavior changes. Likewise, socioeconomic disadvantage constrains the ability of all adults to engage in health-promoting behaviors. Inequities and their consequences also point to questions about the possible benefits of public health interventions designed to reduce dementia risk at the population level, such as by promoting changes in access to resources (e.g., education, housing) or health behaviors (e.g., encouraging physical activity) or by altering the environment (e.g., improving access to exercise venues).

Scientific answers to these questions are urgently needed to support evidence-based, easily transferable, and timely interventions to ameliorate the starkly disparate effects of dementia. Because early interventions are key, rigorous yet rapid research methods that produce findings that can be translated to meet the needs of varied groups and regions will be extremely valuable. Methodological issues are discussed on Chapter 8, but we note here that resources available to support researchers in engaging diverse communities in basic research and intervention development and evaluation include guidebooks developed by the Centers for Disease Control and Prevention and others (see, e.g., Alzheimer's Association and Centers for Disease Control and Prevention, 2019; Portacolone et al., 2020; Ejiogu et al., 2011; Quiñones et al., 2020; Gershon et al., 2020; Streitz et al., 2020).

Having surveyed the landscape of research related to reducing the risk of dementia, the committee identified high-priority research needs in this domain in six broad areas. These areas are summarized in Conclusion 2-1; Table 2-1 provides detailed directions for research in each area.

> CONCLUSION 2-1: For health care and public health professionals to take advantage of modifiable factors to prevent Alzheimer's disease and related dementias or reduce or delay their symptoms, research is needed in six broad areas:
> 1. The causal effects of social factors on the incidence and rate of progression of dementia, including factors from multiple domains (socioeconomic resources, social network, structural drivers of exposure); at multiple levels (individual, family, and community); and at multiple life-course periods (e.g., childhood, early to mid-adulthood, old age).
> 2. The effects of health-related behaviors and their management over the life course.
> 3. Modifiable drivers of racial/ethnic inequality in dementia incidence, as well as other dimensions of inequality (e.g., geography).
> 4. The mechanisms through which socioeconomic factors influence brain health, including physiologic changes, behavioral mechanisms, and medical care pathways.
> 5. Detailed understanding of identified risk factors to support more precise recommendations to individuals about decision making and inform population-level policies for altering social contexts, modifying the environment, or changing social policies/systems to promote brain health.
> 6. Effective means of communicating the magnitude and degree of potential risk and protective factors to support informed decision making.

TABLE 2-1 Detailed Research Needs

1 and 2: Causal Effects of Social Factors and Health-Related Behaviors Over the Life Course	• Identification of causal social and behavioral risk factors versus those that are attributable to noncausal structures; understanding of the influence of confounding reverse causation and selection bias on apparent associations between established risk factors and dementia • Identification of specific dimensions of complex social exposures or behaviors that are relevant to dementia risk, such as aspects of education (e.g., attainment, quality, context), social support (instrumental, emotional, informational), or physical activity (aerobic vs. strength, duration, intensity), as well as of when in the life span they must be modified to have an effect • Studies of the extent to which the influence of socioeconomic resources or behaviors is dependent on context and capacity to utilize a resource • Research to improve understanding of how dementia develops across the life span and at what age the first behavioral or other manifestations emerge • Identification of study designs that can be used to evaluate alternative possible explanations for observational associations • Identification of the mediators/mechanisms linking social factors and dementia risk, in particular, mechanisms that might be modified • Where feasible, use of randomized controlled trial methodology in the study of behavior change and follow-up for dementia and related outcomes, ensuring that the methodology is sufficiently powered such that it involves large sample sizes, longitudinal interventions, and extended follow-up periods necessary to examine cognitive decline
3: Inequality in Dementia	• Research on how interlocking systems of structural racism create disparities in dementia risk • Study of how the risk factors evaluated in typical research samples operate differentially in underrepresented groups • Examination of sources of resilience that reduce risk in individuals exposed to disproportionate, racially stratified risk factors • Exploration of the effects of individual, interpersonal discrimination on dementia risk and the mechanisms through which those effects may occur • Assessment of how promising interventions to delay or prevent dementia may affect disparities • Monitoring trends and progress in reducing disparities in dementia incidence, care, and outcomes

Continued

TABLE 2-1 Continued

4: Mechanisms Through Which Socioeconomic Factors Operate	• Study of the physiologic changes, behavioral patterns, social resources, and medical care mechanisms underlying connections between socioeconomic factors and dementia risk
5: Interventions Involving Changes in Policies, Systems, or Individual Behaviors	• Development and improvement of interventions to modify identified risk factors and reduce both the overall population incidence of dementia and disparities in its incidence and outcomes • Identification of critical elements of preventive factors that can be translated into policy interventions • Exploration of ways to redesign structural and environmental elements that shape the behavioral patterns of individuals (e.g., to improve access to exercise and healthy food) • Identification of the opportunity costs of proposed interventions
6: Effective Means of Communicating About Risk and Protective Factors	• Research on the tailoring of communication about the quality of evidence regarding suspected risk factors to different communities to help individuals make informed decisions

REFERENCES

Ackermann, R.T., Liss, D.T., Finch, E.A., Schmidt, K.K., Hays, L.M., Marrero, D.G., and Saha, C.A. (2015). Randomized comparative effectiveness trial for preventing type 2 diabetes. *American Journal of Public Health*, 105(11), 2328–2334. https://doi.org/10.2105/AJPH.2015.302641

Alzheimer's Association. (2021). *Special Report: Race, Ethnicity and Alzheimer's in America*. https://www.alz.org/media/Documents/alzheimers-facts-and-figures-special-report.pdf

Alzheimer's Association and Centers for Disease Control and Prevention. (2019). *Healthy Brain Initiative: Road Map for Indian Country*. Chicago, IL: Alzheimer's Association. https://www.cdc.gov/aging/healthybrain/pdf/HBI-Road-Map-for-Indian-Country-508.pdf

Arpino, B., Gumà, J., and Julià, A. (2018). Early-life conditions and health at older ages: The mediating role of educational attainment, family and employment trajectories. *PloS One*, 13(4), e0195320. https://doi.org/10.1371/journal.pone.0195320

Artiga, S., and Orgera, A. (2019, November 12). *Key Facts on Health and Health Care by Race and Ethnicity*. Kaiser Family Foundation. https://www.kff.org/racial-equity-and-health-policy/report/key-facts-on-health-and-health-care-by-race-and-ethnicity

Bailey, Z.D., Feldman, J.M., and Bassett, M.T. (2021). How structural racism works—Racist policies as a root cause of U.S. racial health inequities. *New England Journal of Medicine*, 384(8), 768–773. https://doi.org/10.1056/NEJMms2025396

Barnes, D.E., and Yaffe, K. (2011). The projected effect of risk factor reduction on Alzheimer's disease prevalence. *Lancet Neurology*, 10(9), 819–828. https://doi.org/10.1016/S1474-4422(11)70072-2

Barnes, L.L., Leurgans, S., Aggarwal, N.T., Shah, R.C., Arvanitakis, Z., James, B.D., Buchman, A.S., Bennett, D.A., and Schneider, J.A. (2015). Mixed pathology is more likely in black than white decedents with Alzheimer dementia. *Neurology*, 85(6), 528–534.

Barthold, D., Marcum, Z.A., Gray, S.L., and Zissimopoulos, J. (2020). Alzheimer's disease and related dementias risk: Comparing users of non-selective and M3-selective bladder antimuscarinic drugs. *Pharmacoepidemiology and Drug Safety*, 129(12), 1650–1658. https://doi.org/10.1002/pds.5098

Bowling, A., Pikhartova, J., and Dodgeon, B. (2016). Is mid-life social participation associated with cognitive function at age 50? Results from the British National Child Development Study (NCDS). *BMC Psychology*, 4(1), 58. https://doi.org/10.1186/s40359-016-0164-x

Brewster, K.K., Pavlicova, M., Stein, A., Chen, M., Chen, C., Brown, P.J., Roose, S.P., Kim, A.H., Golub, J.S., Brickman, A., and Galatioto, J. (2020). A pilot randomized controlled trial of hearing aids to improve mood and cognition in older adults. *International Journal of Geriatric Psychiatry*, 35(8), 842–850.

Buchmueller, T.C., Levinson, Z.M., Levy, H.G., and Wolfe, B.L. (2016). Effect of the Affordable Care Act on racial and ethnic disparities in health insurance coverage. *American Journal of Public Health*, 106(8), 1416–1421.

Cacciottolo, M., Wang, X., Driscoll, I., Woodward, N., Saffari, A. Reyes, J., Serre, M.L., Vizuete, W., Sioutas, C., Morgan, T.E., Gatz, M., Chui, H.C., Shumaker, S.A., Resnick, S.M., Espeland, M.A., Finch, C.E., and Chen, J.C. (2017). Particulate air pollutants, APOE alleles and their contributions to cognitive impairment in older women and to amyloidogenesis in experimental models. *Translational Psychiatry*, 7(1), e1022. https://doi.org/10.1038/tp.2016.280

Caunca, M.R., Odden, M.C., Glymour, M.M., Elfassy, T., Kershaw, K.N., Sidney, S., Yaffe, K., Launer, L., and Zeki Al Hazzouri, A. (2020). Association of racial residential segregation throughout young adulthood and cognitive performance in middle-aged participants in the CARDIA study. *JAMA Neurology*, 77(8), 1000–1007. https://doi.org/10.1001/jamaneurol.2020.0860

Celidoni, M., Dal Bianco, C., and Weber, G. (2017). Retirement and cognitive decline: A longitudinal analysis using SHARE data. *Journal of Health Economics*, 56, 113–125. https://doi.org/10.1016/j.jhealeco.2017.09.003

Chatterjee, S., Talwar, A., and Aparasu, R.R. (2020). Anticholinergic medications and risk of dementia in older adults: Where are we now?. *Expert Opinion on Drug Safety*, 19(10), 1251–1267. https://doi.org/10.1080/14740338.2020.1811227

Chen, C., and Zissimopoulos, J. (2018). Racial and ethnic disparities in dementia prevalence and risk factors from 2000 to 2012 in the United States. *Alzheimer's and Dementia Translational Research*, 4(1), 510–520. https://doi.org/10.1016/j.trci.2018.08.009

Child Trends. (2018). *High-Quality Preschool Can Support Healthy Development and Learning.* https://www.childtrends.org/wp-content/uploads/2018/05/PreschoolFadeOut FactSheet_ChildTrends_April2018.pdf

Coogan, P., Schon, K., Li, S., Cozier, Y., Bethea, T., and Rosenberg, L. (2020). Experiences of racism and subjective cognitive function in African American women. *Alzheimer's & Dementia (Amsterdam, Netherlands)*, 12(1), e12067. https://doi.org/10.1002/dad2.12067

Crimmins, E.M., Saito, Y., Kim, J.K., Zhang, Y.S., Sasson, I., and Hayward, M.D. (2018). Educational differences in the prevalence of dementia and life expectancy with dementia: Changes from 2000 to 2010. *Journals of Gerontology, Series B*, 73(suppl_1), S20–S28. https://doi.org/10.1093/geronb/gbx135

Denier, N., Clouston, S., Richards, M., and Hofer, S. (2017). Retirement and cognition: A life course view. *Advances in Life Course Research*, 31, 11–21. https://doi.org/10.1016/j.alcr.2016.10.004

Denny, A., Streitz, M., Stock, K., Joyce, E., Balls-Berry, L.L., Barnes, G., Byrd, G.S., Croff, R., Gao, S., Glover, C.M., Hendrie, H.C., Hu, W.T., Manly, J.J., Moulder, K.L., Stark, S., Thomas, S.B., Whitmer, R., Wong, R., Morris, J.C., and Lingler, J.H. (2020). Perspective on the "African American participation in Alzheimer disease research: Effective strategies" workshop, 2018. *Alzheimer's and Dementia*, 16(12), 1734–1744. https://doi.org/10.1002/alz.12160

Duncan, G.J., and Murnane, R.J., Eds. (2011). *Whither Opportunity? Rising Inequality, Schools, and Children's Life Chances.* New York: Russell Sage Foundation.

Ejiogu, N., Norbeck, J.H., Mason, M.A., Cromwell, B.C., Zonderman, A.B., and Evans, M.K. (2011). Recruitment and retention strategies for minority or poor clinical research participants: Lessons from the Healthy Aging in Neighborhoods of Diversity across the Life Span study. *Gerontologist*, 51(Suppl 1), S33–S45. https://doi.org/10.1093/geront/gnr027

Farina, M.P., Hayward, M.D., Kim, J.K., and Crimmins, E.M. (2020). Racial and educational disparities in dementia and dementia-free life expectancy. *Journals of Gerontology. Series B*, 75(7), e105–e112. https://doi.org/10.1093/geronb/gbz046

Finch, C., and Kulminski, A. (2019). The Alzheimer's disease exposome. *Alzheimer's & Dementia*, 15(9), 1123–1132. https://doi.org/10.1016/j.jalz.2019.06.3914

Floud, S., Balkwill, A., Sweetland, S., Brown, A., Mauricio Reus, E., Hofman, A., Blacker, D., Kivimaki, M., Green, J., Peto, R., Reeves, G., and Beral, V. (2021). Cognitive and social activities and long-term dementia risk: The prospective UK Million Women Study. *Lancet Public Health*, 6(2), e116–e123. https://doi.org/10.1016/S2468-2667(20)30284-X

Frieden, T.R. (2010). A framework for public health action: The health impact pyramid. *American Journal of Public Health*, 100(4), 590–595. https://doi.org/10.2105/AJPH.2009.185652

Fulmer, T., Reuben, D.B., Auerbach, J., and Fick, D.M. (2021). Actualizing better health and health care for older adults. *Health Affairs (Project Hope)*, 40(2), 219–225. https://doi.org/10.1377/hlthaff.2020.01470

Garcia, M., Saenz, J., Downer, B., and Wong, R. (2018). The role of education in the association between race/ethnicity/nativity, cognitive impairment, and dementia among older adults in the United States. *Demographic Research*, 38, 155–168. https://doi.org/10.4054/DemRes.2018.38.6

Garcia, M., Downer, B., Chiu, C-T., Saenz, J., Ortiz, K., and Wong, R. (2021). Educational benefits and cognitive health life expectancies: Racial/ethnic, nativity, and gender disparities. *Gerontologist, 61*(3), 330–340. https://doi.org/10.1093/geront/gnaa112

Gershon, R., Nowinski, C., Peipert, J.D., Bedieti, K., Ustinovich, V., Hook, J., Fox, R., and Weintraub, S. (2020). Use of the NIH Toolbox for assessment of mild cognitive impairment and Alzheimer's disease in general population, African-American and Spanish-speaking samples of older adults. *Alzheimer's & Dementia, 16*(S6). https://doi.org/10.1002/alz.043372

Gielen, A., and Green, L. (2015). The impact of policy, environmental, and educational interventions: A synthesis of the evidence from two public health success stories. *Health Education & Behavior, 42*(1 Suppl), 20S–34S. https://doi.org/10.1177/1090198115570049

Glymour, M.M., and Manly, J.J. (2008). Lifecourse social conditions and racial and ethnic patterns of cognitive aging. *Neuropsychology Review, 18*(3), 223–254.

Griffith, K., Evans, L., and Bor, J. (2017). The Affordable Care Act reduced socioeconomic disparities in health care access. *Health Affairs, 36*(8), 1503–1510.

Guth, M., Artiga, S., and Pham, O. (2020). *Effects of the ACA Medicaid Expansion on Racial Disparities in Health and Health Care*. Kaiser Family Foundation. https://www.kff.org/report-section/effects-of-the-aca-medicaid-expansion-on-racial-disparities-in-health-and-health-care-issue-brief

Hayward, M.D., Farina, M.P., Zhang, Y.S., Kim, J.K., and Crimmins, E.M. (2021). The importance of improving educational attainment for dementia prevalence trends from 2000-2014, among older non-Hispanic Black and White Americans. *Journals of Gerontology. Series B*, gbab015. Advance online publication. https://doi.org/10.1093/geronb/gbab015

Institute of Medicine. (2007). *Ending the Tobacco Problem: A Blueprint for the Nation*. Washington, DC: The National Academies Press. https://doi.org/10.17226/11795

———. (2015). *Cognitive Aging: Progress in Understanding and Opportunities for Action*. Washington, DC: The National Academies Press. https://doi.org/10.17226/21693

Jiang, L., Manson, S.M., Beals, J., Henderson, W., Huang, H., Acton, K., Roubideaux, Y., and the Special Diabetes Program for Indians Diabetes Prevention Demonstration Project. (2013). Translating the Diabetes Prevention Program into American Indian and Alaska Native communities: Results from the Special Diabetes Program for Indians Diabetes Prevention demonstration project. *Diabetes Care, 36*(7), 2027–2034. https://doi.org/10.2337/dc12-1250

Jirout, J., LoCasale-Crouch, J., Turnbull, K., Gu, Y., Cubides, M., Garzione, S., Evans, T.M., Weltman, A.L., and Kranz, S. (2019). How lifestyle factors affect cognitive and executive function and the ability to learn in children. *Nutrients, 11*(8), 1953. https://doi.org/10.3390/nu11081953

Kaiser Family Foundation. (2020). *Premium and Cost-sharing Requirements for Selected Services for Medicaid Adults*. https://www.kff.org/0a320d8

Karp, A., Andel, R., Parker, M., Wang, H-X., Winblad, B., and Fratiglioni, L. (2009). Mentally stimulating activities at work during midlife and dementia risk after age 75: Follow-up study from the Kungsholmen project. *American Journal of Geriatric Psychiatry, 17*(3), 227–236. https://doi.org/10.1097/JGP.0b013e318190b691

Kawas, C.H., Kim, R.C., Sonnen, J.A., Bullain, S.S., Trieu, T., and Corrada, M.M. (2015). Multiple pathologies are common and related to dementia in the oldest-old: The 90+ study. *Neurology, 85*(6), 535–542.

Lines, L., Sherif, N., and Wiener, J. (2014). *Racial and Ethnic Disparities among Individuals with Alzheimer's Disease in the United States*. RTI Press. https://doi.org/10.3768/rtipress.2014.RR.0024.1412

Livingston, G., Sommerland, A., Ortega, V., Costafreda, S., Huntley, J., Ames, D., Ballard, C., Banerjee, S., Burns, A., Cohen-Mansfield, J., Cooper, C., Fox, N., Gitlin, L., Howard, R., Kales, H., Larson, E., Ritchie, K., Rockwood, K., Sampson, E., Samus, Q., Schneider, L., Selbæk, G., Teri, K., and Mukadam, N. (2017). Dementia prevention, intervention, and care. *Lancet, 390*(10113), 2673–2734. https://doi.org/10.1016/S0140-6736(17)31363-6

Livingston, G., Huntley, J., Sommerland, A., Ames, D., Ballard, C., Banerjee, S., Brayne, C., Burns, A., Cohen-Mansfield, J., Cooper, C., Costafreda, S., Dias, A., Fox, N., Gitlin, L., Howard, R., Kales, H., Kivimäki, M., Larson, E., Ogunniyi, A., Orgeta, V., Ritchie, K., Rockwood, K., Sampson, E., Samus, Q., Schneider, L., Selbæk, G., Teri, L., and Mukadam, N. (2020). Dementia prevention, intervention, and care: 2020 report of the Lancet Commission. *Lancet, 396*(10248), 413–446. https://doi.org/10.1016/S0140-6736(20)30367-6

Lourida, I., Hannon, E., Littlejohns, T., Langa, K., Hyppönenm E., Ku´zma, E., and Llewellyn, D. (2019). Association of lifestyle and genetic risk with incidence of dementia. *Journal of the American Medical Association, 322*(5), 430–437. https://doi.org/10.1001/jama.2019.9879

Lövdén, M., Fratiglioni, L., Glymour, M.M., Lindenberger, U., and Tucker-Drob, E.M. (2020). Education and cognitive functioning across the life span. *Psychological Science in the Public Interest, 21*(1), 6–41. https://doi.org/10.1177/1529100620920576

Lu, T., Yan, X., Huang, Y., Zhao, M., Li, M., Ma, K., Yin, J., Zhan, C., and Wang, Q. (2019). Trends in the incidence, treatment, and survival of patients with lung cancer in the last four decades. *Cancer Management and Research, 11*, 943–953. https://doi.org/10.2147/CMAR/S187317

Marden, J.R., Tchetgen Tchetgen, E.J., Kawachi, I., and Glymour, M.M. (2017). Contribution of socioeconomic status at 3 life-course periods to late-life memory function and decline: Early and late predictors of dementia risk. *American Journal of Epidemiology, 186*(7), 805–814. https://doi.org/10.1093/aje/kwx155

Matthews, K.A., Xu, W., Gaglioti, A.H., Holt, J.B., Croft, J.B., Mack, D., and McGuire, L.C. (2019). Racial and ethnic estimates of Alzheimer's disease and related dementias in the United States (2015-2060) in adults aged ≥65 years. *Alzheimer's & Dementia, 15*(1), 17–24. https://doi.org/10.1016/j.jalz.2018.06.3063

Mayeda, E.R., Glymour, M.M., Quesenberry, C.P., and Whitmer, R.A. (2016). Inequalities in dementia incidence between six racial and ethnic groups over 14 years. *Alzheimer's & Dementia, 12*(3), 216–224.

Mayeda, E.R., Glymour, M.M., Quesenberry, C.P., Johnson, J.K., Pérez-Stable, E.J., and Whitmer, R.A. (2017a). Heterogeneity in 14-year dementia incidence between Asian American subgroups. *Alzheimer Disease and Associated Disorders, 31*(3), 181.

———. (2017b). Survival after dementia diagnosis in five racial/ethnic groups. *Alzheimer's & Dementia, 13*(7), 761–769. https://doi.org/10.1016/j.jalz.2016.12.008

McMurtray, A., Clark, D.G., Christine, D., and Mendez, M.F. (2006). Early-onset dementia: Frequency and causes compared to late-onset dementia. *Dementia and Geriatric Cognitive Disorders, 21*(2), 59–64. https://doi.org/10.1159/000089546

Mehta, K., and Yeo, G. (2017). Systematic review of dementia prevalence and incidence in United States race/ethnic populations. *Alzheimer's & Dementia, 13*(1), 72–83. https://doi.org/10.1016/j.jalz.2016.06.2360

Mejia-Arango, S., Aguila, E., López-Ortega, M., Gutiérrez-Robledo, L.M., Vega, M., Drumond Andrade, F., Rote, S., Grasso, S., Markides, K., and Angel, J. (2020). Health and social correlates of dementia in oldest-old Mexican-origin populations. *Alzheimer's & Dementia, 6*(1), e12105. https://doi.org/10.1002/trc2.12105

Milton, L.A., and White, A.R. (2020). The potential impact of bushfire smoke on brain health. *Neurochemistry International, 139*, 104796. https://doi.org/10.1016/j.neuint.2020.104796

Montez, J.K., Hayward, M.D., and Wolf, D.A. (2017). Do U.S. states' socioeconomic and policy contexts shape adult disability? *Social Science & Medicine (1982), 178,* 115–126. https://doi.org/10.1016/j.socscimed.2017.02.012

Montez, H., Hayward, M., and Zajacova, A. (2019). Educational disparities in adult health: U.S. states as institutional actors on the association. *Socius, 5.* https://doi.org/10.1177/2378023119835345

Mortamais, M., Gutierrez, L.A., de Hoogh, K., Chen, J., Vienneau, D., Carrière, I., Letellier, N., Helmer, C., Gabelle, A., Mura, T., and Sunyer, J. (2021). Long-term exposure to ambient air pollution and risk of dementia: Results of the prospective Three-City Study. *Environment International, 148,* 106376.

NASEM (National Academies of Sciences, Engineering, and Medicine). (2017). *Preventing Cognitive Decline and Dementia: A Way Forward.* Washington, DC: The National Academies Press. https://doi.org/10.17226/24782

———. (2019a). *Fostering Healthy Mental, Emotional, and Behavioral Development in Children and Youth.* Washington, DC: The National Academies Press.

———. (2019b). *Roadmap to Reducing Child Poverty.* Washington, DC: The National Academies Press.

National Center for Education Statistics. (1993). *120 Years of American Education: A Statistical Portrait.* https://nces.ed.gov/pubs93/93442.pdf

Nelson, C.A., Scott, R.D., Bhutta, Z.A., Harris, N.B., Danese, A., and Samara, M. (2020). Adversity in childhood is linked to mental and physical health throughout life. *BMJ (Clinical Research Ed.), 371,* m3048. https://doi.org/10.1136/bmj.m3048

Ngandu, T., Lehtisalo, J., Solomon, A., Levälahti, E., Ahtiluoto, S., Antikainen, R., Bäckman, L., Hänninen, T., Jula, A., Laatikainen, T., Lindström, J., Mangialasche, F., Paajanen, T., Pajala, S., Peltonen, M., Rauramaa, R., Stigsdotter-Neely, A., Strandberg, T., Tuomilehto, J., Soininen, H., and Kivipelto, M. (2015). A 2 year multidomain intervention of diet, exercise, cognitive training, and vascular risk monitoring versus control to prevent cognitive decline in at-risk elderly people (FINGER): A randomised controlled trial. *Lancet (London, England), 385*(9984), 2255–2263. https://doi.org/10.1016/S0140-6736(15)60461-5

Nguyen, T.T., Tchetgen Tchetgen, E.J., Kawachi, I., Gilman, S.E., Walter, S., Liu, S.Y., Manly, J.J., and Glymour, M.M. (2016). Instrumental variable approaches to identifying the causal effect of educational attainment on dementia risk. *Annals of Epidemiology, 26*(1), 76.e3. https://doi.org/10.1016/j.annepidem.2015.10.006

Norton, S., Matthews, F.E., Barnes, D.E., Yaffe, K., and Brayne, C. (2014). Potential for primary prevention of Alzheimer's disease: An analysis of population-based data. *Lancet Neurology, 13*(8), 788–794. https://doi.org/10.1016/S1474-4422(14)70136-X

Osborn, R., Doty, M.M., Moulds, D., Sarnak, D.O., and Shah, A. (2017). Older Americans were sicker and face more financial barriers to health care than counterparts in other countries. *Health Affairs (Project Hope), 36*(12), 2123–2132. https://doi.org/10.1377/hlthaff.2017.1048

Park, S., and Chen, J. (2020). Racial and ethnic patterns and differences in health care expenditures among Medicare beneficiaries with and without cognitive deficits or Alzheimer's disease and related dementias. *BMC Geriatrics, 20*(1), 482. https://doi.org/10.1186/s12877-020-01888-y

Patnode, C.D., Perdue, L.A., Rossom, R.C., Rushkin, M.C., Redmond, N., Thomas, R.G., and Lin, J.S. (2020). Screening for cognitive impairment in older adults: Updated evidence report and systematic review for the U.S. Preventive Services Task Force. *Journal of the American Medical Association, 323*(8), 764–785. https://doi.org/10.1001/jama.2019.22258

Plassman, B.L., Langa, K.M., Fisher, G.G., Heeringa, S.G., Weir, D.R., Ofstedal, M.B., Burke, J.R., Hurd, M.D., Potter, G.G., Rodgers, W.L., Steffens, D.C., Willis, RJ., and Wallace, R.B. (2007). Prevalence of dementia in the United States: The Aging, Demographics, and Memory study. *Neuroepidemiology*, 29(1-2), 125–132. https://doi.org/10.1159/000109998

Portacolone, E., Palmer, N.R., Lichtenberg, P., Waters, C.M., Hill, C.V., Keiser, S., Vest, L., Maloof, M., Tran, T., Martinez, P., Guerrero, J., and Johnson, J.K. (2020). Earning the trust of African American communities to increase representation in dementia research. *Ethnicity & Disease*, 30(Suppl 2), 719–734. https://doi.org/10.18865/ed.30.S2.719

Quiñones, A.R., Kaye, J., Allore, H.G., Botoseneanu, A., and Thielke, S.M. (2020). An agenda for addressing multimorbidity and racial and ethnic disparities in Alzheimer's disease and related dementia. *American Journal of Alzheimer's Disease and Other Dementias*, 35, 1533317520960874. https://doi.org/10.1177/1533317520960874

Rohwedder, S., and Willis, R.J. (2010). Mental retirement. *Journal of Economic Perspectives*, 24(1), 119–138. https://doi.org/10.1257/jep.24.1.119

Ruiz-Hernandez, A., Navas-Acien, A., Pastor-Barriuso, R., Crainiceanu, C.M., Redon, J., Guallar, E., and Tellez-Plaza, M. (2017). Declining exposures to lead and cadmium contribute to explaining the reduction of cardiovascular mortality in the U.S. population, 1988–2004. *International Journal of Epidemiology*, 46(6), 1903–1912.

Sajeev, G., Weuve, J., Jackson, J., VanderWeele, T., Bennett, D., Grodstein, F., and Blacker, D. (2016). Late-life cognitive activity and dementia: A systematic review and bias analysis. *Epidemiology*, 27(5), 732–742. https://doi.org/10.1097/EDE.0000000000000513

Schneider, J.A., Arvanitakis, Z., Leurgans, S.E., and Bennett, D.A. (2009). The neuropathology of probable Alzheimer disease and mild cognitive impairment. *Annals of Neurology*, 66(2), 200–208.

Seblova, D., Brayne, C., Machu, V., Kuklová, M., Kopecek, M., and Cermakova, P. (2019). Changes in cognitive impairment in the Czech Republic. *Journal of Alzheimer's Disease*, 72(3), 693–701. https://doi.org/10.3233/JAD-190688

Sharp, E.S., and Gatz, M. (2011). Relationship between education and dementia: An updated systematic review. *Alzheimer Disease and Associated Disorders*, 25(4), 289–304. https://doi.org/10.1097/WAD.0b013e318211c83c

Simon, K., Soni, A., and Cawley, J. (2017). The impact of health insurance on preventive care and health behaviors: Evidence from the first two years of the ACA Medicaid expansions. *Journal of Policy Analysis and Management*, 36(2), 390–417.

Sommers, B.D., Gunja, M.Z., Finegold, K., and Musco, T. (2015). Changes in self-reported insurance coverage, access to care, and health under the Affordable Care Act. *Journal of the American Medical Association*, 314(4), 366–374.

SPRINT-MIND Investigators for the SPRINT Research Group, Williamson, J., Pajewski, N., Auchus, A., Bryan, R.N., Chelune, G., Cheung, A., Cleveland, M., Coker, L., Crowe, M., Cushman, W., Cutler, J., Davatzikos, C., Desiderio, L., Erus, G., Fine, L., Gaussoin, S., Harris, D., Hsieh, M-K., Johnson, K., Kimmel, P., Tamura, M., Launer, L., Lerner, A., Lewis, C., Martindale-Adams, J., Moy, C., Nasrallah, I., Nichols, L., Oparil, S., Ogrocki, P., Rahman, M., Rapp, S., Reboussin, D., Rocco, M., Sachs, B., Sink, K., Still, C., Supiano, M., Snyder, J., Wadley, V., Walker, J., Weiner, D., Whelton, P., Wilson, V., Woolard, N., Wright, J., and Wright, C. (2019). Effect of intensive vs standard blood pressure control on probable dementia: A randomized clinical trial. *Journal of the American Medical Association*, 321(6), 553–561. https://doi.org/10.1001/jama.2018.21442

Stern, Y. (2009). Cognitive reserve. *Neuropsychologia*, 47(10), 2015–2028. https://doi.org/10.1016/j.neuropsychologia.2009.03.004

Thunell, J., Joyce, G., Chen, Y., Barthold, D., Brinton, R., and Zissimopoulos, J. (2021). Drug therapies for chronic conditions and risk of Alzheimer's disease and related dementias: A scoping review. *Alzheimer's & Dementia, 17*, 41–48. https://doi.org/10.1002/alz.12175

Walsemann, K., and Ailshire, J. (2020). Early educational experiences and trajectories of cognitive functioning among U.S. adults in midlife and later. *American Journal of Epidemiology, 189*(5), 403–411. https://doi.org/10.1093/aje/kwz276

Weden, M.M., Shih, R.A., Kabeto, M.U., and Langa, K.M. (2018). Secular trends in dementia and cognitive impairment of U.S. rural and urban older adults. *American Journal of Preventive Medicine, 54*(2), 164–172. https://doi.org/10.1016/j.amepre.2017.10.021

Wei, Y., Wang, Y., Lin, C.K., Yin, K., Yang, J., Shi, L., Li, L., Zanobetti, A., and Schwartz, J.D. (2019). Associations between seasonal temperature and dementia-associated hospitalizations in New England. *Environment International, 126*, 228–233.

Werner, P. (2019). Reflections on quality of care for persons with dementia: Moving toward an integrated, comprehensive approach. *International Psychogeriatrics, 31*(3), 307–308. https://doi.org/10.1017/S1041610219000346

Wilkerson, I. (2020). *Caste: The Origins of Our Discontent*. New York: Random House.

Wolters, F.J., Chibnik, L.B., Waziry, R., Anderson, R., Berr, C., Beiser, A., Bis, J.C., Blacker, D., Bos, D., Brayne, C., Dartigues, J.-F., Darweesh, S.K.L., Davis-Plourde, K.L., De Wolf, F., Debette, S., Dufouil, C., Fornage, M., Goudsmit, J., Grasset, L., Gudnason, V., Hadjichrysanthou, C., Helmer, C., Ikram, M.A., Ikram, M.K., Joas, E., Kern, S., Kuller, L.H., Launer, L., Lopez, O.L., Matthews, F.E., McRae-McKee, K., Meirelles, O., Mosley, T.H., Pase, M.P., Psaty, B.M., Satizabal, C.L., Seshadri, S., Skoog, I., Stephan, B.C.M., Wetterberg, H., Wong, M.M., Zettergren, A., and Hofman, A. (2020). Twenty-seven-year time trends in dementia incidence in Europe and the United States. *Neurology, 95*(5), e519–e531. https://doi.org/10.1212/WNL.0000000000010022

Xu, W., Tan, L., Wang, H.F., Tan, M.S., Tan, L., Li, J.Q., Zhao, Q.F., and Yu, J.T. (2016). Education and risk of dementia: Dose-response meta-analysis of prospective cohort studies. *Molecular Neurobiology, 53*(5), 3113–3123. https://doi.org/10.1007/s12035-015-9211-5

Yaffe, K. (2019). Prevention of cognitive impairment with intensive systolic blood pressure control. *Journal of the American Medical Association, 321*(6), 548–549. https://doi.org/10.1001/jama.2019.0008

Yaffe, K., Falvey, C., Harris, T.B., Newman, A., Satterfield, S., Koster, A., Ayonayon, H., Simonsick, E., and Health ABC Study. (2013). Effect of socioeconomic disparities on incidence of dementia among biracial older adults: Prospective study. *BMJ (Clinical Research Ed.), 347*, f7051. https://doi.org/10.1136/bmj.f7051

Zahodne, L.B., Stern, Y., and Manly, J.J. (2015). Differing effects of education on cognitive decline in diverse elders with low versus high educational attainment. *Neuropsychology, 29*(4), 649–657. https://doi.org/10.1037/neu0000141

Zahodne, L.B., Manly, J.J., Smith, J., Seeman, T., and Lachman, M.E. (2017). Socioeconomic, health, and psychosocial mediators of racial disparities in cognition in early, middle, and late adulthood. *Psychology and Aging, 32*(2), 118–130. https://doi.org/10.1037/pag0000154

Zhang, Z., Gu, D., and Hayward, M.D. (2010). Childhood nutritional deprivation and cognitive impairment among older Chinese people. *Social Science & Medicine (1982), 71*(5), 941–949. https://doi.org/10.1016/j.socscimed.2010.05.013

Zhang, Z., Hayward, M.D., and Yu, Y.L. (2016). Life course pathways to racial disparities in cognitive impairment among older Americans. *Journal of Health and Social Behavior, 57*(2), 184–199. https://doi.org/10.1177/0022146516645925

Zinzi, D.B., Krieger, N., Agénor, M., Graves, J., Linos, N., and Bassett, M.T. (2017). Structural racism and health inequities in the USA: Evidence and interventions. *Lancet*, *389*(10077), 1453–1463. https://doi.org/10.1016/S0140-6736(17)30569-X

Zissimopoulos, J., Tysinger, B., St. Clair, P., and Crimmins, E. (2018). The impact of changes in population health and mortality on future prevalence of Alzheimer's Disease and other dementias in the United States. *Journals of Gerontology: Series B*, *73*(suppl_1), S38–S47. https://doi.org/10.1093/geronb/gbx147

Zuelsdorff, M., Okonkwo, O.C., Norton, D., Barnes, L.L., Graham, K.L., Clark, L.R., Wyman, M.F., Benton, S.F., Gee, A., Lambrou, N., Johnson, S.C., and Gleason, C.E. (2020). Stressful life events and racial disparities in cognition among middle-aged and older adults. *Journal of Alzheimer's Disease*, *73*(2), 671–682. https://doi.org/10.3233/JAD-190439

3

Improving Outcomes for Individuals Living with Dementia

The experiences of people living with dementia are at the heart of the challenge of reducing the negative impacts of the disease. To deepen our understanding of those experiences, the committee began with a close look at the reflections of a number of individuals, made available to us through the work of the advisory panel formed to support this study (see Chapter 1). The paper prepared by the members of this panel summarizes findings from a public call for commentaries that was posted on the project website and also widely distributed, and from a survey conducted by the Alzheimer's Association (Huling Hummel et al., 2020).[1] It includes anonymous first-person accounts, as well as a synthesis of the challenges the advisory panel identified as most important. We accorded these perspectives special weight as we examined the challenges of living with dementia and reviewed the available research, drawing on papers commissioned for this study,[2] academic studies and reports, and presentations to the committee (see Chapter 1).

The chapter begins with a discussion of the challenges identified by the advisory panel. The remaining sections review research in several areas relevant to those challenges: diagnosis of dementia, autonomy and protection from harm, and interventions to improve the experiences of people living

---

[1] The panel's paper is available at https://www.nationalacademies.org/our-work/decadal-survey-of-behavioral-and-social-science-research-on-alzheimers-disease-and-alzheimers-disease-related-dementias.

[2] https://www.nationalacademies.org/event/10-17-2019/meeting-2-decadal-survey-of-behavioral-and-social-science-research-on-alzheimers-disease-and-alzheimers-disease-related-dementias

with dementia. The chapter closes with a discussion of research directions for each of these areas.

PERSPECTIVES ON LIVING WITH DEMENTIA

Prior work offers important insights into possible gaps in research relevant to living with dementia. For example, the 2020 National Research Summit offered recommendations drafted by its Persons Living with Dementia Stakeholder Group (2020). Examples include the call for research on how disparities affect the experience of living with dementia; how finances affect choices about diagnosis, treatment, and research participation; and methods for improving the quality of end-of-life care. In addition to reviewing this prior work, the committee wished to hear directly from individuals living with dementia, and we appreciated the opportunities to integrate the advisory panel's perspectives throughout this study. This small group of people provided us with a snapshot of their own experiences, responded to our questions, and participated in public workshop discussions. The panel also provided a thoughtful summation of the perspectives of a larger group of people living with dementia and family caregivers gathered through the call for commentaries (Huling Hummel et al., 2020). The advisory panel made an invaluable contribution to our understanding, primarily of the perspectives of individuals in the early stages of disease and family caregivers. It is important to note that insights into the experiences of individuals at advanced stages of disease are much less accessible because at those stages, dementia can limit people's capacity to articulate their thoughts and feelings (Reuben, 2019).

The advisory panel identified four themes as primary challenges for persons living with dementia:

1. problems in obtaining an accurate and timely dementia diagnosis,
2. problems in obtaining needed supports and services,
3. communication challenges with doctors and other health care professionals, and
4. fear and loss.

The panel's perspectives on these challenges are summarized below.

Problems in Obtaining an Accurate and Timely Dementia Diagnosis

Respondents to the call for commentaries and members of the advisory panel repeatedly noted frustration with the diagnostic process. They pointed out that many primary care physicians lack the expertise to diagnose dementia accurately, an issue that may be particularly important for the small minority of people who show signs of dementia before age 65. They suggested that many physicians believe that receiving a dementia diagnosis is either inconsequential because there is no remedy or actually harmful to patients. While there may be people who would prefer not to be told, multiple respondents reported that delays in receiving a diagnosis caused harm to themselves or loved ones. Respondents also expressed the view that delays in diagnosis reflect skepticism about reported symptoms ("My doctor did not believe me. My primary physician thought my problems were all due to the high stress of my position."). Other delays resulted from diagnostic uncertainty ("It was difficult at first because with each new doctor I had a different diagnosis."). One respondent reported, "I am a neurologist who retired early.... I sought medical help for my symptoms for 10 years prior to my diagnosis...." Other respondents encountered clinicians who were dismissive because of the lack of effective treatments ("When she pressed her doctor for more definitive diagnosis [after 2 years], she was told by her doctor, 'Why bother, it won't change your treatment approach.'").

Errors and delays in diagnosis carried significant risks, as comments from caregivers suggested: "...Dad was confined to a psychiatric ward for a week after frightening family members with a gun because of terrifying hallucinations ... a neuropsychiatrist finally diagnosed Dad with Lewy body dementia." Delays in diagnosis also can have a significant economic impact, as one respondent noted: "It is important to receive a diagnosis as early as possible so you can leave work before you are fired due to performance issues that dementia inevitably causes. I was fired from my job, but I did not get diagnosed until 5 years later."

Some respondents characterized the diagnostic experience as lacking in empathy: "What the doctor didn't say out loud was, 'Now get out of my office so I can see someone I can actually do something for.'"

Problems in Obtaining Supports and Services

Many respondents reported experiencing a disconnect between diagnosis and assessment and/or referral for services of any kind. One respondent noted, "When I first saw a neurologist he gave me a short test and a prescription, and that was that. He gave me no information about vascular dementia or any other [psychoeducational] resources at all. This is unacceptable for a terminal illness!" Others discovered that available services were inappropriate ("...support services are geared more toward care partners and not for those with the actual disease.") or that potentially beneficial resources were unavailable: "My local ALZ Association will not allow me to participate in support groups or classes 'without being accompanied by someone....' I live alone and do not yet need a caregiver."

Nevertheless, respondents reported that clinicians in some settings worked hard to avoid creating a feeling of abandonment for their clients, connecting people diagnosed with dementia to available supports. New York University, for instance, encourages referral to the Family Support Program when a person receives a diagnosis of dementia and requests permission for a staff member to follow up with patients and family in the week after diagnosis to provide any needed information or referrals. One survey respondent was able to enroll their partner and teenage children in counseling, noting the great benefit of "getting everyone on the same page as to what to expect, and ... showed there was a lot more living to do." Box 3-1 presents the perspective of an advisory panel member on the challenge of finding enrichment activities at an early stage of the disease.

Challenges in Communicating with Doctors and Other Health Care Professionals

Many respondents noted poor communication with health care professionals at the time of diagnosis ("The doctor did all kinds of tests that showed there was nothing wrong with his brain. She basically shrugged and sent us on our way."); poor coordination of care ("Her doctors don't communicate with each other and her dementia diagnosis is not flagged in her records. She has to ask her health care professionals to 'slow down' when giving instructions or explaining things."); and general communication problems ("Communication is non-existent. They are not helpful or,

---

BOX 3-1
Perspective: Programs for Individuals with Early-Onset Dementia

I began experiencing early stage dementia at age 47. My search for programs that would allow me to connect with other individuals with dementia and participate in enrichment activities that would help me maintain my quality of life led me to my local senior center. Unfortunately, this was a huge disappointment. The senior center offers crafts and classes for seniors; however, they refused me membership because I was not yet 55 years old. The local community college, as well as my own university have programs for seniors to audit or take full credit classes for little to no cost. However, they require that I be 65 years of age to participate, so I have been paying full price to take one class each semester in order to keep my mind busy learning new things, which I am told will help develop new pathways in my brain even as others shut down.

SOURCE: Advisory panel member.

frankly, knowledgeable." "My biggest frustration is communicating with my Geriatric Specialist....").

Fear and Loss

Survey respondents described many ways in which dementia brings both fear and loss. Financial concerns were cited frequently. These concerns included worry about being preyed upon financially ("Our accountant estimated that my Dad wrote checks worth tens of thousands of dollars to charities, bogus car warranty companies, scam lotteries and gold coin merchants and nearly lost his home due to non-payment of taxes."). Another respondent stated, "I was forced to take a medical leave because of my symptoms and lost my employee health insurance 3 days before I turned 65, so I would not be entitled to a pension." Many respondents noted the shocking expense of care they would need in the future and their inability to pay for services of sufficient quality to maintain their safety or dignity: "I live in fear of getting worse with no financial options for assisted living or memory care."

Social isolation has long been a problem for older Americans but is significantly exacerbated by dementia. Bias from others and embarrassment about real or potential errors related to cognitive deficits can severely limit social opportunities. Sensitivity to noise can make public gatherings jarring and unpleasant. Cognitive impairment may slow responses in conversation and make old hobbies and sports activities difficult to pursue. As one respondent noted, "I am unable to pursue my hobbies. I would love to still have the right to work in my old job and not get paid for it."

Some respondents addressed how the COVID-19 pandemic has exacerbated the problem of isolation. One said, "I miss my family and I'm very lonely and depressed." Other findings, such as those from a nationwide survey of nursing home residents conducted in July and August 2020 (Montgomery et al., 2020), reinforce the impression that lack of contact was especially hard on older people living away from family.

Box 3-2 describes art programs available during the COVID-19 pandemic.

RESEARCH ON KEY ASPECTS OF LIVING WITH DEMENTIA

Researchers have provided insights relevant to many aspects of the experience of living with dementia, including those described by the advisory panel. The committee reviewed the state of the literature to identify priorities for future research in these areas. We could not address every aspect of life with dementia but identified a set of examples that reflect the diversity of relevant research. In the medical domain, we review challenges

> **BOX 3-2**
> **Perspective: Programs Available During the COVID-19 Pandemic**
>
> The Smithsonian Institution offers special community support activities for those living with dementia. We get together, on Zoom,[a] and we look at different art topics/pieces and discuss what we see, how it moves us, etc. It is quite powerful. Also, prior to the pandemic, the local office of the Alzheimer's Association was meeting once a month with those living with a variety of differing dementias. The organizer also had given us options to attend gallery shows where we could get our own hands dirty in painting. I am looking forward to these tasks returning. They weren't just an opportunity to be in community; they allowed me to feel I could accomplish something new and creative. They helped me define purpose.
>
> ---
>
> [a]Because of the COVID-19 pandemic.
>
> SOURCE: Advisory panel member.

in making and communicating the diagnosis of dementia. In the nonmedical domain, we summarize issues related to decision making, financial vulnerability, and sexuality. A host of other issues, including driving, medication management, and housing choices, are equally important, and we hope the examples discussed here may be used as a template for further work in additional domains.

Diagnosing Dementia[3]

Early and accurate diagnosis of dementia can be difficult. Most types of dementia develop slowly, but different types present different symptoms, and symptoms vary even among individuals experiencing the same type of dementia. Doctors who see patients for limited appointment times in an examining room may not be certain how to interpret symptoms and their relationship to other medical issues the patient may have. The lack of clarity is often very frustrating for patients and families. Clinicians and families also wonder about the ethics of disclosing a diagnosis for which there is limited treatment.

---

[3]This section draws on a paper commissioned by the committee (Bennett, 2020). That paper provides more detail about diagnosis and the types of dementia.

Challenges in Arriving at a Diagnosis

Clinicians use guidelines to identify individuals who meet criteria that apply to a range of dementia diagnoses. The process of diagnosis often includes several steps; it may be initiated in response to concerning symptoms reported by the person or family or to the results of routine screening. Public education campaigns and tools, such as the Alzheimer's Association's 10 Early Signs and Symptoms of Alzheimer's (Alzheimer's Association, n.d.), have heightened awareness of the early signs of dementia, and anecdotal evidence suggests that screening by primary care providers has also become more common.

Although the U.S. Preventive Services Task Force (2020) currently rates the evidence for dementia screening as insufficient, clinicians may opt to screen individual patients using a variety of instruments (see Box 3-3) or through the Medicare Annual Wellness Visit. Cognitive screening is a required component of this visit, but guidelines do not specify how it should be done, and anecdotal evidence suggests that many clinicians do not adhere to the screening requirement (Jacobson and Zissimopoulos, 2020). Guidelines about what should be included in this cognitive screen are urgently needed.

Once cognitive concerns have been identified, the diagnostic evaluation typically involves obtaining a history of decline, usually through interviews with the patient and family and through mental status testing that identifies

---

BOX 3-3
Screening Tools

Brief mental status tests provide objective evidence of impairment in one or more areas of cognition, such as memory, reasoning or judgment, and language. Examples include the Mini-Mental State Examination (MMSE), the Montreal Cognitive Assessment (MoCA), Mini-Cog, and Addenbrooke's Cognitive Examination III (ACE-III) and mini-ACE (Arevalo-Rodriguez et al., 2015; Beishon et al., 2019; Davis et al., 2015; Larner and Mitchell, 2014). Other diagnostic tools that rely on information provided by family members or others who know the patient well address functional impairment as well as cognitive changes. These include the Informant Questionnaire on Cognitive Decline in the Elderly (IQCODE) and AD8 (Chan et al., 2016; Harrison et al., 2016). While it is valuable to have screening for cognitive decline, these tests vary in their ability to detect mild cognitive impairment and dementia, and most are not sensitive to the earliest stages of cognitive decline. Moreover, false positives can occur with any of these tests, which may lead to misdiagnosis.

at least two areas of cognition in which there has been a decline severe enough to impair social or occupational functioning (McKhann et al., 2011; American Psychiatric Association, 2013). Blood tests and neuroimaging studies are used to check for treatable conditions that may cause cognitive impairment that mimics dementia.

Although these basic approaches to diagnosis are well known, studies have suggested that cognitive impairment is significantly underdiagnosed—indeed by one estimate, roughly half the population of individuals who have Alzheimer's disease or a related dementia receive a formal diagnosis (Alzheimer's Association, 2019). Early-stage dementia is least likely to be diagnosed, and Hispanic and non-Hispanic Black people are less likely to receive a diagnosis of mild cognitive impairment than are non-Hispanic White people (NASEM, 2021). Moreover, the effectiveness of diagnostic evaluation is limited by linguistic, educational, and cultural factors that affect the validity of results (Lewis et al., 2021; Jervis et al., 2010, 2018).[4] For example, the results of functional questionnaires are influenced by context. Patients' responses are affected by baseline levels of function, limitations related to motor or sensory changes, and degree of insight. Family members' observational facility and cultural expectations, as well as cultural biases in the questionnaires themselves, also affect results (Jervis et al., 2018). Similarly, scores on cognitive tests are influenced by patients' baseline cognitive performance, mood and effort, sensory and motor changes, and comfort level (which themselves are influenced by education and culture), and by linguistic and cultural biases in the tests themselves.

Diagnosis is complex in part because cognition is not a finite or unitary capacity: the evaluation covers multiple cognitive abilities, such as episodic memory (ability to encode and recall a story and/or list of words), language or semantic memory (capacity for naming and fluency), executive function (such capacities as planning, focusing attention, and self-monitoring needed to direct one's own cognition), and perceptual speed and working memory (ability to hold and manipulate information in short-term memory stores). Moreover, it is common for people's cognitive capacity to decline as they age: a degree of decline is accepted as a normal part of the aging process, although it may be the result of pathologic changes in the brain (Salthouse, 2019).

Cognitive loss occurs on a continuum. Cutpoints along that continuum identify points at which the decline can be classified as impairment, beginning with mild cognitive impairment, in which objective measures of cognition are abnormal but function is preserved, and progressing through stages of severity that increasingly have clinical consequences. Thus, mild

---

[4]Similarly, there is ongoing research examining whether biomarkers of Alzheimer's disease differ by race, particularly among those with APOE 4-positive (Rajan et al., 2019).

cognitive impairment is a change in an individual's cognition significant enough to be recognized as impairment but mild enough that the individual retains independence and functional abilities (Albert et al., 2011). A loss of cognition that impairs function is considered dementia. However, because cognitive impairment is defined primarily in terms of changes over time for the individual, clinicians use information about level of education, occupation, and other aspects of the individual's life to set expectations for performance that can serve as the basis for assessing decline. Like the identification of a degree of decline that interferes with social or occupational functioning, these criteria are subjective and likely to be affected by cultural and other differences across populations, and thus are problematic for researchers and clinicians alike.

Today, dementia and its precursor, mild cognitive impairment, are diagnosed primarily based on clinical symptoms. Often, family members are the first to notice subtle early psychological and cognitive changes in their loved ones and bring them to a clinician's attention. Researchers are beginning to evaluate whether information that can be collected unobtrusively (e.g., from website interactions, smartphones, and wearable devices) can be used to detect cognitive impairment or early dementia.[5] There are also many tests that assess the neuropathology associated with Alzheimer's disease and other forms of dementia, using such modalities as brain scanning technology that can reveal structural changes, deposits, or biochemical changes in the brain, or testing of cerebrospinal fluid for abnormal markers.[6] These tests are valuable for research and can be used clinically to help distinguish one type of dementia from another, although they cannot be used for diagnosis of mild cognitive impairment or dementia, which is based on clinical symptoms, as discussed above. Such tests can detect signs of brain pathology even when no clinical symptoms are evident. Imaging, biomarker, and autopsy studies all indicate that many asymptomatic people have Alzheimer's biomarkers. Not all such individuals will eventually develop dementia, and some biomarkers can be detected many years before any symptoms develop. In individuals with clinical evidence of mild cognitive impairment or dementia, these tests can be valuable in distinguishing Alzheimer's disease from other dementias (e.g., frontotemporal degeneration, Lewy body dementia), and they can also be used to select individuals for trials of preventive strategies. Substantial progress has recently been made in the use of blood tests to measure biomarkers of Alzheimer's disease, but the same limitations apply to these tests (Palmqvist et al., 2020).

---

[5] https://www.betteraging.com/cognitive-aging/new-study-will-research-cognitive-health-using-apple-watch-iphone

[6] https://www.nia.nih.gov/health/biomarkers-dementia-detection-and-research

Researchers seek to identify signs of preclinical change because of the hope that treatments offered earlier, before symptoms are apparent, can increase the chances of improving outcomes for patients. As noted in Chapter 1, however, no disease-modifying treatments have yet been approved for Alzheimer's disease; the pharmacologic treatments that exist address symptoms but not root causes. Biomarker research is nonetheless useful for advancing understanding of the development and progression of disease, differentiating types of dementia, and guiding research to develop new interventions, both to control symptoms better and potentially to address the causes of the disease (Mangialasche et al., 2010; Tan et al., 2014). It is important to note, moreover, that biomarker studies have been conducted largely in convenience samples of predominantly White and highly educated individuals, and even the few epidemiologic studies of biomarkers have had limited representation of individuals from rural communities and minority populations, so the generalizability of their results is limited (Glymour et al., 2018).

It is important to consider as well that if biomarker screenings do become widely used clinically, they will likely raise new questions. As noted above, many people who demonstrate biomarker evidence of Alzheimer's pathology never go on to develop clinical symptoms. Would this group, with normal cognition but positive biomarkers, be considered to have Alzheimer's disease? If biomarker evidence were officially part of the disease definition, would people who meet the clinical criteria for dementia (progressive impairment of cognition and resultant disability) but do not show the currently measured biomarkers for disease be counted in estimates of Alzheimer's prevalence? If biomarkers were used routinely for screening (e.g., of the adult offspring of persons with Alzheimer's disease), what additional challenges might arise?

Perhaps most important are ethical questions about whether or when an asymptomatic individual who has biomarkers for dementia should receive that information. Being told that one may—or may not—develop a potentially devastating and ultimately fatal disease 10 or more years in the future could have profound psychological and other consequences for individuals and their families. And how could the privacy of the information be safeguarded? Would asymptomatic, biomarker-positive individuals lose access to life and long-term care insurance, housing options, employment, or other benefits? Consideration of the potential psychological, financial, and other impacts on such individuals is needed so that sound guidelines can be established. Research on these and related questions is scant; more such research is needed to support the development of guidelines, as well as important decisions regarding policy, insurance coverage, and public health messaging.

Questions About Communicating a Dementia Diagnosis

Even apart from questions about disclosure raised by screening for biomarkers, clinicians may struggle to assess the benefits and liabilities related to making and disclosing a diagnosis of dementia. An early and accurate diagnosis has benefits. A diagnosis may be an eligibility requirement for some services and provide reassurance that unexplained symptoms have a clear cause. It may allow individuals to work with loved ones to revise legal documents, anticipate needed support services, avoid medical and financial risks, and plan for future care while they can still fully participate in decision making. Yet receiving a diagnosis has potential negative ramifications as well. As noted, life and long-term care insurance could be denied to those with a preexisting condition. Access to some living options (e.g., entry into continuing care retirement communities and assisted living facilities) may be denied for those diagnosed with dementia, and even at times for those diagnosed with mild cognitive impairment. In some states, a dementia diagnosis must be disclosed to the department of motor vehicles, triggering evaluations that can lead to revocation or restriction of driving privileges. Finally, the stigma of dementia may affect how individuals feel about themselves and how they are treated in society and within health care settings.

There is relatively sparse guidance for clinicians about disclosing a diagnosis and communicating about care, symptoms, and the progress of disease. The Gerontological Society of America's KAER toolkit[7] has a section on how to disclose a diagnosis, which includes links to videos and external resources. Guidance for patient-centered communication during diagnosis has been suggested, but with variable results thus far (Zaleta and Carpenter, 2010).

Promoting Autonomy and Protecting from Harm

Generally, clinicians are taught to balance autonomy, which would promote disclosure of diagnosis and prognosis, against beneficence, which emphasizes protection from harm. Some clinicians fear the impact of diagnosis on their patients' mental health and well-being, particularly when cognitive deficits limit an individual's ability to process and respond to information. The challenges of communication deepen as dementia progresses, although many people still want to be included in conversations about their care even as their ability to understand and articulate opinions declines. Indeed, supporting individuals living with dementia while protecting their autonomy—recognizing their values and right to make decisions

---

[7]https://www.geron.org/images/gsa/Marketing/KAER/GSA_KAER-Toolkit_2020_Final.pdf

as other adults do while also providing appropriate and graduated levels of protection against harm—is the central ethical challenge posed by dementia.

Assessment of decision-making capacity must be tailored to individual circumstances; it cannot be based simply on the cutpoints for cognitive test results. While research has addressed how to evaluate decisional capacity for research and treatment purposes, there is no standard practice for capacity assessment (Pennington et al., 2018), and available instruments and insights have not been widely adopted in clinical practice. For decisions outside of or adjacent to the medical realm, including those related to housing, finances, and safety matters (guns, sexuality), research is extremely limited. There is a growing literature on assessment of driving capacity, but specialists who can make such assessments are not widely available (see, e.g., Wolfe and Lehockey, 2016; Schultheis et al., 2008).

The tension between autonomy and safety increases as patients' cognitive decline continues and they become more vulnerable. A significant potential threat to dignity comes with overprotection, yet the risk of abuse and neglect grows when protection is insufficient for an individual whose capacity to make decisions that reflect personal values and interests is compromised by disease. People living with dementia, as with some other illnesses, are negatively affected by stigma, both when others see and treat them disrespectfully and when they incorporate societal bias into their own self-image. This self-stigma can diminish self-esteem and self-efficacy (Watson et al., 2007).

Thus, the need to balance respect for autonomy and beneficence, to promote self-advocacy while offering sufficient support, complicates decision making by and for people living with dementia. Adulthood brings with it the right to make decisions in risky domains, including finance, sexuality and relationships, medical care, driving, gun access, and many others. The committee cannot cover every potentially risky domain in this report, but we review issues related to finance and sexuality for persons living with dementia in order to analyze the nature of the challenges, explore potential solutions, and generate areas for research.[8] These two domains represent burdens that are both common and serious for people living with dementia and their family caregivers. In addition, we perceive a gap in the research regarding how to promote independence while also providing appropriate protection. Better guidance to help clinicians, people with dementia, and families navigate these complex issues is sorely needed. Finally, we see

---

[8]One key area in which people living with dementia are at risk is the use of physical restraints, which, although it has become less common in institutional settings such as nursing homes, remains an issue with untrained caregivers in the community. See, e.g., https://www.ncbi.nlm.nih.gov/pmc/articles/PMC7058582; https://www.ncbi.nlm.nih.gov/pmc/articles/PMC2564468 for more on this issue.

in that evidentiary gap the potential for improvement in alleviating the challenges of dementia by developing better interventions, guidelines, and policies.

Financial Decisions and Potential for Abuse

Decisional capacity is a cornerstone of autonomy. Those who can weigh risks and benefits make their own decisions, while those who cannot adequately assess risks have decisions made on their behalf by others. Prematurely limiting the decision-making authority of persons with dementia robs them of their rights and dignity. At the same time, however, protecting someone who has become vulnerable is an ethical responsibility. Two key points regarding decisional capacity are worth noting. First, a diagnosis of dementia does not automatically mean a person has lost the right or ability to make decisions. Dementia is a progressive illness, and people in earlier stages can clearly express and act upon their lifelong values and preferences. Second, capacity is decision-specific, meaning a person may be capable of making some decisions but not others. In many individuals, the capacity to make financial decisions fades earlier than other cognitive skills. People may be able to make values-based medical decisions or select a health care proxy when they can no longer handle complex financial transactions. Yet because of loss of insight, which often occurs in early stages of dementia, they may not be willing to relinquish financial decision making, with substantial consequences. Once it has been determined that a person with dementia cannot make a specific decision, it becomes the responsibility of a surrogate to support the person with dementia in decision making based on the person's values and previously expressed preferences, if known.

Those whose cognitive impairment undermines their decisional capacity are at increased risk for abuse of various kinds. Older people hold a substantial percentage of financial assets in the United States; net worth for those older than age 65 is roughly 20 times that for those under 35 (Sawhill and Pulliam, 2019). Financial capacity, defined as "the ability to independently manage one's financial affairs in a manner consistent with personal self-interest," can be one of the earliest deficits of cognitive function, even before a diagnosis of dementia (Widera et al., 2011). An individual may lose a lifetime's savings just when those funds are needed for long-term care, precisely because at that time they have become vulnerable to exploitation. In one large sample, 4.7 percent of older people reported suffering financial exploitation. The cost of such abuse in the United States is challenging to measure because much of it appears to go unreported; estimates vary from $3 billion to as much as $30 billion annually (Stanger, 2015; see also Government Accountability Office, 2020).

Financial exploitation targeting older people with cognitive impairment occurs in many forms. A typical example is a phone call in which the caller claims to represent an Internet service provider who has discovered a problem with the recipient's computer. The caller promises to fix the problem quickly and requests bank account information for direct billing, but instead uses that information to empty the victim's bank account.[9] Older people who live alone, especially those with dementia, can be particularly vulnerable to such scams when their opportunities for human contact are limited.

Sadly, financial abuse by family members or others well known to the victim, including new "friends" who hope to extract money, is even more common than anonymous scams (Spreng et al., 2016). Financial exploitation of older people with dementia often goes unreported. In cases of abuse by family members, the person with dementia may resist reporting to the police for fear of the consequences for a loved one. Those with more advanced dementia may be unaware of the theft or unable to act on their knowledge because of isolation and inability to access help.

Making wise financial choices requires many skills, including good judgment about who is a trustworthy person, as well as basic math skills. A person needs to estimate a reasonable price for goods or services and needs sufficient memory or record keeping skills to know, for instance, whether they have recently donated to an alumni association or other philanthropy. Experts recommend that clinicians educate patients and family members about the prevalence of scams and the risks of lost financial capacity, as well as ways to identify warning signs of exploitation (Marson, 2013).

There is no single, widely used tool for measuring financial capacity. One model measures cognitive skills, such as mental math, as well as social skills, such as the ability to identify a scam (Spreng et al., 2016). This approach requires a specially trained person to administer the test and takes roughly 30 minutes to complete. An instrument for assessing the capacity to make financial decisions has also been developed (Lichtenberg et al., 2015). Assessments that require expert clinicians and take considerable time to administer may be too costly or inaccessible for many people, although many expert clinicians perform such assessments on a fee-for-service basis, which is not covered by insurance.

Financial vulnerability for older people with cognitive impairment is not a new problem; the legal system has long offered remedies, particularly through the guardianship process. The process of obtaining a guardian can be expensive, time-consuming, and stressful and therefore is used rarely relative to the frequency of dementia. The process typically requires that the

---

[9] Catherine Christian, Chief of the Elder Abuse Unit of the NYC District Attorney's Office, personal interview with Tia Powell, October 10, 2018.

family submit an evaluation to a judge, with a request that the person be declared incompetent and that a family member be named guardian, with authority to access all accounts and disburse funds on the person's behalf. This has traditionally been an all-or-nothing process, in which the person with dementia either retains full decision-making rights or loses them all to a surrogate.

There are many impediments to the smooth functioning of the guardianship process. It is challenging to compel a person to undergo evaluation, and such evaluations can be expensive. The process may be traumatic for the family or disrupt relationships, particularly when dementia has brought impairment of insight or other emotional symptoms. It is not always easy to identify a suitable guardian, and not all guardians discharge their duties as hoped. The criteria for guardianship are generally quite stringent, to protect autonomy, but as one legal scholar and bioethicist has pointed out, the standard guardianship process fails to protect those in the middle, who have neither full capacity nor an utter absence of it (Arias, 2013). In practice, many families "muddle through," relying on the support they can find from clinicians and financial and legal advisors, and adapting to circumstances. An intermediate step of limited guardianship that offers oversight but permits the person with dementia some participation in financial decision making is one recommended approach (Arias, 2013). This approach aligns well with the ethical obligation to balance freedom and supervision in a fashion that promotes inclusion where possible and permits protection as needed, matching the degree of cognitive impairment with the level of authority of the guardian.

The Consumer Financial Protection Bureau has developed educational materials for banking industry professionals, including tools for identifying unusual banking behavior, such as large money orders sent overseas (Consumer Financial Protection Bureau, 2016). Families often set up joint accounts to oversee a person with dementia's financial affairs, but such accounts can also make exploitation easy. These accounts allow the family member or other trusted person full access, but the joint holder can use the incapacitated older person's funds for any purpose, including ones not sanctioned by or in the interest of the person with dementia. Upon the death of one member of a joint account, the funds are owned wholly by the co-holder of the account, which may exclude other family members from an intended inheritance. The move to online banking has enabled some family members to access the account of a person with dementia using that person's credentials; this practice is convenient but does not protect against unwarranted use of funds. Some experts recommend "convenience accounts," in which a designated person can use the account to pay bills but will not inherit the funds. Another useful tool is "read only" access in which a third party can monitor banking activity and alert the bank about suspicious behavior but cannot make withdrawals (Consumer Financial Protection Bureau, 2016).

Sexual Behavior, Risk, and Dementia

Sexual intimacy in the context of dementia is overshadowed by many unhelpful cultural biases, including those involving older people, gender norms, and those with disabilities. Many younger people assume that older people either do not or should not have sexual feelings, and the same incorrect beliefs are often applied to people with disabilities, including cognitive disabilities such as dementia. Moreover, older people with a same-sex orientation may have lived closeted lives, so that even close family members are unaware of their lifelong preferences. The fact is that older people vary markedly in their sexual interests and behaviors, just as other people do, with some remaining sexually active into their 80s and beyond. Aging does not eliminate loneliness or the wish for intimacy, physical touch, and companionship—all reasons why people of any age engage in sexual behaviors. In any case, as with other decisions, a diagnosis of dementia does not in itself prove that someone lacks the capacity to make choices about sexual relationships.

It is also important to note that while most people with dementia live in the community, people with dementia represent more than half of the population of nursing homes. In these institutions, normally private behavior is rarely private.[10] In the past, moreover, nursing homes often prohibited even consensual sexual activity among residents. Standards have evolved in the direction of greater freedom in this regard, although nursing facilities vary significantly in their policies and practices (Ward et al., 2005), and even when facilities have more accepting policies, family members may object and ask staff to prevent relationships among residents. Yet nursing home staff rarely receive training in how to respond to sexual approaches either among residents or to themselves by residents. Sexualized approaches to staff or female residents by male residents, either verbal or physical, are far more likely to be seen as problematic and more likely to result in punitive actions, including rejection from a facility or transfer to a more restrictive section. Women with dementia are more likely to be seen as lacking sexual impulses, and as generally more vulnerable and in need of protection (Ward et al., 2005).

Certainly, sexual behaviors can include risks to both physical safety and dignity for any person, but it is possible, indeed obligatory, to assess risks in individual cases. The presumption should be that sexual behavior among adults, irrespective of a diagnosis of dementia, is a normal and expected expression of self, and that willing and capable participation can

---

[10]https://www.cdc.gov/nchs/fastats/alzheimers.htm

be assessed. These decisions are of an essentially private nature, and the intervention of others poses a significant threat to dignity and the freedom to act as other adults do. Thus, the starting point for decisions about sexual behavior is that they remain the province of the person with dementia unless there are compelling reasons, not based on bias, to think otherwise. When sexual behavior is unwanted by the person to whom it is directed, such as a staff member at a nursing home, respectful, nonpunitive reactions, such as distraction and redirection, are appropriate. If the person with dementia is viewed as being unwilling or otherwise at risk—for instance, because of a predatory or disinhibited partner—intervention by family members, institutions, or even legal authorities may be appropriate, yet must still be approached in a way that preserves dignity. Dementia also can result in uninhibited sexual self-stimulation, which can be disturbing for staff and other residents, as well as undermine the dignity of the person. Distracting and removing the person to a private setting are the best options; restraints and sedation should be avoided unless strictly necessary. Little research or evidence-based training is available to help address this issue.

Possible and appropriate interventions regarding the sexual behavior of persons with dementia fall on a spectrum. When both participants have full capacity, no intervention is ethically justifiable within this intensely private domain. A next step along the spectrum would resemble the sort of inquiry a concerned friend would make of a person who does not have cognitive impairment but appears to be making an unwise choice. For persons with cognitive impairment associated with dementia, an assessment of their decisional capacity is warranted and is indeed a mark of excellence in nursing homes. As the cognitive deficits of dementia advance, a person may no longer be capable of expressing or acting upon a choice. At this stage, a protective role is ethically justified and comes to the fore.[11]

Resources for Assessing and Supporting Decisions

Although dementia can undermine a person's ability to make decisions based on lifelong values, this decline in capacity occurs gradually and affects domains unevenly. As in many aspects of living with dementia, a person may be able to extend autonomy by learning about challenges that dementia is likely to bring as the disease progresses and recording advance directives about medical choices, finances, sexual relationships, and other

---

[11] An issue that touches on both sexual and financial decision making is marriage undertaken by or with a person who has cognitive impairment. Such a marriage offers the possibility of support in the face of the isolation and loneliness that are common among older people and those living with dementia, but there is also the possibility of exploitation, as well as distress for adult children and other family members. This is another area that has not been well studied.

issues. Such documents as the MOLST (Medical Orders for Life-Sustaining Treatment) are important for directing medical care after a person loses capacity. Unfortunately, no one can realistically predict every challenge or devise an advance directive that will provide adequate guidance for every situation that may arise.

As dementia progresses, a person may still retain a strong sense of self but lose insight or have impaired judgment about risks. Risks associated with driving and gun safety may be misjudged by a person with advancing cognitive impairment. These two activities involve risks not only to the person with dementia but also to others, both in the family and in the local community. The ethical viability of removing a person's right to make decisions increases as the danger to self and others increases and as the judgment of the person declines.

Clinicians are often asked by family members for help in assessing various types of decisional capacity (including for financial decisions, as discussed above). Yet many physicians lack the appropriate expertise to fill this role, and a comprehensive exam cannot be accomplished during a brief medical appointment. Assessments of capacity also can be quite variable (Stocking et al., 2008). Neuropsychological evaluations can elucidate the impact of impaired cognition on decisions but require considerable time, expense, and expertise (Gurrera et al., 2006). Although most clinicians cannot perform a detailed neuropsychological evaluation—or an assessment of driving skills or financial capacity—they should be able to determine when such evaluations are needed and refer the patient to a professional with the requisite skills. Unfortunately, no single evaluation or type of specialist can assess a person's capacity to make choices about money, sexual contact, driving, and the wide range of important challenges a person with dementia faces. And as noted, at a given stage of disease, a person may retain the ability to make choices that reflect lifelong values and interests in some domains but not others. This complexity greatly increases the difficulty of finding the right resources to help guide those with dementia and their family caregivers as they navigate potentially risky life choices.

Limited research has been conducted to establish standard tools and methods for assessing different sorts of capacity or to identify ways of making such resources broadly available and easy to administer. The assessment resources available today are not standardized, can be difficult to obtain, and are often expensive and time-consuming. Additional research to develop tools for assessing and supporting decision-making capacity for people living with dementia, aimed at primary care providers, social workers, and others involved in providing care, could help address this gap. Readily accessible educational programs about challenges in decision making for people with dementia and family caregivers, adapted for different cultural groups and languages, might also be helpful.

Interventions to Alleviate the Impact of Dementia

Although the clinical manifestations of different types of dementia vary, particularly at early stages of disease, the similarities are more pronounced as the diseases progress in severity and patients develop more complications. Characteristic symptoms appear during the various stages of the disorder, especially among those with Alzheimer's disease, as shown in Table 3-1. However, biological, sociodemographic, and clinical markers that predict disease progression and the rate of decline are lacking and are a topic for future research.

TABLE 3-1 Progression of Dementia Symptoms

Functional Status	Cognitive Changes	Behavioral Issues	Complications
Mild Cognitive Impairment (preclinical)			
	Report by patient or caregiver of memory loss; objective signs of memory impairment; mild construction, language, or executive dysfunction		
Early, Mild Dementia (typically 1 to 3 years from onset of symptoms)			
Impairment that affects capacity to manage finances, driving, and medications	Decreased insight, short-term memory deficits, poor judgment	Social withdrawal, mood changes: apathy, depression	Poor financial decisions, adverse effects related to medication errors
Middle Stage, Moderate Impairment (typically 2 to 8 years from onset)			
Difficulty with instrumental activities of daily living and some activities of daily living (ADLs), changes in gait and balance	Further declines in memory, getting lost in familiar areas, repeating questions	Apathy, depression, restlessness, anxiety, wandering	Need for assisted living facility, weight loss due to inability to prepare meals, falls
Late, Severe Impairment (typically 6 to 12 years from onset)			
Severe difficulty with ADLs, including continence; problems with mobility, swallowing	Little or unintelligible verbal output, loss of remote memory, inability to recognize family/friends	Motor or verbal agitation, aggression, apathy, depression, sundowning	Pressure sores, contractures, aspiration, pneumonia, weight loss due to forgetting to or refusing to eat

SOURCE: Adapted from American Geriatrics Society (2020). See also Droogsma et al. (2015).

Clinicians often use medicines to try to decrease the symptoms of certain dementias or reduce the emotional and psychological complications, with results that are modest at best (Gaugler et al., 2020; Fink et al., 2020). These medications, whose indications vary by type of dementia, are not addressed in this report because they fall outside the realm of social and behavioral approaches to reducing the impacts of dementia.

Nonpharmacologic interventions include both single- and multicomponent approaches. Although some types of dementia (e.g., frontotemporal degeneration) and situations (e.g., early-onset dementia) may require specific nonpharmacologic interventions, most general interventions are applicable to the majority of persons with dementia and their family caregivers, particularly in the more advanced stages of disease. Interventions may focus on persons living with dementia, caregivers (see Chapter 4), or both. Others are directed at helping the community better support families living with dementia and may be provided by community-based organizations or by health systems, as discussed in Chapter 5. This section reviews objectives for the care of people living with dementia and the evidence for approaches to some of the key challenges.

Goals for the Care of Persons Living with Dementia

Individuals at each stage of dementia have distinct needs, abilities to respond to interventions, and potential quality-of-life outcomes. For example, a positive outcome for people living with mild dementia might be that with added support, they can continue to work or volunteer for longer than would otherwise have been the case. For those living with severe dementia, the goal may be to identify in-home care that allows them to live with family and avoid moving to a nursing home. Needs vary with stage of disease and circumstances, but the areas in which persons living with dementia are likely to need care and support include (NASEM, 2021, p. 9)

- detection and diagnosis;
- assessment of symptoms to inform planning and deliver care, including financial and legal planning;
- information and education;
- medical management;
- support in activities of daily living;
- support for care partners and caregivers;
- communication and collaboration;
- coordination of medical care, long-term services and supports, and community-based services and supports;
- a supportive and safe environment; and
- advance care planning and end-of-life care.

A taxonomy of goals for dementia care (Table 3-2) provides a closer look at what is needed in some of these areas. Derived from focus groups of persons living with dementia and caregivers, this taxonomy has been used to guide care (Jennings et al., 2018). Setting goals and measuring attainment of these goals can serve several purposes that improve the care and lives of persons living with dementia. First, this exercise helps individuals identify and work toward personal goals that are meaningful to them. It also facilitates their providers' efforts to plan and organize care to achieve those goals. Defining outcome measures is another important tool for assessing how well a health system is meeting the needs of persons living with dementia (Reuben and Jennings, 2019). Yet while setting goals and measuring their attainment show promise for improving patient-centered outcomes, additional research is needed on such questions as the frequency of such assessments, the added value of integrating them into dementia care interventions, and appropriate responses when the goals of persons with dementia and those of their caregivers are not aligned.

TABLE 3-2 Goals for Dementia Care Identified by Persons with Dementia and Caregivers

Domain	Goals
Medical Care and End-of-Life Care	Receive needed dementia care
	Have doctors who work with us
	Have providers who understand our cultural background and speak our primary language
	Do not take medications with side effects
	Get adequate sleep at night
	Maintain adequate nutrition
	Control pain
	Do not get burdensome medical care
	Stay out of the hospital
	Die peacefully
	Live as long as possible
	Not be a burden to family
Quality of Life—Physical	Be physically safe (e.g., avoids falls, household hazards, or getting lost)
	Not taken advantage of by others
	Do self-care and household activities
	Be in charge of household activities
	Be physically active
	Continue to drive or use other transportation
	Continue to live at home
	Move to a more supportive setting (e.g., move in with family, assisted living, or nursing home)
	Find acceptable long-term care

Continued

TABLE 3-2 Continued

Domain	Goals
Quality of Life—Social and Emotional	Socialize with family and friends
	Maintain relationship with spouse/partner
	Continue to work or volunteer
	Do recreational activities
	Keep mind stimulated; be alert
	Control agitation or aggression; manage behavioral symptoms of dementia
	Manage depression
	Respected for spiritual preferences
Accessing Services and Supports	Feel financial resources are not a barrier to care; find assistance with managing finances
	Have legal issues in order
	Have adequate caregivers
	Find community resources for dementia that offer what I need
	Find culturally appropriate services for dementia
	Increase community awareness and education about dementia
Caregiver Support	Control caregiver's frustration and manage stress
	Receive caregiver support
	Feel confident in managing dementia-related problems
	Have more free time for caregiver; respite care
	Minimize family conflict with managing dementia care
	Maintain caregiver's health

SOURCE: Reprinted with permission from Springer Nature, *Quality of Life Research*, Jennings et al. (2016).

A recent National Academies' report on the challenges of caregiving has also identified a set of principles to guide care and support for people living with dementia (NASEM, 2021, p. 8):

- Person-centeredness: Recognition of persons living with dementia as individuals with their own goals, desires, interests, and abilities.
- Promotion of well-being: The use of social, behavioral, and environmental interventions that holistically address the needs of persons living with dementia, care partners, and caregivers to enhance well-being.
- Respect and dignity: Attention to each person's particular needs and values, which can be achieved by following models for identifying preferences and values, such as values elicitation, shared decision making, respect for dissent, or seeking either assent or informed consent.
- Justice: Treating people with equal need equally so that, for example, all critically ill persons receive critical care, all expectant

mothers receive prenatal care, and the dying receive palliative care. By extension, all persons living with dementia, care partners, and caregivers have equal access and can receive care, supports, and services according to their needs.
- Racial/ethnic, sexual, cultural, and linguistic inclusivity: The availability of racially, ethnically, sexually, culturally, and linguistically appropriate services for all who may need them, especially underserved and underrepresented populations, such as racial/ethnic minorities and LGBTQ individuals.
- Accessibility and affordability: Care, services, and supports for persons living with dementia, care partners, and caregivers that do not impose an unmanageable financial burden on individuals or their families and are available and accessible to all who may need them, including those living in rural communities.

The authors acknowledge that more research is needed to provide more explicit guidance regarding dementia care but note that following these guidelines would "represent a significant advance" over care that is currently widely available (p. 8).

Approaches for Addressing Key Dementia Symptoms

Researchers have explored a variety of strategies for improving the experiences of people living with dementia, including forms of cognitive training; therapies incorporating music, animal companionship, and other approaches; exercise; environmental modification; and others. The committee commissioned a paper that provides an overview of this body of work, based on systematic reviews published from 2016 to 2019 (Gaugler et al., 2020). The authors report that while some interventions may have potential, "conclusions as to efficacy or effectiveness are challenging if not impossible due to how control groups are defined, incomplete reporting of protocols and key intervention characteristics, heterogeneous outcome measures, and lack of clarity related to effect sizes or ... the clinical relevance of reported effects." The authors characterize the lack of conclusive evidence for nonpharmacologic interventions as "frustrating." Described below are some approaches that may hold promise for addressing key dementia symptoms: cognitive decline, functional decline, and behavioral and psychological symptoms.[12]

Addressing cognitive decline Approaches for addressing cognitive decline include forms of cognitive training, as well as exercise and other lifestyle

---

[12] The committee relied on the commissioned paper by Gaugler and colleagues (2020) for the content of this section.

modifications (Gaugler et al., 2020). In general, cognitive interventions, including cognitive training, cognitive rehabilitation, and cognitive stimulation therapy, appear to produce moderate benefits for cognition. Cognitive training includes guided tasks designed to improve memory and thinking. There is evidence that training targeted at specific domains of cognition, such as speed of processing or attention, can bring improvement in that domain. Cognitive rehabilitation is designed to enhance daily living using memory activities and memory-boosting approaches. It has shown limited benefit, particularly compared with other approaches designed to maintain or improve cognition for persons living with dementia. Overall, these approaches appear to have the capacity to strengthen people's capacity for the task they are practicing, but the benefits do not extend to other cognitive challenges.[13]

The evidence for *cognitive stimulation training (CST)* is stronger, and it is the only nonpharmacologic therapy recommended by the National Institute for Health and Clinical Excellence in the United Kingdom. Designed to enhance cognitive and social function, CST is often presented in group settings using such approaches as reminiscence and reality orientation (orienting individuals to the day, date, and weather to place them in "reality"). Reality orientation appears to have moderate benefits for cognition (Chiu et al., 2018). Systematic reviews have shown that CST can help improve cognition and memory, usually for persons with less severe dementia (Aguirre et al., 2013; Bahar-Fuchs et al., 2013; Woods et al., 2012). However, researchers have not yet established whether it is effective in community-based settings (as opposed to residential environments). Moreover, the cognitive benefits do not appear to be lasting, and CST does not affect other important domains, such as mood, behavioral symptoms, or daily function.

A fair amount of research supports the idea that physical activity (including both aerobic and nonaerobic exercise) also has the potential to maintain or enhance cognitive function for people with dementia, or possibly delay dementia symptoms (see, e.g., Duan et al., 2018; Farina et al., 2014; Groot et al., 2016; Karssemeijer et al., 2017; Liang et al., 2018; Lim et al., 2019). Although existing research does not provide a clear picture as to which interventions are most consistently efficacious at preventing cognitive decline, emerging work points to the possible benefits of a multicomponent approach that takes advantage of several mechanisms, such as nutrition, exercise, cognitive training, and social activity (Kivipelto et al., 2018).

Addressing functional decline Decline in such functions as self-care activities is a core symptom of dementia and is directly linked to such adverse

---

[13] https://www.thelancet.com/pdfs/journals/lancet/PIIS0140-6736(20)30367-6.pdf

events as falls and greater dependence on help from others. Functional decline that results in dependence is caused in part by neuropathological changes, but contextual factors also play a role. For example, cluttered, loud, or poorly lighted environments; information that is communicated ineffectively; lack of structures to support medication management; and overly complex tasks all may increase challenges for people living with dementia (Gitlin et al., 2020). These contextual factors are modifiable.

The available evidence suggests that several types of interventions are modestly beneficial in ameliorating functional decline. These include occupation-based and cognitive interventions; physical activity that features aerobic exercise, resistance training, or flexibility training or activities that combine all three; modification of the home environment; and family caregiver skills training programs. Approaches that provide education for caregivers and equip them with strategies for managing behavioral challenges, offer physical activity, and modify the home environment show promise (Gaugler et al., 2020).

There is also some evidence that technological assists can be beneficial. Remaining in their homes through the course of their illness is important to many persons with dementia. Such emerging tools as assessment and monitoring technologies, assistive devices, therapeutic devices, and caregiver supportive technologies show promise for supporting these individuals (Moyle, 2019) (see also the discussion of the use of technology to support caregiving in Chapter 5). Currently, many of these technologies (e.g., smart home technologies; artificial intelligence, including the Internet of Things; wearable devices that monitor activities; robotics; medication reminders) are most appropriate for those in the early stages of disease, but some facilitate physical functions, such as feeding and transferring from bed to chair, and may be helpful for those who are in more advanced stages. Some of these technologies are currently available, while others (e.g., self-driving cars) are in development or being tested.

Addressing behavioral and psychological symptoms Behavioral and psychological symptoms can be very distressing for people living with dementia and their families, and often drive the decision to seek residential care (Gaugler et al., 2009). Interventions to alleviate these symptoms include tailoring activities to the interests of the individual and providing education, skill building, and support to family caregivers (Gaugler et al., 2020) (see also the discussion of approaches for addressing these symptoms in Chapter 4). Emerging evidence points to possible benefits of multidisciplinary care and to the possible reduction of aggressive and agitated behaviors through massage, music therapy, and touch therapy. Cognitive and sensory stimulation, music therapy, animal therapy, and psychotherapeutic approaches (e.g., cognitive-behavioral therapy) show potential for reducing depressive symptoms and anxiety, as well as enhancing overall quality of life and mood (e.g., Kishita et al., 2020; Hu et al., 2018; Liang et al., 2018; Lorusso and Bosch, 2018; Peluso et al., 2018; Tay et al., 2019; van der Steen et al., 2018; Wood et al., 2017; Yen and Lin, 2018; Zhang et al., 2017; Aguirre et al., 2013; Fukushima et al., 2016; Garcia-Casal et al., 2017). In general, these approaches appear to be more beneficial than pharmacologic treatment in managing behavioral and psychological symptoms and to have fewer negative consequences (Watt et al., 2019).

RESEARCH DIRECTIONS

The committee's exploration of research intended to improve the experiences of individuals living with dementia points to key gaps in knowledge across the areas discussed in this chapter. Looking first at screening and diagnosis, we identified needs related to disclosure of diagnostic information and predictive measures, as well as the use of biomarkers and their value in clinical practice, including the ramifications, both positive and negative, for asymptomatic persons who could be notified that they have these specific markers of disease. There is a need for psychometric research on the accuracy of screening and diagnostic tools and approaches (e.g., what combinations of historical information about the person's symptoms, cognitive testing, laboratory tests, and neuroimaging are most accurate), as well as qualitative research on the impact on persons receiving a dementia diagnosis.

We also reviewed research needs related to the support and dignity of people living with dementia. We examined decision making from varied perspectives and identified needs for both qualitative and quantitative research related to the needs of persons at all stages of dementia. Research on how to strengthen protections while respecting autonomy will need to be interdisciplinary, including both ethicists and legal experts along with clinicians and researchers. Research to examine the impact of dementia on decision-making capacity can support the development and testing of interventions with the potential to mitigate such adverse consequences as stigma and improve protection from abuse.

Gaps in the development of nonpharmacologic interventions to slow or prevent cognitive decline, decrease behavioral and psychological symptoms, and increase comfort and well-being for those living with dementia were also evident from our review. Although several interventions (e.g., exercise and cognitive stimulation therapy) have shown promise, few have been studied in adequately powered or pragmatic trials and with diverse groups. Such research is needed to justify broad dissemination.

Finally, we reflected on the nature of the research available in these domains. Much of the research on interventions for people living with dementia is primarily observational or conducted using conventional rather than pragmatic trials. As discussed in Chapter 2 (see the section on "Interpreting the Evidence"), observational studies provide insight but are not conclusive in determining the effectiveness of interventions. Interpreting observational data is challenging because it can be difficult to disentangle factors that may confound evidence about the factor under study or to identify causation. For example, the effect of physical activity on cognitive decline may depend on when in the life course exercise is initiated, when it is assessed, and the type and amount of exercise involved. Clinical trials are needed to provide more valid answers to such questions. However, conventional clinical trials aimed at demonstrating efficacy may not provide sufficient insight into what is achievable in real-world settings, such as health care systems.

Related is the need for improved measures that can be used in assessing outcomes relevant to persons living with dementia and their family caregivers throughout the course of the disease. Consistent, shared definitions of outcomes of interest and ways to measure them can support efforts to synthesize research from varied domains in this complex area. For example, the goal of supporting people living with dementia in remaining at home through as much of their illness as possible is valued by clinicians, social workers, and families, and a wide array of interventions may contribute to meeting that goal. Use of consistent measures, such as number of days spent at home, across studies would be a valuable aid to harmonizing research, thereby increasing the ability to compare the effectiveness of interventions implemented in different studies. Psychometric research, including qualitative studies to identify meaningful goals for measurement, as well as validation studies, are needed to create instruments that are patient-centered and capture what matters most to those living with dementia and their caregivers over the course of disease. These issues are discussed further in Chapter 8.

The committee identified priority areas for research related to the experiences of individuals living with dementia in two domains: diagnosis and decision-making support, and support for well-being and quality of life. The priority areas for research in each of these domains are summarized in Conclusions 3-1 and 3-2; Tables 3-3 and 3-4, respectively, provide detailed directions for research in each area of these domains.

> CONCLUSION 3-1: Research in the following areas related to diagnosis and decision-making support has the potential to substantively improve the experience of individuals living with dementia by supporting their dignity and well-being:
> - Improved screening and diagnosis to identify persons living with dementia, including guidance for clinicians that also addresses issues related to disclosure.
> - Development of guidance to support ethical and responsible decision making by and for people living with dementia.

TABLE 3-3 Detailed Research Needs: Diagnosis and Decision-Making Support

1: Improved Screening and Diagnosis	• Social science research addressing the use of biomarkers, including accuracy in unselected populations, clinical utility, and the positive and negative implications of disclosure to patients and families. • Studies of screening, including the comparative effectiveness of different approaches; evidence-based guidance on whom and when to screen; and improved accuracy of screening approaches, particularly for minority and less-educated populations. • Improved coordination of resources for patients once diagnosed, including medical care, information, social supports, and community resources. • Public education strategies to heighten awareness of impaired cognition and the need for diagnostic evaluation. • Evaluation of dementia education programs for health care providers.
2: Support for Ethical and Responsible Decision Making	• Development and evaluation of approaches to including persons with dementia in conversations about their preferences and care, and guidance for adapting communication as the severity of disease increases. • Improved guidance on balancing the goals of autonomy and safety for the person living with dementia and others who could be harmed, as well as training for clinicians and others in applying this guidance. • Improved education for families about the types of decisions affected by dementia. • Improved methods (e.g., shorter, less expensive, more accurate) for assessing capacity for various types of decision making. • Improved guidance for advance care planning for health care, financial management, housing, and other nonmedical choices. • Improved methods for predicting disease progression and survival, including digital markers.

CONCLUSION 3-2: Research in the following areas has the potential to advance the development of interventions to support the well-being and quality of life of people living with dementia.
- Development and validation of outcome measures that reflect the perspectives of people living with dementia, their family caregivers, and communities.
- Improved design and evaluation of nonpharmacologic interventions to slow or prevent cognitive and functional decline, reduce or ameliorate behavioral and psychological symptoms, improve comfort and well-being, and adequately and equitably serve diverse populations.

TABLE 3-4 Detailed Research Needs: Support for Well-Being and Quality of Life

1: Development and Validation of Outcome Measures	• Identification of outcomes of interest that apply across contexts (e.g., health care system, community, residential care) to support alignment of research. • Development and validation of person-centered and caregiver-centered outcome measures and outcomes that reflect positive aspects of dementia and dementia care. • Leveraging of existing data sources, such as claims data. • Identification and development of outcomes that effectively capture well-being and health-related quality of life across all stages of disease and symptomatology. • Development of outcome measures that can be communicated by persons living with dementia when they have capacity and by family caregivers or other proxies when they no longer have capacity.
2: Improved Design and Evaluation of Nonpharmacologic Interventions	• Clinical and pragmatic trials to test the efficacy and effectiveness of promising but unproven nonpharmacologic interventions. • Research on methods of dissemination and adaptation of interventions to varied contexts and populations.

Research focused on the priorities identified above has the potential to substantially improve the comfort and dignity of the experience of living with dementia. However, we close this chapter with the observation that the need is great and that it was not possible to explore adequately every possible opportunity for meaningful improvement. Among the important areas for which we were unable to establish the basis for explicit conclusions within the time allotted for this study are the impact of implicit and explicit bias and stigma against people living with dementia and their family caregivers on their well-being; the needs of people living with dementia who do not have family caregivers; and the needs of specific subpopulations of people living with dementia, including LGBTQ, African American, Latinx, and America Indian/Alaska Native populations. We emphasize that we in no way wish to discourage research in these areas.

REFERENCES

Aguirre, E., Woods, R., Spector, A., and Orrell, M. (2013). Cognitive stimulation for dementia: A systematic review of the evidence of effectiveness from randomised controlled trials. *Ageing Research Reviews*, 12(1), 253–262. https://doi.org/10.1016/j.arr.2012.07.001

Albert, M.S., DeKosky, S.T., Dickson, D., Dubois, B., Feldman, H.H., Fox, N.C., Gamst, A., Holtzman, D.M., Jagust, W.J., Petersen, R.C., Snyder, P.J., Carrillo, M.C., Thies, B., and Phelps, C.H. (2011). The diagnosis of mild cognitive impairment due to Alzheimer's disease: Recommendations from the National Institute on Aging-Alzheimer's Association workgroups on diagnostic guidelines for Alzheimer's disease. *Alzheimer's & Dementia*, 7(3), 270–279. https://doi.org/10.1016/j.jalz.2011.03.008

Alzheimer's Association. (n.d.). *10 Early Signs and Symptoms of Alzheimer's*. https://www.alz.org/alzheimers-dementia/10_signs

———. (2019). *2019 Alzheimer's Disease Facts and Figures*. https://www.alz.org/media/documents/alzheimers-facts-and-figures-2019-r.pdf

American Geriatrics Society. (2020). *Geriatrics at Your Fingertips*. https://geriatricscareonline.org/ProductAbstract/geriatrics-at-your-fingertips-2020/B052

American Psychiatric Association. (2013). *Diagnostic and Statistical Manual of Mental Disorders* (5th ed.). https://doi.org/10.1176/appi.books.9780890425596

Arevalo-Rodriguez, I., Smailagic, N., Roqué i Figuls, M., Ciapponi, A., Sanchez-Perez, E., Giannakou, A., Pedraza, O.L., Bonfill Cosp, X., and Cullum, S. (2015). Mini-Mental State Examination (MMSE) for the detection of Alzheimer's disease and other dementias in people with mild cognitive impairment (MCI). *Cochrane Database of Systematic Reviews*, *2015*(3), CD010783. https://doi.org/10.1002/14651858.CD010783.pub2

Arias, J. (2013). A time to step in: Legal mechanisms for protecting those with declining capacity. *American Journal of Law and Medicine*, *39*, 134–159.

Bahar-Fuchs, A., Clare, L., and Woods, B. (2013). Cognitive training and cognitive rehabilitation for mild to moderate Alzheimer's disease and vascular dementia. *Cochrane Database of Systematic Reviews*, *2013*(6), CD003260. https://doi.org/10.1002/14651858.CD003260.pub2

Beishon, L.C., Batterham, A.P., Quinn, T.J., Nelson, C.P., Panerai, R.B., Robinson, T., and Haunton, V.J. (2019). Addenbrooke's Cognitive Examination III (ACE-III) and mini-ACE for the detection of dementia and mild cognitive impairment. *Cochrane Database of Systematic Reviews*, *12*(12):CD013282. https://doi.org/10.1002/14651858.CD013282.pub2

Bennett, D.A. (2020). *Defining Different Types of Dementia*. Paper prepared for the National Academies of Sciences, Engineering, and Medicine's Committee on Decadal Survey of Behavioral and Social Science Research on Alzheimer's Disease and Alzheimer's Disease-Related Dementias. https://www.nationalacademies.org/event/10-17-2019/meeting-2-decadal-survey-of-behavioral-and-social-science-research-on-alzheimers-disease-and-alzheimers-disease-related-dementias#sectionEventMaterials

Chan, Q.L., Xu, X., Shaik, M.A., Chong, S.S., Hui, R.J., Chen, C.L., and Dong, Y. (2016). Clinical utility of the informant AD8 as a dementia case finding instrument in primary healthcare. *Journal of Alzheimer's Disease*, *49*(1), 121–127. https://doi.org/10.3233/jad-150390

Chiu, H.Y., Chen, P.Y., Chen, Y.T., and Huang, H.C. (2018). Reality orientation therapy benefits cognition in older people with dementia: A meta-analysis. *International Journal of Nursing Studies*, *86*, 20–28. https://doi.org/10.1016/j.ijnurstu.2018.06.008

Consumer Financial Protection Bureau. (2016). *Recommendations and Report for Financial Institutions on Preventing and Responding to Elder Financial Exploitation*. https://201603_cfpb_recommendations-and-report-for-financial-institutions-on-preventing-and-responding-to-elder-financial-exploitation.pdf

Davis, D.H., Creavin, S.T., Yip, J.L., Noel-Storr, A.H., Brayne, C., and Cullum, S. (2015). Montreal Cognitive Assessment for the diagnosis of Alzheimer's disease and other dementias. *Cochrane Database of Systematic Reviews*, *2015*(10), CD010775. https://doi.org/10.1002/14651858.CD010775.pub2

Droogsma, E., van Asselt, D., and De Deyn, P.P. (2015). Weight loss and undernutrition in community-dwelling patients with Alzheimer's dementia. From population based studies to clinical management. *Zeitschrift fur Gerontologie und Geriatrie,* *48*(4), 318–324. https://doi.org/10.1007/s00391-015-0891-2

Duan, Y., Lu, L., Chen, J., Wu, C., Liang, J., Zheng, Y., Wu, J., Rong, P., and Tang, C. (2018). Psychosocial interventions for Alzheimer's disease cognitive symptoms: A Bayesian network meta-analysis. *BMC Geriatrics*, *18*(1), 175. https://doi.org/10.1186/s12877-018-0864-6

Farina, N., Rusted, J., and Tabet, N. (2014). The effect of exercise interventions on cognitive outcome in Alzheimer's disease: A systematic review. *International Psychogeriatrics*, 26(1), 9–18. https://doi.org/10.1017/S1041610213001385

Fink, H.A., Linskens, E.J., MacDonald, R., Silverman, P., McCarten, R., Talley, K., Forte, M., Desai, P., Nelson, V., Miller, M., Hemmy, L., Brasure, M., Taylor, B., Ng, W., Ouellette, J., Sheets, K., Wilt, T., and Butler, M. (2020). Benefits and harms of prescription drugs and supplements for treatment of clinical Alzheimer-type dementia. *Annals of Internal Medicine*, 172(10), 656–668. https://doi.org/10.7326/M19-3887

Fukushima, R.L.M., do Carmo, EG., Pedroso, R.D.V., Micali, P.N., Donadelli, P.S., Fuzaro Junior, G., Venancio, R.C.dP., Viola, J., and Costa, J.LR. (2016). Effects of cognitive stimulation on neuropsychiatric symptoms in elderly with Alzheimer's disease: A systematic review. *Dementia & Neuropsychologia*, 10(3), 178–184. https://doi.org/10.1590/S1980-5764-2016DN1003003

Garcia-Casal, J.A., Loizeau, A., Csipke, E., Franco-Martin, M., Perea-Bartolome, M.V., and Orrell, M. (2017). Computer-based cognitive interventions for people living with dementia: A systematic literature review and meta-analysis. *Aging & Mental Health*, 21(5), 454–467. https://doi.org/10.1080/13607863.2015.1132677

Gaugler, J.E., Fang, Y., Krichbaum, K., and Wyman, J. (2009). Predictors of nursing home admission or persons with dementia. *Medical Care*, 47(2), 191–198. https://doi.org/10.1097/MLR.0b013e31818457ce

Gaugler, J., Jutkowitz, E., and Gitlin, L.N. (2020). *Non-Pharmacological Interventions for Persons Living with Alzheimer's Disease: Decadal Review and Recommendations*. Paper prepared for the National Academies of Sciences, Engineering, and Medicine's Committee on Decadal Survey of Behavioral and Social Science Research on Alzheimer's Disease and Alzheimer's Disease-Related Dementias. https://www.nationalacademies.org/event/10-17-2019/meeting-2-decadal-survey-of-behavioral-and-social-science-research-on-alzheimers-disease-and-alzheimers-disease-related-dementias

Gitlin, L., Jutkowitz, E., and Gaugler, J.E. (2020). *Dementia Caregiver Intervention Research Now and into the Future: Review and Recommendations*. Paper prepared for the National Academies of Sciences, Engineering, and Medicine's Committee on Decadal Survey of Behavioral and Social Science Research on Alzheimer's Disease and Alzheimer's Disease-Related Dementias. https://www.nationalacademies.org/event/10-17-2019/meeting-2-decadal-survey-of-behavioral-and-social-science-research-on-alzheimers-disease-and-alzheimers-disease-related-dementias

Glymour, M.M., Brickman, A.M., Kivimaki, M., Mayeda, E.R., Chêne, G., Dufouil, C., and Manly, J.J. (2018). Will biomarker-based diagnosis of Alzheimer's disease maximize scientific progress? Evaluating proposed diagnostic criteria. *European Journal of Epidemiology*, 33(7), 607–612. https://doi.org/10.1007/s10654-018-0418-4

Government Accountability Office. (2020). *Elder Justice: HHS Could Do More to Encourage State Reporting on the Costs of Financial Exploitation*. https://www.gao.gov/assets/gao-21-90.pdf

Groot, C., Hooghiemstra, A.M., Raijmakers, P.G., van Berckel, B.N., Scheltens, P., Scherder, E.J., van der Flierad, R., and Ossenkoppele, R. (2016). The effect of physical activity on cognitive function in patients with dementia: A meta-analysis of randomized control trials. *Ageing Research Reviews*, 25, 13-23. https://doi.org/10.1016/j.arr.2015.11.005

Gurrera, R., Moye, J., Karel, M., Azar, A., and Armesto, J. (2006). Cognitive performance predicts treatment decisional abilities in mild to moderate dementia. *Neurology*, 66(9), 1367–1372. https://doi.org/10.1212/01.wnl.0000210527.13661.d1

Harrison, J.K., Stott, D.J., McShane, R., Noel-Storr, A.H., Swann-Price, R.S., and Quinn, T.J. (2016). Informant Questionnaire on Cognitive Decline in the Elderly (IQCODE) for the early diagnosis of dementia across a variety of healthcare settings. *Cochrane Database of Systematic Reviews*, 2016(11). https://doi.org/10.1002/14651858.CD011333.pub2

Hu, M., Zhang, P., Leng, M., Li, C., and Chen, L. (2018). Animal-assisted intervention for individuals with cognitive impairment: A meta-analysis of randomized controlled trials and quasi-randomized controlled trials. *Psychiatry Research*, 260, 418–427. https://doi.org/10.1016/j.psychres.2017.12.016

Huling Hummel, C., Pagan, J.R., Israelite, M., Patterson, E., Van Buren, B., and Woolfolk, G. (2020). *A Summary of Commentaries Submitted by Those Living with Dementia and Care Partners*. Paper prepared for the National Academies of Sciences, Engineering, and Medicine's Committee on Decadal Survey of Behavioral and Social Science Research on Alzheimer's Disease and Alzheimer's Disease-Related Dementias. https://www.nationalacademies.org/our-work/decadal-survey-of-behavioral-and-social-science-research-on-alzheimers-disease-and-alzheimers-disease-related-dementias#sl-three-columns-b93dcbe8-e082-4170-9bfc-a8cae8ef0445

Jacobson, M., and Zissimopoulos, J. (2020). *The Role of Medicare's Annual Wellness Visit in the Assessment of Cognitive Health*. Pilot project, Center for Aging and Health Research, National Bureau of Economic Research. https://www.nber.org/programs-projects/projects-and-centers/center-aging-and-health-research/7783-role-medicares-annual-wellness-visit-assessment-cognitive-ealth?page=1&perPage=50

Jennings, L.A., Palimaru, A., Corona, M., Cagigas, X., Ramirez, K., Zhao, T., Hays, R.D., Wenger, N.S., and Reuben, D.B. (2016). Patient and caregiver goals for dementia care. *Quality of Life Research*, 3, 685–693.

Jennings, L.A., Ramirez, K., Hays, R.D., Wenger, N.S., and Reuben, D.B. (2018). Personalized goal attainment in dementia care: Measuring what persons with dementia and their caregivers want. *Journal of the American Geriatrics Society*, 66(11), 2120–2127. https://doi.org/10.1111/jgs.15541. PMID:30298901

Jervis, L.L., Fickenscher, A., Beals, J., Manson, S.M., and Arciniegas, D. (2010). Predictors of performance on the MMSE and the DRS-2 among American Indian elders. *Journal of Neuropsychiatry and Clinical Neurosciences*, 22(4), 417–425. https://doi.org/10.1176/jnp.2010.22.4.417

Jervis, L.L., Cullum, C.M., Cox, D., and Manson, S.M. (2018). Dementia assessment in American Indians. In G. Yeo, L.A. Gerdner, and D. Gallagher-Thompson (Eds.), *Ethnicity and the Dementias* (3rd ed., pp. 108–123). New York: Routledge.

Karssemeijer, E.G.A., Aaronson, J.A., Bossers, W.J., Smits, T., Olde Rikkert, M.G.M., and Kessels, R.P.C. (2017). Positive effects of combined cognitive and physical exercise training on cognitive function in older adults with mild cognitive impairment or dementia: A meta-analysis. *Ageing Research and Reviews*, 40, 75–83. https://doi.org/10.1016/j.arr.2017.09.003

Kishita, N., Backhouse, T., and Mioshi, E. (2020). Nonpharmacological interventions to improve depression, anxiety, and quality of life (QoL) in people with dementia: An overview of systematic reviews. *Journal of Geriatrics Psychiatry and Neurolology*, 33, 28–41. https://doi.org/10.1177/0891988719856690

Kivipelto, M., Mangialasche, F., and Ngandu, T. (2018). Lifestyle interventions to prevent cognitive impairment, dementia and Alzheimer disease. *National Review of Neurology*, 14(11), 653–666. https://doi.org/10.1038/s41582-018-0070-3. PMID: 30291317

Larner, A.J., and Mitchell, A.J. (2014). A meta-analysis of the accuracy of the Addenbrooke's Cognitive Examination (ACE) and the Addenbrooke's Cognitive Examination-Revised (ACE-R) in the detection of dementia. *International Psychogeriatrics/IPA, 26*(4), 555–563.

Lewis, J.P., Manson, S.M., Jernigan, V., and Noonan, C. (2021). Making sense of a disease that makes no sense: Understanding Alzheimer's disease and related disorders among caregivers and providers in Alaska. *Gerontologist, 61*(3), 363–373. https://doi.org/10.1093/geront/gnaa102

Liang, J.H., Xu, Y., Lin, L., Jia, R.X., Zhang, H.B., and Hang, L. (2018). Comparison of multiple interventions for older adults with Alzheimer disease or mild cognitive impairment: A PRISMA-compliant network meta-analysis. *Medicine, 97*(20), e10744. https://doi.org/10.1097/md.0000000000010744

Lichtenberg, P., Stoltman, J., and Flicker, L. (2015). A person-centered approach to financial capacity assessment: Preliminary development of a new rating scale. *Clinical Gerontologist, 38*, 49–67. http://doi.org/10.1080/07317115.2014.970318

Lim, K.H., Pysklywec, A., Plante, M., and Demers, L. (2019). The effectiveness of Tai Chi for short-term cognitive function improvement in the early stages of dementia in the elderly: A systematic literature review. *Clinical Interventions in Aging, 14*, 827–839. https://doi.org/10.2147/cia.s202055

Lorusso, L.N., and Bosch, S.J. (2018). Impact of multisensory environments on behavior for people with dementia: A systematic literature review. *Gerontologist, 58*(3), e168–e179. https://doi.org/10.1093/geront/gnw168

Mangialasche, F., Solomon, A., Winblad, B., Mecocci, P., and Kivipelto, M. (2010). Alzheimer's disease: Clinical trials and drug development. *Lancet Neurology, 9*(7), 702–716. https://doi.org/10.1016/S1474-4422(10)70119-8

Marson, D. (2013). Clinical and ethical aspects of financial capacity in dementia: A commentary. *American Journal of Geriatric Psychiatry, 21*(4), 382–390. https://doi.org/10.1097/JGP.0b013e31826682f4

McKhann, G.M., Knopman, D.S., Chertkow, H., Hyman, B.T., Jack, Jr., C.R., Kawas, C.H., Klunk, W.E., Koroshetz, W.J., Manly, J.J., Mayeux, R., Mohs, R.C., Morris, J.C., Rossor, M.N., Scheltens, P., Carrillo, M.C., Thies, B., Weintraub, S., and Phelps, C.H. (2011). The diagnosis of dementia due to Alzheimer's disease: Recommendations from the National Institute on Aging-Alzheimer's Association workgroups on diagnostic guidelines for Alzheimer's disease. *Alzheimer's & Dementia, 7*(3), 263–269. https://doi.org/10.1016/j.jalz.2011.03.005

Montgomery, A., Slocum, S., and Stanik, C. (2020). *Experiences of Nursing Home Residents during the COVID-19 Pandemic.* Altarum. https://altarum.org/sites/default/files/uploaded-publication-files/Nursing-Home-Resident-Survey_Altarum-Special-Report_FINAL.pdf

Moyle, W. (2019). The promise of technology in the future of dementia care. *Nature Reviews Neurology, 15*, 353–359. https://doi.org/10.1038/s41582-019-0188-y

National Academies of Sciences, Engineering, and Medicine. (2021). *Meeting the Challenge of Caring for Persons Living with Dementia and Their Care Partners and Caregivers: A Way Forward.* Washington, DC: The National Academies Press. https://doi.org/10.17226/26026

Palmqvist, S., Janelidze, S., Quiroz, Y.T., Zetterberg, H., Lopera, F., Stomrud, E., Su, Y., Chen, Y., Serrano, G.E., Leuzy, A., Mattsson-Carlgren, N., Strandberg, O., Smith, R., Villegas, A., Sepulveda-Falla, D., Chai, X., Proctor, N.K., Beach, T.G., Blennow, K., Dage, J.L., Reiman, E.M., and Hansson, O. (2020). Discriminative accuracy of plasma phospho-tau217 for Alzheimer disease vs other neurodegenerative disorders. *Journal of the American Medical Association, 324*(8), 772–781. https://doi.org/10.1001/jama.2020.12134

Peluso, S., De Rosa, A., De Lucia, N., Antenora, A., Illario, M., Esposito, M., and De Michele, G. (2018). Animal-assisted therapy in elderly patients: Evidence and controversies in dementia and psychiatric disorders and future perspectives in other neurological diseases. *Journal of Geriatric Psychiatry and Neurology*, 31(3), 149–157. https://doi.org/10.1177/0891988718774634

Pennington, C., Davey, K., Meulen, R., Coulthard, E., and Kehoe, P. (2018). Tools for testing decision-making capacity in dementia. *Age and Ageing*, 47(6), 778–784. https://doi.org/10.1093/ageing/afy096

Persons Living with Dementia Stakeholder Group. (2020). *National Research Summit on Care, Services and Support for Persons Living with Dementia*. https://aspe.hhs.gov/system/files/pdf/263846/PLwDRecom20.pdf

Rajan, K., Barnes, L., Wilson, R., Weuve, J., McAninch, E., and Evans, D. (2019). Apolipoprotein E genotypes, age, race, and cognitive decline in a population sample. *Journal of the American Geriatric Society*, 67(4), 734–740. https://doi.org/10.1111/jgs.15727

Reuben, D.B. (2019). The voices of persons living with dementia. *American Journal of Geriatric Psychology*, 28(4), 443–444. https://doi.org/10.1016/j.jagp.2019.11.005

Reuben, D.B., and Jennings, L.A. (2019). Putting goal-oriented patient care into practice. *Journal of the American Geriatrics Society*, 67(7), 1342–1344. https://doi.org/10.1111/jgs.15885

Salthouse, T.A. (2019). Trajectories of normal cognitive aging. *Psychology and Aging*, 34(1), 17–24. https://doi.org/10.1037/pag0000288

Sawhill, I., and Pulliam, C. (2019). Six facts about wealth in the United States. *Middle Class Memos*. Brookings Institution. https://www.brookings.edu/blog/up-front/2019/06/25/six-facts-about-wealth-in-the-united-states

Schultheis, M., DeLuca, J., and Chute, D., Eds. (2008). *Handbook for the Assessment of Driving Capacity*. Elsevier Academic Press. https://doi.org/10.1016/B978-0-12-631255-3.X0001-X

Spreng, R.N., Karlawish, J., and Marson, D.C. (2016). Cognitive, social and neural determinants of diminished decision-making and financial exploitation risk in aging and dementia: A review and new model. *Journal of Elder Abuse and Neglect*, 28(45), 320–344.

Stanger, T. (2015, September 29). Financial elder abuse costs $3 billion a year. Or is it $36 billion? *Consumer Reports*. https://www.consumerreports.org/cro/consumer-protection/financial-elder-abuse-costs--3-billion-----or-is-it--30-billion-

Stocking, C., Hougham, G., Danner, D., Patterson, P., Whitehouse, P., and Sachs, G. (2008). Variable judgments of decisional capacity in cognitively impaired research subjects. *Journal of the American Geriatrics Society*, 56(10), 1893–1897. https://doi.org/10.1111/j.1532-5415.2008.01922.x

Tan, C.C., Yu, J.T., and Tan L. (2014). Biomarkers for preclinical Alzheimer's disease. *Journal of Alzheimer's Disease*, 42(4), 1051–1069. https://doi.org/10.3233/JAD-140843

Tay, K.W., Subramaniam, P., and Oei, T.P. (2019). Cognitive behavioural therapy can be effective in treating anxiety and depression in persons with dementia: A systematic review. *Psychogeriatrics*, 19(3), 264–275. https://doi.org/10.1111/psyg.12391

U.S. Preventive Services Task Force. (2020, February 25). *Cognitive Impairment in Older Adults: Screening*. Final Recommendation Statement. https://www.uspreventiveservicestaskforce.org/uspstf/recommendation/cognitive-impairment-in-older-adults-screening

van der Steen, J.T., Smaling, H.J., van der Wouden, J.C., Bruinsma, M.S., Scholten, R.J., and Vink, A.C. (2018). Music-based therapeutic interventions for people with dementia. *Cochrane Database of Systematic Reviews*, 7, Cd003477. https://doi.org/10.1002/14651858.CD003477.pub4

Ward, R, Vass, A., Aggarwal, N., Garfield, C., and Cybyk, B. (2005). A kiss is still a kiss? The construction of sexuality in dementia care. *Dementia*, 4(1), 49–72.

Watson, A.C., Corrigan, P., Larson, J.E., and Sells, M. (2007). Self-stigma in people with mental illness. *Schizophrenia Bulletin*, *33*(6), 1312–1318. https://doi.org/10.1093/schbul/sbl076

Watt, J.A., Goodarzi, Z., Veroniki, A.A., Nincic, V., Khan, P.A., Ghassemi, M., Thompson, Y., Tricco, A.C., and Straus, S.E. (2019). Comparative efficacy of interventions for aggressive and agitated behaviors in dementia: A systematic review and network meta-analysis. *Annals of Internal Medicine*. https://doi.org/10.7326/M19-0993

Widera, E., Steenpass, V., Marson, D., and Sudore, R. (2011). Finances in the older patient with cognitive impairment. *Journal of the American Medical Association*, *305*(7), 698–706. https://doi.org/10.1001/jama.2011.164

Wolfe, P.L., and Lehockey, K.A. (2016). Neuropsychological assessment of driving capacity. *Archives of Clinical Neuropsychology*, *31*(6), 517–529. https://doi.org/10.1093/arclin/acw050

Wood, W., Fields, B., Rose, M., and McLure, M. (2017). Animal-assisted therapies and dementia: A systematic mapping review using the Lived Environment Life Quality (LELQ) Model. *American Journal of Occupational Therapy*, *71*(5), 7105190030. https://doi.org/10.5014/ajot.2017.027219

Woods, B., Aguirre, E., Spector, A.E., and Orrell, M. (2012). Cognitive stimulation to improve cognitive functioning in people with dementia. *Cochrane Database of Systematic Reviews*, *2*, CD005562. https://doi.org/10.1002/14651858.CD005562.pub2

Yen, H.Y., and Lin, L.J. (2018). A systematic review of reminiscence therapy for older adults in Taiwan. *Journal of Nursing Research*, *26*(2), 138–150. https://doi.org/10.1097/jnr.0000000000000233

Zaleta, A.K., and Carpenter, B.D. (2010). Patient-centered communication during the disclosure of a dementia diagnosis. *American Journal of Alzheimer's Disease & Other Dementias*, *25*(6), 513–520. https://doi.org/10.1177/1533317510372924

Zhang, Y., Cai, J., An, L., Hui, F., Ren, T., Ma, H., and Zhao, Q. (2017). Does music therapy enhance behavioral and cognitive function in elderly dementia patients? A systematic review and meta-analysis. *Ageing Research Reviews*, *35*, 1–11. https://doi.org/10.1016/j.arr.2016.12.003

4

Caregivers: Diversity in Demographics, Capacities, and Needs

The first person to recognize subtle or significant changes in a person's understanding and experience of the world is generally not a health care professional but a family member, coworker, or friend. Common early changes associated with dementia include trouble managing finances and/or medications, difficulty driving and/or way finding, mood changes, memory lapses, and repetitious speech, all of which are more likely to be apparent outside of the medical setting. While some may recognize their loved one's difficulties as possible signs of early-stage dementia, others may perceive these changes as ordinary aspects of aging. For those many persons who are developing cognitive impairment while living alone and who have limited contact with family, such changes may go undetected for longer.

This chapter discusses the work of the family members and others who support people living with dementia. These caregivers, who are generally unpaid, may be family members, friends, neighbors, or coworkers. The term "family caregivers" is used here to include the potentially large network of those who provide support and to distinguish them from those who are connected to the person with dementia through the formal health and direct care systems. The chapter provides an overview of the crucial work that family caregivers provide and their diverse demographics, experiences, and needs for support and training. It summarizes the current state of research on interventions to support caregivers, focusing on care transitions, the potential and actual use of technology, and symptom control.

Many people with dementia never receive a diagnosis, but family members and others provide support and care regardless. Even for those whose dementia has been identified, family caregivers are often uncertain how they should help. It may be difficult for them to find resources and educate themselves about the disease. Family members must navigate complex health systems and put care plans in place. They search the Internet and/or call friends who have provided care for a loved one with dementia, hoping to learn how to support their own loved one and themselves. Cultural norms, access to resources, education, and an understanding of dementia can influence the family caregiver's perception of the challenges of dealing with dementia, but there is no doubt the challenges are considerable.

To better understand the challenges facing family caregivers, the committee explored what is known about the care they and others provide. We also sought insight into caregivers' perspectives on their experiences and the supports that would benefit them most. We are indebted to the advisory panel that supported this study (see Chapter 1) for their contributions to our understanding. In addition, we examined the available research on and reviews of interventions and programs to support family caregivers and existing policies that can bolster such supports. Finally, we relied on a paper by Gitlin and colleagues (2020) commissioned for this study.

RELIANCE ON FAMILY CAREGIVERS

The early and middle phases of dementia typically last much longer than the final stage (see Chapter 3); most family caregiving occurs during those earlier phases, but caregiving can become more intense as the dementia progresses. During the earlier phases, people living with dementia typically remain in their homes, and if they receive care, it is in the home or in other community settings. All people turning 65—not just those with dementia—have a 70 percent chance of needing long-term care for some period of time, and half of this care is unpaid (Johnson, 2019). For those with dementia, 85 percent of care in the United States is provided by unpaid family members (O'Shaughnessy, 2014). Many family members embrace caregiving and view it as part of their identity, as well as a source of satisfaction, but because the United States lacks an adequate and dependable system for identifying and financing long-term services and supports, some family members find that they have no real choice.

In the United States, and indeed globally, there is a societal expectation that family members will provide care to their loved ones with dementia if they can, although cultural expectations and resources affect these decisions. In short, family caregivers fill a very substantial gap in care. This has been true historically, is the case currently, and will be the case into the future (Gitlin et al., 2020; Gitlin and Wolff, 2012). It is also true around the world—in low-, middle-, and high-income countries; in families of all socioeconomic levels; and among all racial/ethnic groups (World Health Organization, 2017).

The need for family caregivers is increasing as the population ages, and even as the pool of those who could provide such care is shrinking (NASEM, 2016). People over 80 make up one of the fastest-growing segments of the population (Ortman et al., 2014) and the group most likely to require help (Ortman et al., 2014). At the same time, the population of those who can provide care will shrink as a result of changes in family structure and social norms, including lower fertility rates and smaller families, as well as higher rates of childlessness, never-married status, female participation in the formal workforce, and divorce (Redfoot et al., 2013). These overlapping shifts affect women in particular, who make up two-thirds of family caregivers (Kasper et al., 2014), creating a perfect storm in which more people will live longer with dementia and need support while fewer family members will be there to help. Indeed, many of those living with dementia will be living alone.

In 2011, 92 percent of people over 65 in the United Sates were living in the community, not in a facility, according to the National Health and Aging Trends Study (Toth et al., 2020). Of those receiving assistance with basic and instrumental activities of daily living,[1] nearly all relied on some help from family or friends, and almost two-thirds relied exclusively on these unpaid caregivers (Friedman et al., 2015). Results of the companion National Study on Caregiving indicate that in 2011, an estimated 17.7 million individuals were caregivers for an older adult who resided at home, in the community, or in a residential care setting (other than a nursing home) (Freedman and Spillman, 2014). Nearly one-half of these caregivers (8.6 million) provided care to a high-need older adult, defined as an older adult who had dementia and/or who needed assistance with three or more activities of daily living (e.g., bathing, eating, getting in and out of bed) (NASEM, 2016; Spillman et al., 2014).

The economic value of this caregiving is extraordinary. In 2018, caregivers of people living with dementia provided an estimated 18.5 billion hours of unpaid assistance, valued at $290 billion (Alzheimer's Association, 2019). It has been estimated that families cover (through a combination of unpaid care and spending on care) 70 percent of the average cost ($225,140) incurred in the course of an individual's illness (Jutkowitz et al., 2017); the remainder is paid for by Medicare and Medicaid. (See Chapters 6 and 7 for more on these issues.)

---

[1] Clinicians use the terms "activities of daily living" (such basic tasks as personal hygiene, dressing, feeding, and moving independently) and "instrumental activities of daily living" (activities that support independent living, such as cooking, cleaning, transportation, and managing finances) to characterize the functioning of people living with dementia.

Family caregivers may provide care for relatively short periods or for many years. They may devote a few or many hours each day or week to providing care. According to 2011 data from the National Study of Caregiving, the median number of years a family caregiver provided care was 5 years, and nearly 70 percent provided care for 2 to 10 years (NASEM, 2016). "Caregiving trajectories" is a term researchers use to characterize the way the caring role evolves over time, depending on the care needed and the setting in which it occurs (Gitlin and Wolff, 2012; Peacock et al., 2014; Penrod et al., 2011). One important role for caregivers is coordinating transitions across all settings, providing communication that links different providers, as their family members may move back and forth from home to hospital to rehabilitation or skilled nursing facilities.

Family caregivers are most often spouses, adult children, or siblings, although other relatives, neighbors, friends, members of a shared faith community, and others also provide care without pay. As noted above, even though many fewer families now include women who are not employed outside the home than in the past, females remain the main source of caregiving (Sharma et al., 2017):

- One-third of family caregivers are 65 or older.
- Two-thirds are women, and two-thirds live with the person who has dementia.
- One-fourth provide care both to an aging relative with dementia and to children under the age of 18.

Most caregivers still need income and must juggle their caregiving with work schedules and other responsibilities, including child care (NASEM, 2016; DePasquale et al., 2016).

Family caregivers reflect the country's diversity. As the U.S. population becomes both more diverse and older, the percentages and numbers of older people and people with dementia in minority communities are increasing. As discussed in Chapter 1, available data show that members of minority populations are more likely to develop dementia relative to their non-Hispanic White counterparts. Rates of family caregiving vary modestly across racial/ethnic groups, according to survey data, with caregiving being most common among Hispanic populations (Family Caregiver Alliance, 2019). Gender and family roles, cultural expectations, and proximity are among the factors that lead to one family member rather than another taking on the caregiver role (Cavaye, 2008). For instance, caregivers in African American families are less likely to be a spouse than are those in non-Hispanic White families (National Alliance for Caregiving and AARP, 2020; Pinquart and Sörensen, 2005). Caregivers for LGBTQ people living with dementia are less likely to be formal family members (Frederiksen-Goldsen and Hooyman, 2008).

The specific help provided by family caregivers varies significantly, depending on the age of both caregiver and care receiver, the nature of their relationship, the stage of dementia, other comorbidities, and cultural context. Table 4-1 lists the range of supports caregivers provide for older adults (not just those living with dementia). For a person living with early-stage dementia, assistance may include organizing medical referrals to clarify diagnosis and prognosis, financial planning, help in identifying work and disability options for those still working, and emotional support with such challenges as declines in function or the stigma of dementia. For those living with midphase dementia, care may include all of the above plus more assistance handling bills and finances; transportation and advocacy for medical appointments; assistance with groceries, food preparation, and medications; and housing upkeep, modification, and repairs. As dementia progresses, a person will also require care that is more intimate and physical, including toileting, bathing, dressing, and feeding. Caregiving at this later stage requires longer hours and engagement with more difficult tasks.

TABLE 4-1 What Family Caregivers Do for Older Adults

Domain	Caregiver's Activities and Tasks
Household Tasks	• Help with bills, deal with insurance claims, and manage money • Home maintenance (e.g., install grab bars, ramps, and other safety modifications; repairs, yardwork) • Laundry and other housework • Prepare meals • Shopping • Transportation
Self-care, Supervision, and Mobility	• Bathing and grooming • Dressing • Feeding • Supervision • Management of behavioral symptoms • Toileting (e.g., getting to and from the toilet, maintaining continence, dealing with incontinence) • Transferring (e.g., getting in and out of bed and chairs, moving from bed to wheelchair) • Help getting around inside or outside
Emotional and Social Support	• Provide companionship • Discuss ongoing life challenges with care recipient • Facilitate and participate in leisure activities • Help care recipient manage emotional responses • Manage family conflict • Troubleshoot problems

Continued

TABLE 4-1 Continued

Domain	Caregiver's Activities and Tasks
Health and Medical Care	• Encourage healthy lifestyle • Encourage self-care • Encourage treatment adherence • Manage and give medications, pills, or injections • Operate medical equipment • Prepare food for special diets • Respond to acute needs and emergencies • Provide wound care
Advocacy and Care Coordination	• Seek information • Facilitate person and family understanding • Communicate with doctors, nurses, social workers, pharmacists, and other health care and long-term services and supports (LTSS) providers • Facilitate provider understanding • Locate, arrange, and supervise nurses, social workers, home care aides, home-delivered meals, and other LTSS (e.g., adult day services) • Make appointments • Negotiate with other family member(s) regarding respective roles • Order prescription medicines • Deal with insurance issues
Surrogacy	• Handle financial and legal matters • Manage personal property • Participate in advanced planning • Participate in treatment decisions

SOURCE: Excerpted from NASEM (2016, p. 81). Copyright 2016 by the National Academy of Sciences. All rights reserved.

Spouses, daughters, and those residing with the person living with dementia are more likely to provide this level of care (Kasper et al., 2015).

FAMILY CAREGIVERS' PERSPECTIVES

The advisory panel appointed to support the committee provided valuable insights from family caregivers about the challenges they face (Huling Hummel et al., 2020; see Chapter 3 for discussion of the advisory panel's insights about the experiences of people living with dementia). The paper prepared by the panel summarizes the members' own perspectives and those of others who participated in a call for commentaries that yielded further insights into the challenges caregivers face (see Chapters 1 and 3). Like the people living with dementia who responded to this call, caregivers reported frustration with delays in obtaining a diagnosis for their loved ones, and many observed a lack of competence and empathy in the health care professionals involved throughout the diagnostic process. One contributor commented, "No doctor would take the time to explain what is possibly expected and how the disease works."

Caregivers reported considerable difficulties in identifying and obtaining services. Many reported frustration with government offices on aging (see Chapter 5), such as when the local office was unable to link families with paid providers. The challenge of finding paid care providers in rural areas was noted in particular. One respondent stated that the community in which she had lived for 44 years "does little" to support her husband or her. Other respondents reported their own successful efforts to create needed resources previously unavailable in their community, such as helping a local adult day service incorporate materials and programming in different languages. Some caregivers had words of praise for compassionate employers, who offered flexibility to take time off for caregiving. Nonetheless, many reported experiencing stress related to managing conflicts with their work schedules and demands.

Like persons with dementia (see Chapter 3), many caregivers faulted clinicians for the poor quality of communication about what to expect as dementia progressed and limited efforts to connect those with dementia to services and resources. Caregivers observed that many clinicians even lacked basic education about dementia. Another said, in reference to communication with doctors, "non-existent—they are not helpful or frankly knowledgeable." One caregiver's father had dementia without memory loss, which delayed diagnosis. During a frustrating period of going from clinician to clinician, they went to a neurologist, who "did all kinds of tests that showed there was nothing wrong with his brain. She basically shrugged and sent us on our way."

Caregiver respondents to the call for commentaries noted multiple significant stressors associated with their role. Isolation, lack of relief, economic concerns, and sorrow were common themes. Comments included, "I seem to always be on call 24/7," and "I don't socialize anymore. I don't take vacation without her." One respondent wrote, "I had to essentially give up any interests and hobbies and focus on working and just getting through each day. I've lost weight, am now anxious, don't sleep well, and am fearful about our financial situation." Other respondents also voiced concern about finances, including the high risk of scams aimed at those with cognitive impairment, the high cost of care, and the lack of useful insurance for dementia care.

Caregivers who contributed their perspectives to the advisory panel's work also reported positive experiences. Examples included finding a sense of meaning and importance in their caregiving work, as well as happy experiences shared with their loved ones, including working on puzzles and games; playing with a grand- or great-grandchild; and happily sharing birthday cake, whether or not the person living with dementia recognized the birthday.

RESEARCH ON FAMILY CAREGIVING

The perspectives reported above provided a valuable backdrop for the committee's exploration of the available research on the caregiving experience, the positive and negative effects on caregivers themselves, and the interventions that might support caregivers. There is an extensive literature on how the physical and mental status of caregivers is affected by caregiving, and how the nature of these effects varies according to the functional status of the care recipient, the hours worked, and the intensity of the work (Carpentier et al., 2010; Peacock et al., 2014; Penrod et al., 2011). Most recently, the National Academies of Sciences, Engineering, and Medicine released the report *Meeting the Challenge of Caring for Persons Living with Dementia and Their Care Partners: A Way Forward*, which, as discussed later in this chapter, identifies two categories of interventions for which there is evidence of benefit (NASEM, 2021). A number of prior National Academies reports—including *Families Caring for an Aging America* (NASEM, 2016) and *Care Interventions for Individuals with Dementia and Their Caregivers* (National Academies of Sciences, Engineering, and Medicine [NASEM], 2018)—provide relevant information. The focus here is on evidence about the caregiving experience and support and interventions for caregivers.

The Caregiving Experience

A substantial body of evidence documents both positive and detrimental effects of providing care for a person living with dementia (Gitlin et al., 2020; NASEM, 2016).[2] This section briefly examines the caregiving experience and how it varies across groups and activities, and how the COVID-19 pandemic has brought new challenges for caregivers.

The caregiving experience is highly varied, as would be expected given the broad range of people, activities, and hours involved. The experience also evolves along with the stage of dementia, creating a trajectory of needs and impacts. Researchers have shown that family caregivers may experience significant stress that is apparent throughout the course of the disease: worry and anxiety that begin in the earlier stages, depression and distress

---

[2]The discussion here relies on a paper commissioned for this study (Gitlin et al., 2020) and an in-depth study of caregiving in the United States, referenced above, carried out by an earlier National Academies committee (NASEM, 2016).

in later stages, and complicated grief when their loved one dies (NASEM, 2016; Ornstein et al., 2019). Physical strain associated with caregiving, sleep disturbance, financial hardship, and the challenge of caring for an individual who requires near-constant supervision are particularly associated with caregiver stress (Gitlin et al., 2020).

Caregivers also experience higher rates of physical illness and hospitalization, as well as reduced attention to their own health, compared with their noncaregiving counterparts. They experience financial losses from missing work, cutting back work hours, or leaving their employment, losses that affect their earnings, social security payments, benefits, and future work opportunities (NASEM, 2016). Social isolation and cognitive decline have also been reported among caregivers (Jutkowitz et al., 2017; Pinquart and Sörensen, 2003; Sörensen et al., 2006).

On the other hand, positive outcomes of family caregiving may include increased self-confidence, lessons in dealing with difficult situations, strengthened bonds with the family member receiving care, and confidence that that person is receiving good care (NASEM, 2016).

Focused research on caregiver stress offers insights into how the caregiving experience is different for different groups. For instance, spouses providing care report greater stress levels relative to adult child caregivers (Gaugler et al., 2015), while caregivers who believe the care recipient is suffering physically or psychologically are more likely to experience depression (Schulz et al., 2008). A study of African American caregivers found that, compared with other caregivers, they devoted more of their hours of care to relatives with high degrees of disability. African American caregivers also faced greater financial strain, yet they reported experiencing more gains from caregiving and were less likely to report emotional difficulties (Fabius et al., 2020). African American caregivers in this study received more help from others and from government and community resources. They also reported significantly smaller decreases in desired activities, such as visiting with family and friends.

Recent work among older American Indians echoes these findings and draws attention to the importance of accounting for race in addressing caregiver needs and proposed supports (Schure et al., 2015; Conte et al., 2015; Spencer et al., 2013; Goins et al., 2011). The research regarding American Indian and African American communities offers important insight, yet studies of the experience of minority caregivers are unacceptably few in number, a gap noted at the Dementia Summit and in a range of other reviews (National Institute on Aging, 2020; NASEM, 2021).

Caregiver stress affects the recipient of care as well. For example, one study showed that an individual cared for by a highly stressed caregiver is 12 percent more likely than a counterpart to enter a nursing home within a year, and 17 percent more likely to do so in 2 years

(Spillman and Long, 2007). There is also evidence that individuals being cared for by caregivers who are experiencing stress related to their own unmet needs are in turn more likely to have unmet care needs (Beach and Schulz, 2017), with high levels of caregiver stress having been linked to substandard care and the risk of neglect (Beach and Schulz, 2017). Another study found that such factors as anxiety, stress, and unmet care needs were associated with earlier mortality in care recipients, although the authors note that more fine-grained studies of this issue are needed (Schulz et al., 2021).

COVID-19 has brought new challenges. It will take time to adequately assess the full impact of the pandemic on those living with dementia and their caregivers. However, accounts from the United States and other nations indicate that the experience of being a family caregiver became significantly more challenging as a result of the pandemic (see, e.g., D'Cruz and Banerjee, 2020; Greenberg et al., 2020; Alzheimer's Association, 2020). Chapter 1 notes the devastating impact of the pandemic on the elderly and on residents of nursing homes and other care facilities. Caregivers have been called upon to devise new ways of acquiring food and medicine and monitoring the health of family members with dementia without putting them at risk through normal human contact. Crucial services caregivers have provided for nursing home residents, including advocating for services, helping with feeding, organizing medical care, monitoring quality of care, and providing crucial human contact and affection, have all been compromised by COVID-based restrictions on visitation that have radically increased the isolation of people living in nursing homes (see Chapter 6).

At the same time, anecdotal evidence indicates that both formal and informal sources of support and respite (e.g., other family members, paid caregivers, day care programs) have become less accessible to caregivers during the pandemic. Data collection and research to document and analyze this evolving situation will be critical for protecting vulnerable populations and identifying lessons that can be useful in future public health emergencies. COVID has highlighted the terrible impact of health inequities on American communities in several ways. Those who were least likely to be able to work from home and maintain social distancing either at work or at home were more likely to contract COVID and were also disproportionately members of minority groups. COVID hit communities with large non-White populations brutally, with significantly higher rates of infection, hospitalization, and mortality that also hit the family caregivers in those communities especially hard (see Chapters 2 and 5 for more discussion of systemic factors and social determinants of health).

Researchers who study family caregivers often rely on qualitative studies using surveys and similar tools (NASEM, 2016; Whitlatch and Orsulic-Jeras, 2018). However, researchers find the study of family caregivers challenging for reasons that include limitations of the available data, wide variation in the nature of family caregiving and the kinds of supports needed, and the multiple ways of defining people who provide care outside of institutional settings. There are as yet no firmly established assumptions and methods to guide researchers so their results can be easily synthesized, as discussed further in Chapter 8 (NASEM, 2016).

Caregiver Capacity and Screening

The care provided by family members is so vital that it is difficult to raise the issue of assessing its quality. Nevertheless, the challenges of caregiving can be enormous, and most family caregivers likely take on this role gradually, with limited opportunities to understand in advance the full scope of what it may entail. Providing care for a person with dementia draws on a wide range of skills and competencies, including patience, empathy, and communication skills. Also required is the capacity to provide support for complex emotional and behavioral issues and to carry out nursing and related medical tasks. Furthermore, caregivers may be called upon to understand and navigate complex health care and long-term care options and to take on legal responsibilities.

Unfortunately, the limited available evidence suggests that few caregivers receive formal preparation for this role, and more than half report carrying out medical or nursing tasks without preparation, although many express a desire to receive training (NASEM, 2016; Burgdorf et al., 2020). One survey showed that family caregivers—often without training—carried out the functions of geriatric case managers, medical record keepers, paramedics, and patient advocates, filling gaps in a system that does not systematically meet those needs (Bookman and Harrington, 2006).

At present, few tools are available for assessing the nature and quality of care provided by family caregivers. Quality measures used in health care are intended to evaluate paid workers and institutions and hold them accountable. Institutions must report data related to quality measures, accept inspection, and provide remedies for any problems identified, and they face such negative consequences as reduced payments or loss of licensure. This model is inappropriate for family caregivers, who are neither paid nor licensed, and no entity has responsibility for inspecting private homes where care is provided unless abuse has been reported.

Not all family caregivers have had the opportunity to acquire the skills, tools, and education that might enhance the care they provide. Caregivers who lack understanding of the symptoms and trajectory of the disease their loved one is experiencing or strategies for addressing common problems may both experience and cause unnecessary stress, or even put their loved one at risk. For instance, a 2019 study found that family caregivers' well-intentioned efforts may complicate interactions with health care professionals, such as when symptoms or care needs are less evident to a provider because of a caregiver's efforts to mitigate them (Häikiö et al., 2019). More disturbing, an Internet search for "dementia restraints" provides an anecdotal indication of potential problems. Although it has been well established that the use of physical restraints for dementia patients is harmful—both dangerous and degrading—many such products are sold, and advertisements encourage their use by stressed caregivers.

While educational resources are available for family caregivers, there is limited systematic information about access to or use of these resources across groups and geographic regions. A few studies have examined available training and resources, focusing primarily on outcomes for caregivers rather than care recipients (e.g., Sousa et al., 2016; Parker et al., 2008; Hepburn et al., 2001). Because dementia symptoms may emerge gradually over a period of years, it is likely to take time for the disease to be recognized and for a family member to identify as a caregiver and begin to seek support (Peterson et al., 2016). While caregivers may be open to new

---

BOX 4-1
Examples of Resources for Family Caregivers

Resources available to family caregivers include websites that offer collections of instructional videos; research summaries; and other information, including information about advocacy organizations and community supports, such as day or respite care (see Chapter 5).

Independent associations and advocacy groups. These groups offer online educational resources on such topics as the warning signs of dementia, stages of dementia, legal and financial planning, and when and how to intervene in response to dementia-related behavior. One example is the Family Caregiver Alliance, a national nonprofit network that offers guidance on physical care (e.g., bathing, dental care, dressing and grooming), as well as strategies for communicating with individuals with brain impairment and strategies caregivers can use to control frustration.[a] Other organizations that offer resources for family caregivers include the Alzheimer's Association, the BrightFocus Foundation, and Help for

information, they may not know that such information is available at all, or where and how to seek it. Those with limited Internet access and expertise cannot easily take advantage of the abundance of web-based information. Box 4-1 provides examples of the sorts of resources that are publicly available to caregivers of individuals living with dementia.

SUPPORTS FOR FAMILY CAREGIVERS

Comprehensive approaches to dementia care (discussed in Chapter 6) have focused on the key role of family caregivers and the need to provide support for them explicitly (Gitlin et al., 2020). As suggested above, caregivers need many different kinds of support, and their needs vary with the stage of the care recipient's disease, as shown in Figure 4-1. It is also important to note that most supports for caregivers are available only once their loved one has received a diagnosis of dementia. As discussed in Chapters 2 and 3, there are significant barriers to obtaining a timely and accurate diagnosis, a problem that significantly affects the ability of caregivers to access even those supports that are available. Nevertheless, various types of supports have been developed. This section reviews the status of research on interventions to support caregivers and considers promising directions for future development addressing three key issues: care transitions, the use of technology to support caregiving, and approaches for addressing behavioral and psychological symptoms of dementia.

Alzheimer's Families.[b] Some universities offer free online training resources; an example is the University of California, Los Angeles (UCLA) Caregiver Training Video series, which includes guidance on how caregivers should respond to such dementia-related behaviors as aggression, agitation and anxiety, and resistance to taking medications.[c]

State and local resources. Offered by departments of health and other relevant agencies and entities, resources include informational and instructional programs on providing care for individuals with dementia, strategies for self-care, and referrals to other resources. Wisconsin's website for caregivers is one example.[d]

---

[a]https://www.caregiver.org/about-family-caregiver-alliance-fca
[b]https://www.alz.org/help-support/resources/care-training-resources; https://www.brightfocus.org/alzheimers/article/caregiver-training-what-you-need-know; https:// www.helpforalzheimersfamilies.com/learn/alzheimers-education
[c]https://www.uclahealth.org/dementia/caregiver-education-videos
[d]https://www.dhs.wisconsin.gov/dementia/families.htm; https://aging.lacity.org/caregiver-resources

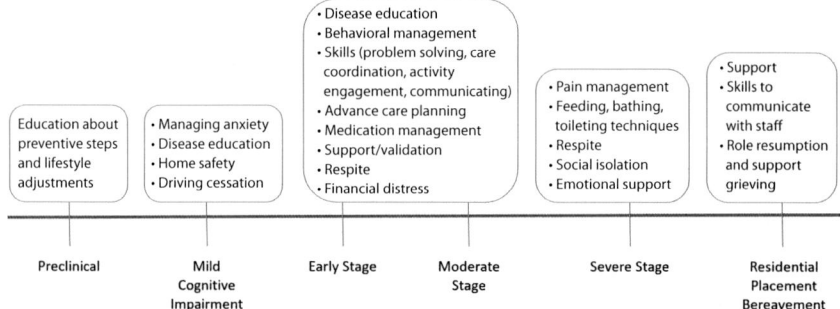

FIGURE 4-1 Caregiver needs by stage of disease.
SOURCE: Gitlin et al. (2020), adapted from Gitlin and Hodgson (2018).

Intervention Research

Interventions to support caregivers have been studied for decades, and work conducted in the past decade or so has included robust and methodologically sound trials. Examples include the National Institute on Aging / National Institute of Nursing Research REACH (Resources for Enhancing Alzheimer's Caregiver Health) initiatives (Phases I and II), which examined six caregiver interventions: psychoeducational group counseling, individual counseling, skills training, problem solving, technology-based education, and supportive programs (Gitlin et al., 2020).

The authors of the review of intervention research commissioned for this study (Gitlin et al., 2020) assessed research reviews published between 2000 and 2019 and identified 4,112 articles that met their inclusion criteria.[3] The authors found that there is evidence for the efficacy of many different types of interventions designed to support family caregivers, including psychoeducation, counseling, problem solving, skill building, social support, and respite. These interventions demonstrate benefits for caregivers' own health behaviors, depressive symptoms, self-confidence, well-being, and perception of burden.

Gitlin and colleagues found that the programs for which there is evidence of effectiveness share several characteristics: they are based on needs assessments and are tailored to meet specific unmet needs; and they include multiple components, such as counseling, education, stress, mood management, and skill building. The studies reviewed also reveal that caregivers have preferences about how they wish to receive support.

However, Gitlin and colleagues identify important limitations of this

---

[3] See Gitlin et al. (2020) for detailed discussion of the literature review.

body of work. In general, effect sizes in the studies are small, so further research is needed to confirm and expand on the findings. Few of the studies shed light on the mechanisms by which the interventions may yield benefits or on factors that may moderate their results, particularly how effects may vary across groups and circumstances. Gitlin and colleagues also found a paucity of caregiver intervention studies assessing caregivers' experiences with dementia stages other than the moderate, middle stage of clinical dementia symptoms or addressing longer-term effects on caregivers' health or well-being. They note a lack of diversity among study participants, which further limits the applicability of the findings. Moreover, none of the studies address financial distress, physical burden, or social isolation—three key documented sources of stress for family caregivers.

Gitlin and colleagues also looked at studies examining the implementation and scaling of interventions in order to assess their effectiveness when delivered in a community or health care system. Such implementation studies are crucial to determine which interventions will actually show benefit once moved from research settings to real-world environments. Of 1,130 implementation studies the authors located, only 28 met their inclusion criteria.

From their review of the available literature, Gitlin and colleagues conclude that evidence points to "an impressive array of interventions" (p. 33) that may improve family caregivers' psychosocial well-being. Most promising are strategies targeting caregivers of persons in the moderate stages of disease that offer education; strategies for coping, managing behavioral symptoms, and problem solving; and counseling. Benefits to caregivers are most pronounced with respect to health and health care behaviors. A number of the translational studies also show that implementation can be effective. Strategies that appear to contribute to effectiveness include engaging stakeholders, providing staff coaching, adapting a program to fit local circumstances, and integrating the intervention into daily workflows.

Overall, however, Gitlin and colleagues present a somber view of the existing research on caregiver interventions and call for significant changes to improve the quality and scale of this work. Their conclusions are similar to those presented in the paper on interventions for individuals living with dementia commissioned by the committee (Gaugler et al., 2020; discussed in Chapter 3). The existing research related to caregivers, Gitlin and colleagues found, has "many methodological (but fixable) flaws, small effect sizes, a failure to address unmet needs of families across the disease trajectory, and a failure to examine outcomes of importance to different stakeholders" (p. 3). They note a lack of attention to fidelity—the extent to which the delivered intervention matches the original protocol or model—in the studies they examined, as well as inadequate characterization of samples and inconsistent labeling of the interventions. These flaws limit researchers' ability to make useful comparisons across studies.

As the committee was completing its work, the National Academies released the above-referenced report assessing evidence on care-related interventions for people with dementia and their caregivers, which provides additional insights (NASEM, 2021). The authoring committee for that report relied on an Agency for Healthcare Research and Quality (AHRQ) systematic review of randomized controlled trial evidence on care interventions for persons living with dementia and their caregivers, as well as other evidence. The report notes positive developments in intervention research for dementia caregivers, and specifically the start of a crucial shift from focusing on the mere prevention of harm to the promotion of well-being and inclusion. However, the report's authors express "disappointment that the AHRQ systematic review did not uncover a stronger, more convincing evidence base" (NASEM, 2021). The AHRQ review identified two categories of interventions for which there is low-strength evidence of benefit: (1) collaborative care models, and (2) the REACH II multicomponent intervention and associated adaptations. The committee that produced that report concluded that the evidence is sufficient to justify implementation of these two types of interventions in community settings.

Focus on Three Key Issues: Care Transitions, Use of Assistive Technology, and Approaches for Addressing Behavioral and Psychological Symptoms

To illustrate the complexity of the issues faced by family caregivers and the potential for progress, this section focuses on the three issues of care transitions, the use of technology to support caregiving, and approaches for addressing behavioral and psychological symptoms of dementia.

Care Transitions

Transitioning an individual with dementia from one care setting to another—for instance, from home to hospital, nursing home, or emergency room—is often stressful for the person living with dementia and the family (Boltz et al., 2015; Shankar et al., 2014). Care transitions are associated with increased risk for significant adverse events, such as falls, delirium, treatment errors, and mortality (Callahan et al., 2012). Moreover, such

> **BOX 4-2**
> **Perspective: Challenges in Managing Transitions**
>
> At age 82, my father, who had been diagnosed with Alzheimer's 6 years earlier, had recently transitioned from assisted living to the memory care floor of the facility in which he had lived for most of a year. He developed a kidney stone, which was not immediately diagnosed because he had difficulty describing his discomfort, and was hospitalized. He needed to use a urinary catheter while in the hospital, and to remain in bed or in the lounge chair next to the bed. The catheter was uncomfortable, and he tried repeatedly to remove it, so the hospital staff placed large, padded mittens on his hands. Finding those both frustrating and humiliating, and also feeling physically well and eager to move, he was not willing to stay seated. The staff placed restraints on him, which he found maddening, and tried moving his lounge chair to the nursing station so that he could be under observation and have company. They also used sedatives to keep him calm. While expressing sympathy at our concern, the busy staff had neither time nor inclination to discuss alternatives.
>
> Once he was returned to the memory care floor of his assisted living facility, he needed individual oversight because he was disoriented by the hospitalization—possibly experiencing delirium—and was at high risk of falling. We learned that the facility did not have sufficient staff to provide that additional care. The two options were hiring supplementary care or moving him to a nursing home. Needing immediate coverage while we arranged ongoing 24-hour care (a substantial cost beyond the monthly charges for the memory care floor), we asked a professional driver who had worked with Dad for several years—taking him on regular outings—to remain with him during the first day. Dad was very fond of this man, who had experience working with elderly clients but no training as a caregiver. Concerned that Dad would fall while using the toilet, this man engaged with Dad physically, but he lacked training to do this safely. Dad fell against the bathroom sink, cracking two ribs. The driver did not immediately report the incident, perhaps not recognizing that Dad was injured. Dad was not able to describe his pain and again he was not diagnosed right away, but ultimately returned to the hospital, where he experienced delirium and received antipsychotic medication. His decline after the second hospitalization was precipitous, and he moved home to receive hospice care within the month.
>
> SOURCE: National Academies' staff member.

transitions often reflect poor communication and may be unnecessary (see Box 4-2).

A systematic review examined interventions to help caregivers delay transitions in care, finding that despite the importance of the issue, it has not been well studied. These researchers identified only seven papers that met their inclusion criteria. The available studies that did meet those criteria pointed to possible ways of delaying or avoiding transitions, such as a program involving a combination of individual and family counseling and telephone assistance in problem solving that was able to delay nursing home placement among participants by more than 1.5 years (Mittelman et al., 2006). However, very little evidence has been accumulated to answer questions about when transition is appropriate, how caregivers and family members can determine what setting is best based on the individual's and family's preferences and needs, or what support and education caregivers need. There is virtually no research on how well the options available in communities align with the values, needs, and wishes of people with dementia and their caregivers.

Use of Technology to Support Caregiving

Technological assistance in a wide variety of forms is increasingly available to support caregiving. These include multiple smartphone apps, including those designed to provide assistance in tracking medications, appointments, and documents, as well as supports for community building and encouragement for stressed individuals (American Seniors Housing Association, 2021). Yet while such technology offers intriguing options for improving care, it also may exacerbate the digital divide given the severely limited access to online technology in many communities, including sparsely populated rural and low-income urban areas. Until it is available to all, then, technology based on Internet access will increase options for those with better resources and leave those without such resources further behind. Moreover, some of these apps cost money, while others are free to use yet may sell the user's data to support targeted advertising. Accordingly, AARP has produced a review article assessing several apps that offer users an array of choices (Saltzman, 2019).

A related issue is the widespread use of electronic medical records, which in the past decade has changed virtually every aspect of health care, including caregiving. Caregivers may now access the health information of persons living with dementia as their surrogate decision makers, but the ease and degree of this access vary by institution and system (Wolff et al., 2018), and appropriate protections for access to and use of this information may remain unclear to both providers and families, so this is an area that merits further study.

Technology may offer other valuable ways to ease the family caregiver's stress. For example, a caregiver whose loved one does not require constant supervision can use cameras to monitor for falls, departure from home at unsafe hours, difficulty preparing or consuming food, or other risks. Nonetheless, these devices must be placed strategically to gather appropriate information while minimizing unwarranted intrusions on privacy. For instance, bathroom falls are extremely common among people living with

> **BOX 4-3**
> **Perspective: One Family's Caregiving Dilemma**
>
> Mr. M is a 97-year-old man with dementia and few comorbidities. He walks slowly and carefully, feeds himself, and lives alone in his own home. He is widowed and has several adult children who live in different cities. Mr. M has always been independent and not especially social; he repeatedly expresses contentment with living in his own home. He receives in-home services, including meals, a few hours weekly of housekeeping, and a person who comes to walk with him most days. The family has installed a video camera in the home that documented difficulties using appliances, failure of helpers to arrive, and other challenges. Recently, a neighbor alerted the family that their father was leaning against the neighbor's garage at 7 AM. A review of camera footage aimed at the front door revealed that he had left the home at 11 PM, and his activities in the ensuing 8 hours are unknown. His vision is poor, and it would have been difficult for him to walk safely in the neighborhood at night.
>
> Mr. M returned home unharmed, but the family caregivers now wonder whether he should move to a skilled nursing facility. The siblings disagree about how to weigh their father's safety against his liberty. Mr. M has no memory of this nighttime excursion and continues to express contentment at home. What are the options for this family, facing a common, serious caregiving dilemma? The family is tech-savvy and is installing more cameras to help protect their father. They are now exploring additional technology to send alerts to caregivers when the door opens outside of specified hours. What they would do should that alert be received remains a matter of debate.
>
> SOURCE: Committee member.

dementia, but monitoring safety in this context without unduly intruding on privacy is challenging. Accordingly, many prefer to place a bathroom camera so that it monitors only the floor, thus balancing privacy and safety concerns. More research also is needed on such new technologies as voice-activated devices (e.g., Amazon Echo and its artificial intelligence program Alexa) to identify and validate how they can be used to support individuals with dementia and their caregivers. Box 4-3 describes one family's experience using technology to provide additional oversight of a family member at risk.

New technology is also being applied to old devices. Toileting is a significant challenge for family caregivers, in part because of taboos about this intimate physical activity, and in part because a smaller caregiver may be physically unable, even if willing, to safely help a larger person with such activities as toileting and bathing. Difficulties related to toileting increase the likelihood of a transition out of the home and into a skilled nursing facility. For these reasons, some now consider the use of bidets and toilet-bidets that can handle both elimination and hygiene. Although somewhat expensive, these devices, commonly used in Asia, can be cost-effective if they delay nursing home placement for a reasonable period. Research on their use for people with dementia has been quite limited, however (Cohen-Mansfield and Biddison, 2005).

Yet while some activities are more easily accomplished with such technological assistance, others remain better suited to a person-to-person approach. Even as the use of technology to support people living with dementia is increasing, some worry that its use may create other risks, such as by reducing human touch—an important component of providing care for which technology cannot substitute (Prescott and Robillard, 2020). Human connection is crucial for both the care recipient and the caregiver, uniquely eliciting emotion and connection between them (see, e.g., Vernon et al., 2019; Fauth et al., 2012). There is also concern that technology will replace family and professional care, perhaps eventually displacing those with the skills required to support people living with dementia. Given the anticipated decrease in the numbers of both family and paid caregivers, however, the loss of jobs is less likely than a shortage of those who can fill them.

Approaches for Addressing Behavioral and Psychological Symptoms of Dementia

Behavioral and psychological symptoms of dementia are common: 97 percent of people with dementia have at least one such symptom (Scales et al., 2018; see also Chapter 3). These symptoms are challenging for individuals living with dementia and their caregivers, and are a frequent reason for transferring a loved one with dementia from home to an institutional setting or from one institution to another. Individuals with persistent symptoms may experience multiple disruptive transitions because of the challenges they can present to caregivers and the limited availability of effective and safe treatments. Such symptoms are sometimes treated with antipsychotic medications that increase patients' risks of negative outcomes, including falls, cardiovascular events, and death (Kristensen et al., 2018). These and other pharmacological treatments are intended for use only after safer measures have failed, but are still used frequently. It is critical to train family caregivers in how to use safer measures, including gently redirecting their loved ones and limiting or delaying bathing and other stressful activities. Other nonpharmacologic approaches include changes to the environment; sensory treatments, such as massage and aromatherapy; psychosocial treatments, such as reminiscence and music therapy; and protocols for intimate care, such as bathing. However, the evidence base for such approaches is currently limited, ranging from modest (validation therapy) to moderate (music therapy, exercise) (Scales et al., 2018). (See also Chapter 3.)

RESEARCH DIRECTIONS

There is evidence that many interventions to support family caregivers can provide benefit, but there are also important gaps in the existing research. Overall, the consensus from recent scholarly reviews is that interventions to support caregivers show promise, but much work is needed to advance the necessary implementation science so that effective, large-scale interventions can be available more widely. A significant portion of the available studies lack the methodological rigor that would support wide dissemination. There are also important aspects of the caregiving experience and its effects on both caregivers and people living with dementia that have not yet been documented and studied. Caregivers are exceptionally diverse—by race and ethnicity, income, education, gender, sexual orientation, and geography—yet the current research does not reflect this diversity. There is growing recognition that, to know whether they are asking the right questions and developing the right interventions, researchers will need to intensify their efforts to recruit diverse study participants (Dilworth-Anderson et al., 2020). There is a need for improved ways of collecting data about family caregiving and for conducting well-designed research studies of high-priority questions. The committee identified high-priority research needs in four areas related to family caregiving, summarized in Conclusion 4-1; Table 4-2 lists detailed research needs in each of these areas.

CONCLUSION 4-1: Research in the following four areas has the potential to substantially improve the experience of family caregivers:
1. Identification of the highest-priority needs for resources and support for family caregivers, particularly assessment of how caregivers' needs vary across race and ethnicity, and community.
2. Means of identifying the assets that family caregivers bring to their work, as well as their needs for supplemental skills and training and other resources to enhance their capacity to provide care while maintaining the safety and well-being of both the recipients of their care and themselves.
3. Continued development and evaluation of innovations to support and enhance family caregiving and address the practical and logistical challenges involved.
4. Continued progress in data collection and research methods.

TABLE 4-2 Detailed Research Needs

1: Meeting Highest-Priority Needs	• Improved description of family caregivers, with attention to the heterogeneity and disparities within the group, including such caregiver characteristics as age, ethnicity, education, skills, wealth, social capital, and geographic location, with attention to future projections of available caregivers, long-distance caregivers, and culturally diverse caregivers. • Improved understanding of the number and distribution of people living with dementia who do not have family caregivers, and ways to identify their unmet needs and design appropriate interventions. • Improved understanding of the changing needs of caregivers throughout the stages of dementia and the life course of caregivers. • Assessment of caregivers who balance multiple caring roles and the effects of the stress they experience. • Ways to identify the caregivers in greatest need and provide them with adequate support. • Expansion of the concept and measurement of caregiver needs to incorporate stresses associated with medical and nursing tasks and navigation of a complex landscape of long-term care supports and services. • Training for physicians, nurses, direct care providers, and other team members in identifying caregiver stresses and providing information about relevant resources to assist them. • Examination of systemic barriers to communication between providers and caregivers and navigation of the health care system. • Assessment of practices and experiences related to dementia diagnosis and care, including questions about caregiver access to the electronic health record and provider responsibility for identifying needs and impairments.
2: Caregiver Screening and Assessment	• Identification of caregiver strengths and deficits across different populations and development of supports that are culturally relevant. • Examination of the connections between caregiver education and training and access to resources and outcomes for patients. • Design of an evaluation of effective, accessible educational materials for caregivers. • Research into technological approaches to assessment and training, including web-based education, use of smartphones, etc. Improved access to Internet-based resources is essential to address the "digital divide." • Improved understanding of family dynamics and networks, family functioning and well-being, division of labor, and role definitions and their links to better outcomes.

TABLE 4-2 Continued

3: Intervention Development and Evaluation	• Assessment of the efficacy of interventions for caregivers who vary by age, ethnicity, education, skills, wealth, social capital, and geography, as well as ways to integrate them routinely into care plans. • Study of the alignment of interventions with identified unmet needs of people living with dementia and caregivers, including housing options, transportation, social connection/isolation, money management, and protection from financial abuse. • Improved understanding of care coordination, reduction of poorly managed care transitions, and identification of appropriate placements. • Development and evaluation of strategies for fostering supportive contact between family caregivers and nursing home residents. • Development and improvement of technological interventions to support people living with dementia and their caregivers in ways that limit privacy intrusions while enhancing freedom and safety, including computer and smartphone applications, as well as physical devices that assist with such high-stress caring activities as toileting and bathing. • Development and evaluation of interventions for persons with dementia living alone and/or without family or friend caregivers.
4: Data Collection and Research Methods	• Development of methods for collecting actionable and relevant context- and setting-specific data on the challenges faced by caregivers and the related stresses. • Improved study designs to facilitate adaptation beyond the research setting. • Implementation studies for improved understanding of how to scale up effective interventions from research settings to the real world. • Improved measurement of objective (physiological) outcomes and their relationship to subjective measures.

REFERENCES

Alzheimer's Association. (2019). *2019 Alzheimer's Disease Facts and Figures*. https://www.alz.org/media/documents/alzheimers-facts-and-figures-2019-r.pdf

———. (2020). *Coronavirus (COVID-19) and Dementia: Tips for Public Health Community*. https://www.alz.org/professionals/public-health/coronavirus-(covid-19)-and-dementia-tips-for-publ

American Seniors Housing Association. (2021, February 9). *16 Caregiver Apps You Should Use in 2020*. https://www.whereyoulivematters.org/best-caregiver-apps

Beach, S.R., and Schulz, R. (2017). Family caregiver factors associated with unmet needs for care of older adults. *Journal of the American Geriatrics Society*, 65(3), 560–566. https://doi.org/10.1111/jgs.14547

Boltz, M., Chippendale, T., Resnick, B., and Galvin, J.E. (2015). Anxiety in family caregivers of hospitalized persons with dementia: Contributing factors and responses. *Alzheimer Disease and Associated Disorders*, 29, 236–241. https://doi.org/10.1097/WAD.0000000000000072

Bookman, A., and Harrington, M. (2006). Family caregivers: A shadow workforce in the geriatric health care system? *Journal of Health Politics, Policy and Law*, 32(6), 1005–1041.

Burgdorf, J.G., Arbaje, A.I., and Wolff, J.L. (2020). Training needs among family caregivers assisting during home health, as identified by home health clinicians. *Journal of the American Medical Directors Association*, 21(12), 1914–1919.

Callahan, C.M., Arling, G., Tu, W., Rosenman, M.B., Counsell, S.R., Stump, T.E., and Hendrie, H.C. (2012). Transitions in care for older adults with and without dementia. *Journal of the American Geriatrics Society*, 60(5), 813–820. https://doi.org/10.1111/j.1532-5415.2012.03905.x

Carpentier, N., Bernard, P., Gernier, A., and Guberman, N. (2010). Using the life course perspective to study the entry into the illness trajectory: The perspective of caregivers of people with Alzheimer's disease. *Social Science and Medicine*, 70(10), 1501–1508.

Cavaye, J.E. (2008). *From Dawn to Dusk: A Temporal Model of Caregiving: Adult Carers of Frail Parents*. Paper presented at CRFR Conference, Understanding Families and Relationships over Time, October 28, 2008, University of Edinburg. https://oro.open.ac.uk/27974/1/CRFR%20Conf%20Paper%20October%202008%20Final.pdf

Cohen-Mansfield, J., and Biddison, J. (2005). The potential of wash-and-dry toilets to improve the toileting experience of nursing home residents. *Gerontologist*, 45(5), 694–699.

Conte, K.P., Schure, M.B., and Goins, R.T. (2015). Correlates of social support in older American Indians: The Native Elder Care Study. *Aging & Mental Health*, 19(9), 835–843. https://doi.org10.1080/13607863.2014.967171

D'Cruz, M., and Banerjee, D. (2020). Caring for persons living with dementia during the COVID-19 pandemic: Advocacy perspectives from India. *Frontiers in Psychiatry*, 11, 603231. https://doi.org/10.3389/fpsyt.2020.603231

DePasquale, N., Davis, K.D., Zarit, S.H., Moen, P., Hammer, L.B., and Almeida, D.M. (2016). Combining formal and informal caregiving roles: The psychosocial implications of double- and triple-duty care. *Journals of Gerontology, Series B*, 71(2), 201–211. https://doi.org/10.1093/geronb/gbu139

Dilworth-Anderson, P., Moon, H., and Aranda, M.P. (2020). Dementia caregiving research: Expanding and reframing the lens of diversity, inclusivity, and intersectionality. *Gerontologist*, 60(5), 797–805. https://doi.org/10.1093/geront/gnaa050

Fabius, C., Wolff, J., and Kasper, J. (2020). Race differences in characteristics and experiences of black and white caregivers of older Americans. *Gerontologist*, 60(7), 1244–1253.

Family Caregiver Alliance. (2019). *Caregiver Statistics: Demographics*. https://www.caregiver.org/resource/caregiver-statistics-demographics

Fauth, E., Hess, K., Piercy, K., Norton, M., Corcoran, C., Rabins, P., Lyketsos, C., and Tschanz, J. (2012). Caregivers' relationship closeness with the person with dementia predicts both positive and negative outcomes for caregivers' physical health and psychological well-being. *Aging & Mental Health*, 16(6), 699–711. https://doi.org/10.1080/13607863.2012.678482

Frederiksen-Goldsen, K., and Hooyman, N.R. (2008). Caregiving research, services, and policies in historically marginalized communities: Where do we go from here? *Journal of Gay & Lesbian Social Services*, 18(3–4), 129–145.

Freedman, V.A., and Spillman, B.C. (2014). Disability and care needs among older Americans. *Milbank Quarterly*, 92(3), 509–541.

Friedman, E.M., Shih, R.A., Langa, K.M., and Hurd, M.D. (2015). U.S. prevalence and predictors of informal caregiving for dementia. *Health Affairs (Project Hope)*, 34(10), 1637–1641. https://doi.org/10.1377/hlthaff.2015.0510

Gaugler, J.E., Reese, M., and Mittelman, M. (2015). Effects of the Minnesota adaptation of the NYU Caregiver Intervention on depressive symptoms and quality of life for adult child caregivers of persons with dementia. *American Journal Geriatric Psychiatry*, 23, 1179–1192. https://doi.org/10.1016/j.jagp.2015.06.007

Gaugler, J., Jutkowitz, E., and Gitlin, L.N. (2020). *Non-Pharmacological Interventions for Persons Living with Alzheimer's Disease: Decadal Review and Recommendations*. Paper prepared for the National Academies of Sciences, Engineering, and Medicine, Decadal Survey of Behavioral and Social Science Research on Alzheimer's Disease and Alzheimer's Disease-Related Dementias. https://www.nationalacademies.org/event/07-08-2020/meeting-3-decadal-survey-of-behavioral-and-social-science-research-on-alzheimers-disease-and-alzheimers-disease-related-dementias-and-workshop-4

Gitlin, L., and Hodgson, N. (2018). *Better Living with Dementia* (1st Edition). Academic Press. https://doi.org/10.1016/C2016-0-01912-5

Gitlin, L., and Wolff, J. (2012). Family involvement in care transitions of older adults: What do we know and where do we go from here? *Annual Review of Gerontology and Geriatrics*, 31(1), 31–64.

Gitlin, L., Jutkowitz, E., and Gaugler, J.E. (2020). *Dementia Caregiver Intervention Research Now and into the Future: Review and Recommendations*. Paper prepared for the National Academies of Sciences, Engineering, and Medicine, Decadal Survey of Behavioral and Social Science Research on Alzheimer's Disease and Alzheimer's Disease-Related Dementias. https://www.nationalacademies.org/event/10-17-2019/meeting-2-decadal-survey-of-behavioral-and-social-science-research-on-alzheimers-disease-and-alzheimers-disease-related-dementias

Goins, R.T., Spencer, S.M., McGuire, L.C., Goldberg, J., Wen, Y., and Henderson, J.A. (2011). Adult caregiving among American Indians: The role of cultural factors. *Gerontologist*, 51(3), 310–320. https://doi.org/10.1093/geront/gnq101

Greenberg, N.E., Wallick, A., and Brown, L.M. (2020). Impact of COVID-19 pandemic restrictions on community-dwelling caregivers and persons with dementia. *Psychological Trauma*, 12(S1), S220–S221.

Häikiö, K., Sagbakken, M., and Rugkåsa, J. (2019). Dementia and patient safety in the community: A qualitative study of family carers' protective practices and implications for services. *BMC Health Services Research*, 19, 635. https://www.ncbi.nlm.nih.gov/pmc/articles/PMC6728989

Hepburn, K.W., Tornatore, J., Center, B., and Ostwald, S.W. (2001). Dementia family caregiver training: Affecting beliefs about caregiving and caregiver outcomes. *Journal of the American Geriatric Society*, 49(4), 450–457.

Huling Hummel, C., Pagan, J.R., Israelite, M., Patterson, E., Van Buren, B., and Woolfolk G. (2020). *A Summary of Commentaries Submitted by Those Living with Dementia and Care Partners*. Paper prepared for the National Academies of Sciences, Engineering, and Medicine's Committee on Decadal Survey of Behavioral and Social Science Research on Alzheimer's Disease and Alzheimer's Disease-Related Dementias. https://www.nationalacademies.org/our-work/decadal-survey-of-behavioral-and-socialscience-research-on-alzheimers-disease-and-alzheimers-disease-related-dementias#sl-threecolumns- b93dcbe8-e082-4170-9bfc-a8cae8ef0445

Johnson, R. (2019). *What is the Lifetime Risk of Needing and Receiving Long-Term Services and Supports?* Washington, DC: Urban Institute and Office of the Assistant Secretary for Planning and Evaluation. https://aspe.hhs.gov/basic-report/what-lifetime-risk-needing-and-receiving-long-term-services-and-supports

Jutkowitz, E., Kane, R.L., Gaugler, J.E., MacLehose, R.F., Dowd, B., and Kuntz, K.M. (2017). Societal and family lifetime cost of dementia: Implications for policy. *Journal of the American Geriatrics Society, 65*(10), 2169–2175. https://doi.org/10.1111/jgs.15043

Kasper, J., Freedman, V., and Spillman, B. (2014). *Disability and Care Needs of Older Americans by Dementia Status: An Analysis of the 2011 National Health and Aging Trends Study*. U.S. Department of Health and Human Services. http://aspe.hhs.gov/report/disability-and-care-needs-olderamericans-dementia-status-analysis-2011-national-healthand-aging-trends-study

Kasper, J., Freedman, V., Spillman, B., and Wolff, J. (2015). The disproportionate impact of dementia on family and unpaid caregiving to older adults. *Health Affairs, 34*(10), 1642–1649.

Kristensen, R., Norgaard, A., Jensen-Dahm, C., Gasse, C., Wimberley, T., and Waldemar, G. (2018). Polypharmacy and potentially inappropriate medication in people with dementia. *Journal of Alzheimer's Disease, 63*(1), 383–394.

Mittelman, M.S., Haley, W.E., Clay, O.J., and Roth, D.L. (2006). Improving caregiver well-being delays nursing home placement of patients with Alzheimer disease. *Neurology, 67*(9), 1592–1599. https://doi.org/10.1212/01.wnl.0000242727.81172.91

NASEM (National Academies of Sciences, Engineering, and Medicine). (2016). *Families Caring for an Aging America*. Washington, DC: The National Academies Press. https://doi.org/10.17226/23606

———. (2018). *Considerations for the Design of a Systematic Review of Care Interventions for Individuals with Dementia and Their Caregivers: Letter Report*. Washington, DC: The National Academies Press. https://doi.org/10.17226/25326

———. (2021). *Meeting the Challenge of Caring for Persons Living with Dementia and Their Care Partners and Caregivers: A Way Forward*. Washington, DC: The National Academies Press. https://doi.org/10.17226/26026

National Alliance for Caregiving and AARP. (2020). *Caregiving in the United States, 2020: The "Typical" African American Caregiver*. Washington, DC. https://www.caregiving.org/wp-content/uploads/2020/05/AARP1316_CGProfile_AfricanAmerican_May7v8.pdf

National Institute on Aging. (2020). *Dementia Care Summit Gaps and Opportunities*. https://www.nia.nih.gov/research/summit-gaps-opportunities

Ornstein, K., Wolff, J., Bollen-Lund, E., Rahman, O-K., and Kelley, A. (2019). Spousal caregivers are caregiving alone in the last years of life. *Health Affairs, 36*(6). https://doi.org/10.1377/hlthaff.2019.00087

Ortman, J.M., Velkoff, V.A., and Hogan, H. (2014). *An Aging Nation: The Older Population in the United States*. Washington, DC: U.S. Census Bureau. http://www.census.gov/prod/2014pubs/p25-1140.pdf

O'Shaughnessy, C. (2014). *National Spending for Long-Term Services and Supports (LTSS), 2012*. National Health Policy Forum, Paper 284. https://hsrc.himmelfarb.gwu.edu/sphhs_centers_nhpf/284

Parker, D., Mills, S., and Abbey, J. (2008). Effectiveness of interventions that assist caregivers to support people with dementia living in the community: A systematic review. *International Journal of Evidence-Based Healthcare*, 6(2), 137–172.

Peacock, S., Hammond-Collins, K., and Forbes, D.A. (2014). The journey with dementia from the perspective of bereaved caregivers: A qualitative descriptive study. *BMC Nursing*, 13(1), 42–52.

Penrod, J., Hupcey, J.E., Baney, B.L., and Loeb, S.J. (2011). End-of-life caregiving trajectories. *Clinical Nursing Research*, 20(1), 7–24.

Peterson, K., Hahn, H., Lee, A.J., Madison, C., and Atri, A. (2016). In the Information Age, do dementia caregivers get the information they need? Semi-structured interviews to determine informal caregivers' education needs, barriers, and preferences. *BMC Geriatrics*, 16, 164. https://doi.org/10.1186/s12877-016-0338-7

Pinquart, M., and Sörensen, S. (2003). Associations of stressors and uplifts of caregiving with caregiver burden and depressive mood: A meta-analysis. *Journals of Gerontology Series B*, 58(2), 112–128.

———. (2005). Ethnic differences in stressors, resources, and psychological outcomes of family caregiving: A meta-analysis. *Gerontologist*, 45(1), 90–106. https://doi.org/10.1093/geront/45.1.90

Prescott, T., and Robillard, J. (2020). Are friends electric? The benefits and risks of human-robot relationships. *iScience*, 24(1), 101993. https://doi.org/10.1016/j.isci.2020.101993

Redfoot, D., Feinberg, L., and Houser, A. (2013). The aging of the baby boom and the growing care gap: A look at future declines in the availability of family caregivers. http://www.aarp.org/content/dam/aarp/research/public_policy_institute/ltc/2013/baby-boom-and-the-growing-care-gap-insight-AARP-ppi-ltc.pdf

Saltzman, M. (2019). *These Apps for Caregivers Can Help You Get Organized, Find Support*. AARP. https://www.aarp.org/home-family/personal-technology/info-2019/top-caregiving-apps.html

Scales, K., Zimmerman, S., and Miller, S. (2018). Evidence-based nonpharmacological practices to address behavioral and psychological symptoms of dementia. *Gerontologist*, 58(S1), S88–S102.

Schulz, R., McGinnis, K., Zhang, S., Martire, L., Hebert, R., Beach, S., Zdaniuk, B., Czaja, S., and Belle, S. (2008). Dementia patient suffering and caregiver depression. *Alzheimer Disease and Associated Disorders*, 22(2), 170–176. https://doi.org/10.1097/WAD.0b013e31816653cc

Schulz, R., Beach, S.R., and Friedman, E.M. (2021). Caregiving factors as predictors of care recipient mortality. *American Journal of Geriatric Psychiatry*, 29(3), 295–303. https://doi.org/10.1016/j.jagp.2020.06.025

Schure, M.B., Conte, K.P., and Goins, R.T. (2015). Unmet assistance need among older American Indians: The Native Elder Care Study. *Gerontologist*, 55(6), 920–928. https://doi.org/10.1093/geront/gnt211

Shankar, K.N., Hirschman, K.B., Hanlon, A.L., and Naylor, M.D. (2014). Burden in caregivers of cognitively impaired elderly adults at time of hospitalization: A cross-sectional analysis. *Journal of the American Geriatrics Society*, 62, 276–284. https://doi.org/10.1111/jgs.12657

Sharma, N., Chakrabati, S., and Grover, S. (2017). Gender differences in caregiving among family-caregivers of people with mental illnesses. *World Journal of Psychiatry*, 6(1), 7–17. https://doi.org/10.5498/wjp.v6.i1.7

Sörensen, S., Duberstein, P., Gill, D., and Pinquart, M. (2006). Dementia care: Mental health effects, intervention strategies, and clinical implications. *Lancet Neurology, 5*(11), 961–973. https://doi.org/10.1016/S1474-4422(06)70599-3

Sousa, L., Sequeira, C., Ferré-Grau, C., Neves, P., and Lleixà-Fortuño, M. (2016). Training programmes for family caregivers of people with dementia living at home: Integrative review. *Journal of Clinical Nursing, 25*(19–20), 2757–2767.

Spencer, S.M., Goins, R.T., Henderson, J.A., Wen, Y., and Goldberg, J. (2013). Influence of caregiving on health-related quality of life among American Indians. *Journal of the American Geriatrics Society, 61*(9), 1615–1620. https://doi.org/10.1111/jgs.12409

Spillman, B.C., and Long, S.K. (2007). *Does High Caregiver Stress Lead to Nursing Home Entry?* Washington, DC: Urban Institute and Office of the Assistant Secretary for Planning and Evaluation. https://aspe.hhs.gov/basic-report/does-high-caregiver-stress-lead-nursing-home-entry

Spillman, B., Wolff, J., Freedman, V.A., and Kasper, J.D. (2014). *Informal Caregiving for Older Americans: An Analysis of the 2011 National Health and Aging Trends Study.* Office of the Assistant Secretary for Planning and Evaluation. https://aspe.hhs.gov/report/informal-caregiving-older-americans-analysis-2011-national-study-caregiving

Toth, M., Martin Palmer, L., Bercaw, L., Johnson, R., Jones, J., Love, R., Voltmer, H., and Karon, S. (2020). *Understanding the Characteristics of Older Adults in Different Residential Settings: Data Sources and Trends.* Washington, DC: RTI International and Office of the Assistant Secretary for Planning and Evaluation. https://aspe.hhs.gov/basic-report/understanding-characteristics-older-adults-different-residential-settings-data-sources-and-trends

Vernon, E.K., Cooley, B., Rozum, W., Rattinger, G.B., Behrens, S., Matyi, J., Fauth, E., Lyketsos, C.G., and Tschanz, J.T. (2019). Caregiver-care recipient relationship closeness is associated with neuropsychiatric symptoms in dementia. *American Journal of Geriatric Psychiatry, 27*(4), 349–359. https://doi.org/10.1016/j.jagp.2018.11.010

Whitlatch, C.J., and Orsulic-Jeras, S. (2018). Meeting the informational, educational, and psychosocial support needs of persons living with dementia and their family caregivers. *Gerontologist, 58*(1), S58–S73. https://doi.org/10.1093/geront/gnx162

Wolff, J.L., Kim, V.S., Mintz, S., Stametz, R., and Griffin, J.M. (2018). An environmental scan of shared access to patient portals. *Journal of the American Medical Informatics Association, 25*(4), 408–412. https://doi.org/10.1093/jamia/ocx088

World Health Organization. (2017). *Global Action Plan on the Public Health Response to Dementia 2017–2025.* http://apps.who.int/iris/bitstream/handle/10665/259615/9789241513487-eng.pdf;jsessionid=1FCE8E87E676952FDE11910F8851B120?sequence=1

5

The Role of the Community

The experiences of individuals living with dementia and their families are shaped in countless ways by the circumstances in which they live. Chapter 2 reviews the interacting forces that influence individuals' cognitive health and the ways in which the environment shapes both risk and protective factors across the life span. This chapter looks more closely at the role of the immediate community. There are many kinds of communities; individuals and families are part of multiple overlapping communities, most of which are relevant to the experience of dementia. Traditions, foodways, attitudes about aging, and other attributes of families and cultural groups have important influences on health and well-being. So, too, do characteristics of the physical and built environment and other aspects of the geographic areas in which people live (neighborhoods, towns, cities). More broadly, community has been defined as "any configuration of individuals, families, and groups whose values, characteristics, interests, geography, or social relations unite them in some way," and in general, the term refers both to places and the people who live in them (National Academies of Sciences, Engineering, and Medicine [NASEM], 2017, p. 1).

Looking specifically at the implications for dementia, communities shape the exposures and behaviors that influence dementia risk from early life through adulthood. (See Chapters 1 and 2 for discussion of how interacting experiences and factors influence cognitive health throughout life.) Community context also affects the way people interpret the meaning of the experience of having dementia or living with someone with the disease, the expectations they have of social interactions, and the availability of resources. Thus, the community is a key context in which interventions may improve outcomes for people living with dementia and their families and caregivers. Understanding community context can provide insights into disease progression as well, and cultural traditions, challenges, and local cultural knowledge may facilitate understanding of new ways to see problems and seek answers to them.

What makes it urgent to consider dementia through a community lens is that communities in the United States vary dramatically in both the harms and opportunities their residents experience. This chapter provides an overview of the contexts that fundamentally shape health and quality of life for individuals living with dementia, including a detailed examination of disparities in community characteristics and opportunities, and how those factors can mitigate or exacerbate the challenges of dementia. It also reviews what is known about opportunities at the community level to ameliorate the challenges for individuals, families, and caregivers. The chapter closes with directions for research to improve understanding of the effects of community characteristics on residents' cognitive health and on the experiences of those who develop dementia and their caregivers.

First, to bring to life the profound influence of place and community on people living with dementia and their caregivers, Box 5-1 presents a personal reflection. Each individual story and commentary the committee heard reflected unique circumstances but also widely shared experiences and reactions, and challenges that affect people across the country. While our focus was on research and policy responses to reduce the negative impacts of dementia on individuals and families, experiences in our own circles of family and friends touched by these diseases were another source of insight. Box 5-1 is the account of how one committee member's caregiving experience has been affected by the community context in which her father lives.

DISPARITIES THAT AFFECT THE IMPACT OF DEMENTIA

Communities in the United States vary across multiple dimensions: size; geography and climate; rural, suburban, or urban character; demographic makeup; comparative wealth; cultural perspective; and much more. Some of the differences reflect historical realities that have introduced and sustained profound inequities and injustices. As noted by the authors of a 2017 National Academies' report, such community conditions as concentrated poverty, low housing values, and low high school graduation rates not only reflect the nation's history of structural racism and economic injustice but also are closely linked to poorer health outcomes and poorer conditions for health (NASEM, 2017). In many regions, current conditions reflect the lasting legacy of slavery; the forced relocation of Indigenous groups and other minorities; segregation laws; and other discriminatory events, policies, and

> **BOX 5-1**
> **Dementia Care in Rural America: A Caregiver's Perspective**
>
> I write as a caregiver for my father, a person living with dementia in one of North Carolina's rural counties. My father lives alone on a small farm with his dog. More than 1 in 5 older Americans live in a rural area; 1 in 3 live alone. Rural areas typically have low population densities, few young families, and heavy concentrations of older adults. Dementia-support resources ought to be prevalent in these areas, but as I researched resources for my father, I learned that rural Americans tend to lack access to dementia resources. Older adults in America's rural areas are not generally poorer than their counterparts in urban areas, or less educated, but resources for living with dementia have become concentrated in towns and cities. As a result of this lack of access, a rural resident with dementia often has more severe life impairment and less independence, as compared to an urban resident with dementia *at the same stage of disease.* This essay explains how that might happen.
>
> Many resources are lacking for rural residents with dementia. My father, typifying many rural older adults, lives 1 mile from his nearest neighbor and 27 miles from the nearest small town. There is no public transportation in the county. Persons with dementia drive their cars long distances for essentials such as grocery stores, banks, doctor visits, or to pick up medications. When a person with dementia should no longer drive, s/he becomes wholly dependent on family for errands. Because younger family members have migrated to cities, drivers are in short supply. Experiences that support quality of life and intellectual stimulation for urban persons with dementia are virtually non-existent in my father's county, including lectures, concerts, arts, social clubs, or technical support for Internet use. The county lacks the sorts of public places where older adults who live in cities gather, such as coffee shops, parks, fitness centers, and shopping malls. The underfunded senior center is open 1 day a week. Meals on Wheels service is available, but as in many rural counties, a case of frozen meals is delivered once a month, depriving the person with dementia from social contact during deliveries (and requiring them to remember to retrieve meals from the freezer and manage reheating). Restaurants do not deliver meals outside town. In addition to self-reliance for transportation, intellectual stimulation, and meals, rural older adults manage more home-maintenance functions than their urban counterparts. They do not enjoy public services such as water, sewer, garbage pickup, road maintenance, snow removal, lawn care, or clean-up after storms. Routine chores such as changing well filters, mowing grass, and hauling garbage fall to persons with dementia, and when dementia disrupts these functions, dependence on family results. Rural residents with dementia lack support resources that enable many urban residents with dementia to maintain independence and quality of life longer, as their disease progresses.
>
> Rural residents with dementia also lack access to health care, a lack which can render them unhealthy and more impaired at an earlier stage of dementia. Like many rural American hospitals in 2021, the hospital in my father's county is bankrupt and expected to close. Hospitals in adjacent cities have refused ambulance transfers. Specialists such as a neurologist, urologist, or cardiologist visit
>
> *Continued*

BOX 5-1 Continued

the town 1 day per month. Tele-medicine videoconferencing technology should help rural residents, but it can be unworkable for older adults who have impairments in hearing, vision, cognition, and memory. A county nurse visits my father a couple of times a year but not when I can participate as carer-informant. On the last visit, when asked about overseas travel (part of the COVID-risk screen), my father terrified the nurse by reporting his return 2 weeks ago, as a missionary to Wuhan, China. True, apart from the key detail that his return was two decades ago. Unlike most rural people with dementia, my father has a professor daughter who can arrange for specialist geriatric-medicine care at her university's medical center, in a city 100 miles away. However, this medical center manages its appointments, co-pays, and instructions for parking through an Internet-based system, which is inaccessible to rural older adults who do not use the Internet. Moreover, university-hospital clinicians communicate under complex privacy regulations and via internal electronic medical-record systems, modern advances which have impeded sharing vital medical information with my father's rural primary care doctor. When persons with dementia must leave their homes for long-term residential care, our rural county's facilities are limited to assisted living plus medical rehabilitation; attractive urban-style continuum-of-care settings are not available. I have observed that, in practice, health care to rural persons with dementia is frequently delivered by law enforcement and fire-and-rescue emergency medical services.

Isolation is a key aspect of rural life that exacerbates impairment for many persons with dementia, particularly those who live alone and those who no longer drive. Many rural residents like my father chose rural life years ago from a personal preference for an uncrowded lifestyle. But times have changed. Internet communication has become essential for countering social isolation, disadvantaging the two-thirds of rural Americans over 65 who have no home broadband, most of whom have never used the Internet.[a] My father has no computer or smartphone, but even if he had these tools and learned to use them, he lives in a rural communications desert lacking cellphone tower coverage and fiber-optic cable for broadband. Internet access is difficult not only for rural persons with dementia but also for rural carers. Churches are a traditional bulwark against isolation, but rural churches tend to be small, understaffed, and underfunded, with congregations who are mostly older adults themselves. My father's tiny church is overwhelmed by the number of dementia cases in the congregation who need pastoral care. Small-town newspapers used to promote social connection for older adults in rural areas, but local newspapers are a thing of the past. My father can no longer enjoy checking for his name in the obituaries each morning. Social isolation is not just unpleasant and understimulating, it is dangerous. There is little surveillance of rural people living with dementia, and therefore food insecurity, neglected home repairs, and falls go undetected. Isolation and loneliness exacerbate vulnerability to elder fraud among persons with dementia. Financial abusers are known to selectively prey on older adults living alone in low population-density rural areas, where escaping detection is easiest. My father, long a sensible, frugal man, gave more than $6,000 to criminal fraudsters last year. He confessed he enjoyed chatting with them on the telephone to pass the time.

> Rural people living with dementia are disadvantaged by factors that can leave them more impaired and less independent than their urban counterparts. Primary among these factors are lack of transportation, inaccessible health care, inadequate rural broadband, and social isolation.
>
> [a] https://www.pewresearch.org/internet/fact-sheet/internet-broadband
> SOURCE: Committee member.

laws. These legacies from the past, along with more recent developments, such as "redlining" of neighborhoods to discourage investment in places where people of color lived, resulted in the displacement of vulnerable populations and the fragmentation of their communities (see, e.g., Fullilove and Wallace, 2011). These issues are well documented elsewhere but are a critical backdrop for understanding how the impacts of dementia vary from place to place in the United States (e.g., Riley, 2018; Bailey et al., 2017; NASEM, 2017; Lewis et al., 2020; Jervis et al., 2018). This section looks first at how the characteristics of disadvantaged communities may influence cognitive health and then at the amplifying impact of racism on such effects.

Links Between Community Characteristics and Cognitive Health

Research on the disparities in health outcomes associated with this history has established links between structural inequities evident at the community level and such basic indicators of population health as infant mortality and life expectancy, as well as diseases that are part of the pathway to dementia (e.g., stroke and diabetes) (see Chapter 2 for more information) (Goins et al., 2021; Lewis et al., 2020; Jervis et al., 2018). These inequities include such factors as poor housing conditions, higher levels of chronic stress and trauma, limited neighborhood cohesion, and segregation (NASEM, 2017). Other research has linked factors that have been associated with dementia risk, such as educational attainment; adult stress; cardiovascular health; and exposure to air pollution; and community characteristics including poverty, crime rate, social cohesion, rurality, and quality of transportation networks (Leventhal and Brooks-Gunn, 2000; Hill et al., 2005; Lawrence et al., 2017; Nieuwenhuijsen, 2018).

Research has shown the relevance of community context for health across the life course. For example, work on children's development has shown how interactions among complex neurobiological processes and characteristics of the physical and social environment shape the health and even the brains of developing children from before they are born. Indeed, these factors also affect reproductive health and thus the development of young people's future offspring (NASEM, 2019a). Maternal stress, nutrition, environmental toxins, prenatal care, and other factors have all been linked to neurocognitive development, particularly the development of language, executive function, and memory (Sherman, 2014).

Researchers have also looked closely at specific community populations to understand how risks and protections function. For example, studies of Mexican American communities have yielded insights about how being a part of such a community can be protective: one longitudinal study, for example, showed that older people who lived in neighborhoods with greater percentages of Mexican American residents had lower rates of cognitive decline (Sheffield and Peek, 2009). Epidemiologists have documented health benefits of social support and cultural preservation among older Mexican Americans in the Southwest, and even suggested that the benefits of social resources could outweigh the harms of socioeconomic disadvantage (Eschbach et al., 2004). Other work has suggested that the social capital benefits of being part of a community (e.g., networks of family and friends) foster resilience that can buffer stresses experienced among immigrant groups in the United States (Alegría et al., 2017). Protections against cross-group tensions and the influence of collective action to improve community conditions have been identified as possible sources of resilience.

More generally, there is evidence that larger social networks and greater levels of social support are associated with improved overall cognition (Kelly et al., 2017). Emotional social support has been associated with lower incidence of cognitive impairment and improved functioning (Yin et al., 2020; Ellwardt et al., 2013).

Nevertheless, the interactive effects of neighborhood characteristics are not fully understood. For example, family support has been strongly associated with self-rated mental health, but the relationship among neighborhood social cohesion and resources, language, and other sociodemographic factors and cognitive health merits further study (National Latino and Asian American Study;[1] Mulvaney-Day et al., 2007). Moreover, segregated neighborhoods also have the potential to isolate individuals from broader community resources, and promote alienation and social stagnation. Research is needed to determine their role in the cognitive health of immigrants and racial/ethnic minority groups in the United States (Alegría et al., 2017).

Little research has directly explored how major features of communities influence the development of dementia, the experience of living with dementia, and its impact on caregivers. The work that is available points to associations between disparities in the prevalence of dementia and such measures of neighborhood disadvantage as income and education level,

---

[1] https://www.massgeneral.org/mongan-institute/centers/dru/research/past/nlaas

housing quality, and employment (Powell et al., 2020). Some research on environmental stressors and exposures illustrates the specific connections among social stratification (by race and ethnicity, gender, socioeconomic status, and rural/urban residence), community stressors and assets, and dementia outcomes (Guo et al., 2019; Wu et al., 2015a, 2015b).

Community stressors potentially place people at greater risk of poor cognitive function and dementia through a variety of mechanisms. The dementia experience (overall quality of life and rate of progression of disease) may be influenced by, for example, how easy it is for individuals to engage in physical activity in the community or to avoid isolation and develop and maintain strong social relationships. Community conditions may also add to caregivers' stress or affect their well-being if, for example, the challenge of providing care is exacerbated by physical distance from or inadequacy of resources and supports.

The mechanisms involved may be physical. For instance, people living in highly segregated neighborhoods are more likely to be exposed to pollutants that exceed thresholds for neurotoxicity and can cause neurodegeneration, thus directly or indirectly influencing diseases that are part of the pathway to dementia. Air pollution is one example. The presence of outdoor particulate air pollutants is associated with higher levels of cognitive impairment in cross-sectional studies and with faster rates of cognitive decline in longitudinal studies. Some recent evidence also documents that community stressors may heighten the negative consequences of particulate air pollutants for dementia risk (Ailshire et al., 2017; Ailshire and Clarke, 2015; Ailshire and Crimmins, 2014; Cacciottolo et al., 2017; Clifford et al., 2016; Power et al., 2016). Both outdoor and indoor particulate air pollutants (perhaps resulting from, e.g., heating/cooking fires) may increase the risk of dementia or influence its symptoms and progression (Saenz et al., 2018; Caldwell et al., 2019; Choi and Matz-Costa, 2018; Dong and Bergren, 2017; Gobbens and van Assen, 2018). Such stressors have been found to have disproportionate effects for racial/ethnic minorities, groups of lower socioeconomic status, and rural residents, although research findings on these disparities are sparse and mixed (Millar, 2020; Rote et al., 2017).

Crime, noise, and neighborhood disorder also affect communities' quality of life, residents' sense of community, and a variety of physical and psychological outcomes (Caldwell et al., 2019; Choi and Matz-Costa, 2018; Dong and Bergren, 2017; Gobbens and van Assen, 2018). Although little research links these aspects of community directly to dementia risk, quality of life for individuals living with dementia, and impacts on caregivers, an abundance of research documents the associations between these neighborhood attributes and self-reported health, frailty, physical health conditions, perceived stress, and emotional well-being (depression, anxiety) (Diez Roux et al., 2016; Cagney et al., 2005; Rodrigues et al., 2021). For example, chronic exposure to community noise in diverse urban environments has been linked to poor cognitive performance, dementia, and Alzheimer's disease (Weuve et al., 2020). Poor communities have greater exposure to damaging noise as well (Agrawal et al., 2008).

The Role of Race and Ethnicity

The above factors may harm the health of residents of any disadvantaged community, urban or rural, in any region. When they intersect with racial/ethnic disparities and structural or direct racism, the effects can be even more detrimental. Many people of color reside in poor communities, independent of their own income level, and residential segregation by race has been historically persistent in many regions of the United States. Black, Latinx, and Native American people are disproportionately likely to live in high-poverty census tracks in the United States. These realities affect health in a number of ways (Williams and Collins, 2001; Solomon et al., 2019; Bailey et al., 2017). Segregated neighborhoods tend to have more limited health care facilities and supermarkets relative to other neighborhoods, for example. They also have fewer parks and green spaces compared with White neighborhoods, which limits opportunities for exercise and socializing (Nardone et al., 2021; South et al., 2015).

Because of residential segregation, people of color are also more likely to be exposed to such environmental hazards as air pollution (Woo et al., 2019; Bravo et al., 2016) and noise pollution (Casey et al., 2017), as well as environmental stressors such as violence (Levy et al., 2020). As noted above, there is reason to believe that these stressors have disproportionate effects on racial/ethnic minorities, among other groups.

Chapter 2 reviews the large body of evidence of connections between educational attainment and cognitive health, and it has long been understood that significant disparities in educational attainment are linked to social and economic disadvantage (see, e.g., Duncan and Murnane, 2011; Gamoran, 2001; Garcia et al., 2018). For numerous reasons, particularly the way public education is funded in the United States, students in disadvantaged and highly segregated communities have historically had more limited educational opportunities relative to their peers in other communities, and these disparities continue to translate to differences in educational attainment and other outcomes. Looking at the association with dementia risk, a 2020 study showed that Black people who had not completed high school had the greatest lifetime burden of dementia because they experienced earlier onset of symptoms (Farina et al., 2020). Evidence that decreasing dementia prevalence may be associated with increases in educational attainment overall supports this connection (Wu et al., 2017; Downer et al., 2019; Hayward et al., 2021). In addition, a recent study showed that between 2000 and 2014, the prevalence of dementia in the United States decreased across racial/ethnic groups, but especially among non-Hispanic Black adults aged 65–74, and that improvements in educational attainment likely contributed to this outcome (Hayward et al., 2021).

Finally, some researchers have explored the effects of poverty and discrimination experienced by members of minority groups on dementia risk and progression (Williams and Earl, 2007; Zuckerman et al., 2008). A hypothesis is that racial and economic stressors in individuals' communities may lead to depressed mood or physiological changes that in turn may increase the risk or severity of dementia (Barnes et al., 2012; Zahodne et al., 2017). The relationship between experiences of discrimination and the development of dementia is an area that deserves further study (Barnes and Bennett, 2014).

There has also been little research directly linking community-level efforts with reductions in dementia-related disparities. There is reason to hope that programs designed to reduce disparities in the social determinants of health may also reduce disparities in dementia through their influence on health behaviors that have been associated with reduced dementia risk, such as eating a healthy diet, engaging in physical exercise, having social connections, and limiting exposure to tobacco and excess alcohol (see Chapter 2). More fundamental approaches to breaking down disparities and barriers, such as increasing the minimum wage, ensuring universal access to health care, and implementing food and housing security programs, could be expected to have benefits for cognitive health (NASEM, 2019b). These important issues are beyond the scope of this report, but research to explore such links will be valuable.

LOOKING THROUGH A COMMUNITY LENS

As discussed in Chapters 2 and 3, cognitive health is influenced throughout the life course by many factors that confer protection or risk, many of which are modifiable. Chapter 2 examines the connections between specific risk factors, such as smoking, cardiovascular health, and social factors (e.g., education and income level), and disparities in cognitive health across population groups. The resources a community affords and the stressors it imposes likely influence not only people's health before they experience cognitive decline but also the experiences they and their caregivers have after diagnosis. As discussed above, these effects are a key reason for stark disparities in dementia prevalence and outcomes.

Figure 5-1 illustrates the dynamic relationship among the experiences of individuals and families and the ways in which community characteristics can influence them. The community environment depicted here includes both conditions that affect people who are living with dementia, such as neighborhood resources, and those that may have an impact throughout the life course, such as air pollution, which may alter brain development and function early in life, conferring risk that is carried forward and may affect cognitive aging and the development of disease (Cacciottolo et al., 2017; Ailshire et al., 2017).

Figure 5-1 illustrates the connections between the community context and the cognitive health and quality of life of people living with dementia, but it is also important to understand that these connections potentially vary in important ways across different types of communities defined by race and ethnicity, socioeconomic status, and rural or urban character. As noted above, racial/ethnic segregation affect how community stressors and resources influence dementia risk and the quality of life for people living with dementia. As the personal narrative at the beginning of the chapter (Box 5-1) illustrates, resources and stressors faced by rural elderly persons living with dementia differ in significant ways from those encountered in urban areas. Communities also differ in their economic resources and how neighborhoods are potentially socioeconomically stratified, illustrating yet another way in which inequality *across* communities influences the connections *within* communities. As yet, researchers have not found clear ways to use a community lens to understand dementia experiences in the population. However, Figure 5-1 points to possible avenues that researchers could pursue to understand the structural origins of dementia.

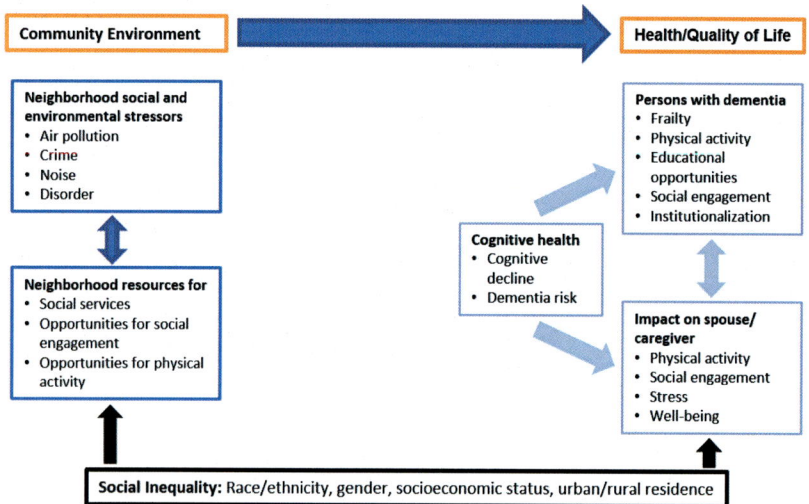

FIGURE 5-1 Outcomes central to the impact of dementia.

An example of the importance of adopting a community lens in dementia research is social isolation, which is common among older adults generally and is strongly associated with dementia. As noted in Chapter 2, it is difficult to know whether social isolation is a cause of cognitive decline, an effect, or both, but it is associated with increased risk of the development of dementia and accelerated disease progression (Wilson et al., 2007; Sundström et al., 2020; Sutin et al., 2020; NASEM, 2020). Social isolation may also influence the well-being of individuals living with dementia and their caregivers (Latham and Clarke, 2016). Among individuals with dementia, greater social isolation may increase the risk for moderate and severe loneliness (Victor et al., 2020), whereas larger social networks with close friends are associated with better cognition among individuals with dementia that may mitigate the effects of loneliness (Balouch et al., 2019). In turn, social networks themselves often reflect inequalities across communities in terms of rural/urban residence, racial/ethnic segregation, and socioeconomic resources.

While the link between loneliness and dementia is not fully understood, hypotheses about the connection between lack of social interaction and loneliness and dementia include the "use it or lose it" theory, which posits that reduced use of the brain for social relationships may lead to atrophy (Hultsch et al., 1999). At the same time, dementia may exacerbate social isolation, such as when a person loses word-finding skills and other attributes that facilitate connection. Loneliness may also compromise the neural system and render individuals more susceptible to the damaging effects of cognitive decline (Wilson et al., 2007). Compared with adults without dementia, adults with dementia may experience increased difficulty dealing with feelings that arise from social isolation and loneliness (Cohen-Mansfield and Perach, 2015). Many other community factors are thought to play a role in cognitive aging and the quality of life experienced by persons living with dementia and their caregivers.

OPPORTUNITIES TO SUPPORT COMMUNITIES

Communities can play a pivotal role in reducing challenges for individuals living with dementia, families, and caregivers. They can strive to support cognitive resilience for older individuals by promoting education and intellectual stimulation earlier in life, for example (Larson, 2010). They can provide parks and recreational facilities, as well as resources that directly serve the elderly, people living with dementia, and caregivers. Overall, however, the research on how communities can improve outcomes related to dementia has not yet firmly established what approaches are most effective and how they can be implemented. This section focuses on opportunities to build the knowledge base for improvements in this regard in the coming decade.

Cultural attitudes and values that are evident at the community level can have significant effects on the experience of living with dementia (Calia et al., 2019). It has been suggested that some cultural groups' negative impressions of dementia can have the effect of stripping people living with the disease of their personhood and keeping them at a distance from resources that support other aging residents (Kitwood, 1998; Gaugler et al., 2019; Grenier et al., 2017). In other settings, acceptance of dementia and a tradition of engagement with declining elders are the norm. In traditional Chinese culture, for example, dementia is an accepted part of the aging process and is not necessarily viewed as requiring specialty care by non–family members (Cipriani and Borin, 2015). People in some Native American communities share this perspective, while others view dementia as a signal of death (Adamsen et al., 2021; Lewis et al., 2020; Kramer, 1996; Cipriani and Borin, 2015).

Recognizing the influences of attitudes and values, some have suggested reframing dementia not as solely a biological disease but as a process integrating biology with the influence of community and culture (Gaugler et al., 2019). This approach is consistent with the social model of disease and helps shift the focus from the limitations of the individual to the ways in which the community either supports or constricts the options of individuals and families.

This section explores some of the types of resources communities afford to individuals living with dementia and their families, issues and disparities that affect the availability of those resources, ways to build community resilience, and examples of innovative living arrangements that are attracting attention.

Types of Resources

Neighborhood resources are community supports that can allow persons with dementia to live active and engaged lives and provide help with the challenges faced by their caregivers (Ng et al., 2018; Clarke et al., 2015). As with stressors, there is evidence that such resources are associated with both the risk of dementia and disease progression. For example, a resource that provides stimulating activities and social interaction may support the maintenance of cognitive reserve that slows cognitive decline and reduces the risk of dementia or helps mitigate the effects of neurotoxicity on disease progression among persons with dementia.

As discussed above, researchers have established individual-level associations between social engagement, social isolation, and loneliness and dementia outcomes (e.g., Liang et al., 2020; Penninkilampi et al., 2018;

Saczynski et al., 2006). Substantially less research has assessed the effects of the variety of resources available in the community, such as religious institutions, adult day care centers, or residential care facilities (Clarke et al., 2015; Du Toit et al., 2019). One reason for this gap may be the lack of data that can be used to explore this issue. Investigators often fail to consider collecting information about the types and numbers of community resources available to and utilized by people living with dementia and their caregivers. This information might be collected by conducting a community needs assessment that includes some discussion with people living with dementia and their caregivers.

A study currently under way at the University of Southern California illustrates the value of this type of research (see University of Southern California, 2020). The researchers have developed a data resource for contextual information that can be linked to large population studies of individuals, such as the Health and Retirement Study or the National Aging and Health Trends Study.[2] The contextual data span key community domains, including social, physical, built, and resource environments, that can be linked to communities in which study participants live. This contextual information offers new conceptually important measures that previously have not been widely considered in dementia studies. For the general category of "resources for social interaction and mental stimulation," for example, measures of libraries, gardens and museums, churches, and community centers will allow an in-depth characterization of this community environment domain. The study is attending to the temporal and spatial scales at which contextual data are available while also developing a new data infrastructure to examine ways in which communities influence the dementia experience.

Other work has suggested the potential benefits of neighborhood access to green space as well, including association with physical activity and opportunities for social contact, that have been identified as protective of cognitive health (James et al., 2015). These are among the few domains to focus on positive attributes rather than harmful factors—an important consideration in addressing the requirements for wellness and satisfaction for those living with dementia.

Other resources include the Area Deprivation Index, a measure of socioeconomic deprivation developed by the Health Resources and Services Administration that provides useful information about urban areas but is less useful for insights about rural areas. Researchers in the United Kingdom have also initiated large-scale studies to examine this issue, with the goal of enhancing opportunities for social engagement in communities

---

[2]https://gero.usc.edu/cbph/cdr/#about

(Swarbrick et al., 2019; Zuelsdorff et al., 2020; Kind and Buckingham, 2018).

A Patchwork of Resources and Supports

Communities across the United States have a range of structures in place to address the needs of people living with dementia and their caregivers. Among other functions, they provide information; link people to agencies and organizations that offer supports and services; and deliver care, services, and supports directly. As discussed above, communities also have features that are indirectly supportive or beneficial, such as parks, religious institutions, and other amenities in which people living with dementia can share. Studies of older adults who live alone indicate that home visitation from nurses, peer visitation to share a meal, and community e-health monitoring with telephone counseling appear to improve health outcomes so that older people can age in place (Ahn et al., 2018; McHugh Power et al., 2016; Jung and Lee, 2017).

The resources and supports provided by communities vary for many reasons. Communities differ in size, in their histories and geographic locations, in the demographic characteristics of their populations, and in many other ways. They also differ in both a political and policy sense: they are located within states and localities each with its own guidelines, regulations, laws, and resources relevant to persons with dementia and their caregivers. Funding streams from both the state and the federal government vary and reach the community in different ways. For example, a federal agency may provide block grants to states for social programs, which allow states autonomy in how to use the funds (often without accountability and guidelines). States, in turn, largely determine how to disperse the funds to their own local communities. Communities themselves vary in the level of funding they have to work with, in their approach to investing in the social and economic well-being of their populations, and in the kinds of regulations they adopt to protect vulnerable groups.

People living in rural communities face challenges and inequities that are comparable to those in urban and suburban communities but may require different responses (Warshaw, 2017). In rural areas, for example, access to resources and care may require traveling long distances and time off from work for individuals living with dementia and their caregivers. Health- and medicine-related needs in rural areas are not well addressed in general, and this has been an underresearched area of public health (NASEM, 2021; Bolin et al., 2015). Researchers have noted that medical care tends to be oriented toward large population centers for economic reasons, and efforts to improve the structure and delivery of care tend to focus on those areas as well (a phenomenon that has been called "structural urbanism" [Probst, 2019]). Nevertheless, older adults living in rural areas have assets and opportunities that can be leveraged in prevention, detection, and care for dementia. For instance, among many Indigenous peoples of America, cultural and traditional teachings and practices passed on by elders can build resilience for communities, and social engagement with family and community has been associated with reduced risk of cognitive decline, as noted above (Alzheimer's Association and Centers for Disease Control and Prevention, 2019).

These issues have not been well studied, but one example of an effort to address the challenges in rural areas is the collocation of health care training programs with residential facilities for older adults, which has facilitated multigenerational learning and exchange (NASEM, 2021). Another is use of mobile respite services to increase access to care in rural areas, which has been tried in Australia (Alzheimer's Australia, 2007).

There are many ways in which support can be provided at the local level to individuals living with dementia and their caregivers. These include providing resources for physical activity (e.g., parks, recreational centers) and for social interaction and mental stimulation (e.g., libraries, museums, dementia-related choral groups), as well as the institutions that provide health care, long-term care in the home or in a facility, and hospice and palliative care (discussed in Chapter 6).

Supplementary resources are difficult to categorize, and the sorts of support they provide overlap. In general, however, such resources provide support for everyday tasks, such as grocery shopping and transportation, and offer adult day care/respite care and other kinds of emotional support and information. It is important to note that funding for community-based programs both varies across communities and fluctuates within communities. Some resources are without cost to residents who have access to them, but others have costs that can be substantial. Thus, many are more accessible to people with higher incomes and levels of education. Moreover, the COVID-19 pandemic has altered the way many of these entities function, with major implications for people nationwide. For example, beginning early in the pandemic, most community-based services were no longer provided in person. Disruption due to the pandemic aside, however, sources of support include the following:

- *Religious institutions.* Many churches, synagogues, mosques, and other religious institutions organize activities for individuals living with dementia and support groups for caregivers.
- *Local agencies that offer or coordinate services for the elderly and provide such functions as checking in on seniors, home assessments, meal services and food delivery, and ride service.* These may be agencies of a city, county, or other jurisdiction or private

nonprofit entities designated by local government to provide these services, often coordinating the use of state or federally funded efforts to support the elderly. A key national resource for communities is the network of Area Agencies on Aging (Administration for Community Living, 2021). The Administration on Aging has also developed a consumer-oriented website to assist people who need services.[3]

- *Senior centers and adult day care centers.* Approximately 10,000 senior centers in the United States provide meal and nutrition programs; health, fitness, and wellness programs; transportation; day care programs; and other services. They typically rely on multiple funding sources, including government funds and funds raised by volunteers and donated by businesses (National Council on Aging, 2015).
- *Private agencies.* For families that can afford their services, geriatric care managers and social workers who are either affiliated with nonprofit organizations or in private practice provide supports that include regular visits with individuals living with dementia; coordination of medical care, other services, and paid caregivers; drivers experienced with elderly clients or those with dementia; and counseling and information for family members struggling with the challenges of being a caregiver.
- *Support groups.* Examples include local Alzheimer's Association chapters and local Alzheimer's agencies, which provide such resources as in-person peer mentoring support groups and 24/7 helplines.
- *Structured living arrangements.* Such arrangements are designed to meet the needs of people living with dementia, either alone or with family caregivers, who do not need or wish to live in a long-term care facility. In some of these arrangements, people live in alternative housing, while in others they remain in their homes but with neighborhood community structures filling gaps. Such arrangements include naturally occurring retirement community supportive service programs (NORC programs), village and green house models, and dementia friendly communities (Greenfield et al., 2012; Graham et al., 2017; Lin, 2017).

As noted earlier, limited research has thus far been conducted on community resources for people living with dementia and their caregivers, nor has there been any systematic collection of data about the nature of and methods for evaluating programs that deliver such supports. Evaluation is

---

[3] https://eldercare.acl.gov/Public/Index.aspx

costly, and where funding is tight, as it is for many community resources, evaluation may seem like a luxury. However, data collection and research to identify the features that make some of these approaches effective, particularly such purposeful innovations as dementia friendly communities, is both essential and lacking (Buckner et al., 2018, 2019; Phillipson et al., 2019).

Building Community Responsiveness and Resilience

To advance beyond the current patchwork of community resources described above, it is important to consider what constitutes a responsive and resilient community that can support people living with dementia in remaining safely at home for as long as possible. One key attribute of such a community is a robust formal network of agencies that provide both medical and social services, such as visiting nurse associations, home care companies, elderly housing, meal distribution programs, and day care and senior centers. Such a community also typically has a network of volunteer groups advocating for the elderly with government authorities. When these two sets of actors join to advocate for government funding and set the agenda for local nonprofit foundations, the conditions for a resilient community exist. When only fee-for-service agencies are present, they may collaborate but in a limited fashion, each focused on its own organizational survival, not necessarily on supporting the agenda of the elderly population in general.

Other entities make important contributions to responsive and resilient communities. Community foundations, for example, fund nonprofit agencies, community initiatives, and other efforts, some of which focus specifically on aging. Foundations can provide leadership to social service delivery agencies and advocacy groups, and potentially galvanize community volunteers, political leaders, and media attention. Many religious organizations are centers for social engagement and volunteerism that have impact beyond their own membership and are important resources in disadvantaged neighborhoods and for racial/ethnic minority groups, but little is known about how such groups support people living with dementia and their caregivers. Local businesses have traditionally been another source of funding and other support. However, corporate consolidations have had an impact on business leaders' involvement with local issues.

Unfortunately, there is fairly scant research on the function of communities with respect to the needs of aging populations, and research on the nonprofit sector rarely focuses on issues associated with aging. Systematic attention to this issue is needed using community-level data about nonprofit entities, interagency interaction, and related topics. Research examining community-based agencies for the elderly and the relationship between what agencies offer and population outcomes is sorely needed;

such research can be supported by linking data about community agencies to Medicare data.

The conduct of such research is hampered, however, by the lack of well-developed conceptual models for how community supports can be beneficial, and an infrastructure for testing hypotheses about the observable relationships between interlinked agencies and community resilience and the outcomes experienced by persons living with dementia. There are community-based programs in operation throughout the country, and it is likely that many, if not most, are providing meaningful supports, but few are well documented and rigorously evaluated. As more data become available and greater attention is focused on these issues, it will be possible to learn more about what differentiates communities that are and are not able to implement multifaceted programs to help frail and isolated subgroups of the population. At present, there is no single social science discipline in which these issues are a recognized focus, so a multidisciplinary, team-based approach would likely be best for this research.

Housing for People Living with Dementia

The majority of people with dementia live in the community, either with others (57%) or on their own (24%). The remainder live in residential care settings, such as assisted living (6%) and nursing homes (13%) (Lepore et al., 2017). But the need for residential care rises as the disease progresses and will grow as the population ages. In a recent nationally representative survey of people aged 60–72, 42 percent said that if they had dementia, they would want to live in a place where they could get help with daily activities and health care. Another 14 percent desired a place where they could get help with daily activities. The remaining 46 percent said they would choose to live in a community-based setting (LeadingAge, 2019).

There is reason for clear concern that people with dementia living at home in the community have substantial unmet needs for care and services, but documentation of these needs and to what extent they are met is scarce. Those who live at home are at higher risk for falls, unmanaged behavioral symptoms, pain, sleep disturbances, and environmental challenges (Gitlin et al., 2014). However, the evidence on the use of home- and community-based services by people with dementia is scant. In addition, there are few reliable measures of the quality of these supports.

Approximately 4.7 million very low-income older adults meet the eligibility requirements for affordable housing, although only about a third of them receive such assistance (Joint Center for Housing Studies of Harvard University, 2019). Waiting lists average 2 to 3 years but may be as long as 10 years. As a result, once older individuals obtain a subsidized unit, they remain there as long as possible. However, services available to these residents tend to be limited, despite evidence that combining services with housing can enable people to remain in the community longer, thus supporting their preferences while also avoiding more costly care settings (Sanders et al., 2015).

At the national level, the BOLD Infrastructure for Alzheimer's Act, passed into law in 2018, is a valuable new resource for localities. This act charged the Centers for Disease Control and Prevention (CDC) with three broad goals: establishing public health centers of excellence in addressing Alzheimer's disease and related dementias, providing funds to support public health departments, and improving data collection and reporting and analysis of data.[4] Together with other CDC initiatives designed to promote healthy aging, this act was designed to strengthen the support infrastructure throughout the country. States have begun receiving grants under the act, although further congressional approval will be needed to fully fund the provisions of the law.[5]

Researchers and local service providers (e.g., Area Agencies on Aging) in the United States and in other countries have devised numerous creative innovations at the community level to serve the needs of people living with dementia and their caregivers. Such efforts have targeted, for example, expanded access to long-term care, training in best practices for interacting with people living with dementia, collaborations to facilitate aging in place, and the provision of transportation. The committee could not systematically survey such innovations but explored several that show promise, recognizing that most are at present accessible primarily in communities with ample resources. While there is some research on these and similar efforts, more systematic evaluation of their functioning and impacts, their implementation challenges, and obstacles to their availability in low-income communities is needed.

Dementia Friendly Communities

Many governmental and advocacy groups are developing initiatives that fall under the umbrella of "dementia friendly communities." Such communities foster understanding of people living with dementia and focus on the assets they bring to the community and ways of engaging them and their caregivers in decisions about care and other issues (Alzheimer's Association, 2016; see also Alzheimer's Association, n.d.). They generally offer education and training for varied members of the community and may also include respite care and other services for family caregivers.

---

[4] https://www.cdc.gov/aging/bold/index.html for more information
[5] https://alzimpact.org/media/serve/id/5a2eb6a350348

Figure 5-2 illustrates one approach to the design of a dementia friendly community.

In the United States, Minnesota was an early adopter of this approach. Its program, ACT on Alzheimer's, became a national model. The White House Conference on Aging in 2015 promoted the development of other, similar initiatives, resulting in the creation of Dementia Friendly America, a "national network of communities, organizations and individuals seeking to ensure that communities across the United States are equipped to support people living with dementia and their caregivers" (Dementia Friendly America, 2021).

The World Dementia Council and the World Health Organization (WHO) are collaborating on a number of initiatives related to dementia friendly communities, many of which are developed by advocates in collaboration with local government. Typical of such interventions is the Dementia Friends program, which has included more than 15 million participants spread across nearly a fifth of all nations. While there is some evidence of participant satisfaction, the nature and duration of any impacts from these programs have not been systematically studied. At the 2019 Tokyo Dementia Summit, WHO announced a new dementia friendly

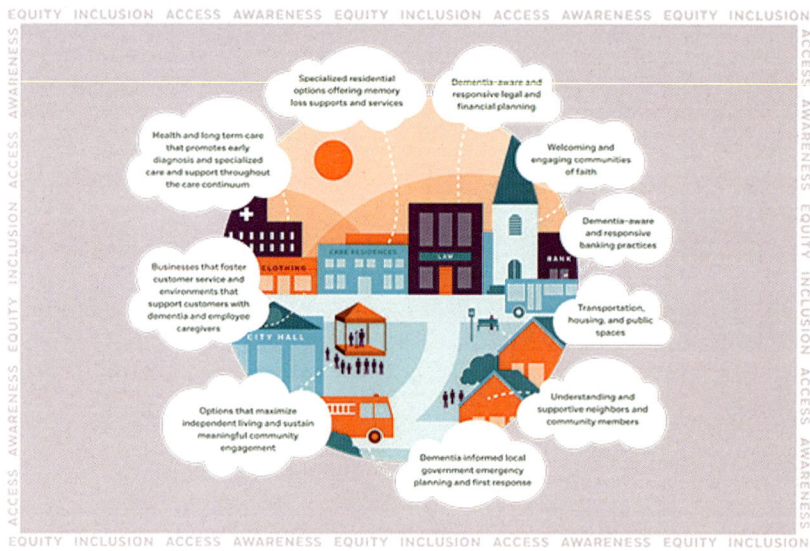

FIGURE 5-2 Elements of a dementia friendly community.
SOURCE: Dementia Friendly America (2021). Reprinted with permission of the Dementia Friendly America initiative at the National Association of Area Agencies on Aging.

toolkit, intended to provide practical tools for planning and implementing dementia-inclusive communities; it is currently being field tested (World Dementia Council, 2019). However, efforts such as the development of this toolkit have been focused largely on the needs of wealthy countries experiencing high levels of population aging rather than the needs of disadvantaged communities.

Research is needed to better understand the essential characteristics of effective dementia friendly communities and their possible effects on such outcomes as quality of life, caregiver stress, and disease progression, as well as possible problems, such as cost and inequitable access. It will also be important to document the interorganizational and social infrastructure and community leadership required to implement the dementia friendly community approach successfully in diverse communities.

Caregiver Support: Washington State

Washington State has developed a multifaceted Family Caregiver Support Program (FCSP) that aims to expand access to long-term care supports and services for state residents. Of the caregivers served, 53 percent are caring for individuals with Alzheimer's disease or dementia (Office of the Assistant Secretary for Planning and Evaluation, 2019). FCSP uses an evidence-based screening tool, the Tailored Caregiver Assessment and Referral System, to assess the needs of family caregivers and determine the types and levels of care they and their care recipients need. Those who complete the assessment are eligible for baseline FCSP services, and caregivers whose scores indicate a higher level of need are granted access to additional supports and services.

The state legislature has increased funding for FCSP, allowing it to lower eligibility thresholds and increase the number of caregivers receiving additional services, which in turn has reduced reliance on Medicaid long-term care services (Witten, 2019). Eligible state workers can also receive payroll deductions to cover the cost of such services as home-delivered meals, adaptive equipment, and training for family caregivers; the value of the benefit can be as high as $36,500 annually.

Aging in Place Challenge Program: Canada

Canada's National Research Council has developed a model for long-term care, the Aging in Place Challenge Program, designed to reduce costs to the Canadian government and shift the focus of nursing homes to those with the highest need. The developers hope to decrease the number of older adults who require nursing home care across Canada by 20 percent by

2031. The program aims to improve the quality of life for older adults and their caregivers and involves collaboration among academic, not-for-profit, and industrial partners.

The Village Movement: Beacon Hill, Boston, Massachusetts

Beacon Hill Village, located in the Beacon Hill district of Boston, is a self-governing community of adults 50 and older who work together to support independence and aging in place. Founded in 1999, Beacon Hill Village was a pioneer in the village movement, in which neighbors collaborate to empower seniors to live in their communities. There are now more than 300 villages; a number of governments, including those of Washington, DC, and New York State, have promoted village movements locally to encourage this volunteer-supported approach to aging in place (Capital Region Collaborative, 2021). Such villages provide programs, activities, and opportunities for community engagement to encourage active, healthy lives as residents grow older.

Researchers studying the movement have reported some positive results, including feelings of improved confidence and perceptions of support among residents helped by a village; reduced likelihood of institutionalization; and the perception that membership in a village was altruistic and had social benefits (Graham et al., 2016; Wurm and Benyamini, 2014; Robertson et al., 2016; Dunkle et al., 2019). Study of a California example of the village approach showed that participants were more likely to remain in their homes and were better able to take care of their homes and themselves (Graham et al., 2017). However, a limitation of these studies is that the vast majority of participants in the village model have been White, wealthy, educated, and female. More research is needed to examine how this model can be transferred to more diverse communities and how effective it is for individuals with advancing dementia.

RESEARCH DIRECTIONS

There is strong evidence that community factors shape the exposures and behaviors that influence dementia risk and the availability of resources for people living with dementia. This evidence reinforces the point that dementia is not just a biological disease but one that reflects the interactions among biological processes and social and cultural influences that occur across the life span. Researchers have not yet fully documented many of the most important direct impacts of community on dementia or produced clear evidence about interventions to counter negative influences on cognitive health at the community level. At the same time, community supports are providing key resources, and innovative approaches to the design of communities in which people living with dementia can thrive show promise. However, limited evidence documents outcomes for these approaches and identifies their essential components, and their application to diverse contexts and populations has yet to be systematically demonstrated.

The committee identified high-priority research needs for building understanding of the effects of community characteristics on the experiences of people living with dementia and the ways in which communities can support these individuals and their caregivers. These research needs fall into four areas, summarized in Conclusion 5-1; Table 5-1 lists detailed research needs in each of these areas.

> CONCLUSION 5-1: Research in four areas is needed to facilitate the development of communities that are well equipped to support people living with dementia and their caregivers and families, allowing those with dementia to live independently for as long as possible and mitigating the negative effects of past and current socioeconomic and environmental stressors:
> 1. Systematic analysis of the characteristics of communities that influence the risk of developing dementia and the experience of living with the disease, with particular attention to the sources of disparities in dementia incidence and disease trajectory.
> 2. Collection of data to document the opportunities and resources available in communities both historically and currently and evaluation of their impact, with particular attention to disparities in population groups' access to resources and including development of the infrastructure needed for data collection.
> 3. Analysis of the community characteristics needed to foster dementia friendly environments, including assessment of alternative community models that foster dementia friendly environments in communities that have different constellations of resources and serve diverse populations.
> 4. Evaluation of innovative approaches to adapting housing, services, and supports so that persons with dementia can remain in the community and out of institutional care.

TABLE 5-1 Detailed Research Needs

1: Community Characteristics That Affect Dementia Risk	• How race and ethnicity, gender, socioeconomic status, urban/rural residence, structural racism, and segregated neighborhoods may influence the development and trajectory of dementia throughout the life span • The impact of exposure to neighborhood-level social and environmental stressors on the health and quality of life of individuals living with dementia • Evidence-based evaluations of structural interventions and policies designed to improve care and quality of life for people with dementia and caregivers, that is, interventions focused not on changing the behaviors of individuals but on the structures that shape behavioral change.
2: Opportunities and Resources	• Development of systematic means of assessing local needs and challenges and identifying gaps that are not well addressed by existing services and supports • Development of a community needs assessment to identify the effects of resources available in the community, such as religious institutions, adult day centers, or residential care facilities, on addressing the needs of individuals living with dementia and their caregivers • Identification of policies that can coordinate federal and state funding efforts to develop effective community supports • Identification of strategies for mobilizing community health and social welfare networks to address dementia disparities for traditionally underserved groups • Development of refined evaluation methods and indicators of effectiveness for interventions aimed at improving accessibility, availability, acceptability, affordability, adequacy, and awareness of services • Interventions to reduce exposure to such community stressors as environmental pollution, crime, and neighborhood disorder • Development/refinement of means of monitoring the accessibility and quality of services and supports for accountability purposes • Identification of models and infrastructures for testing hypotheses about the relationships among interconnected community organizations addressing the needs of individuals living with dementia and their caregivers
3: Characteristics of Dementia Friendly Communities	• Identification of community and cultural values that affect how individuals perceive dementia and of best practices among cultural groups for providing educational materials about dementia and community-based dementia care services • Analysis of emerging data to understand community agencies and analyze utilization of services on the local and national levels, focusing in particular on disparities

TABLE 5-1 Continued

3: Characteristics of Dementia Friendly Communities (continued)	• Refinement of reliable means of measuring the outcomes that community-level policies are designed to foster • Development of improved means of supporting collaboration among and facilitating the development of local organizations and resources • Analysis of structures and approaches for fostering collaboration among and the development of local organizations and resources
4: Innovative Approaches	• Evaluation of innovative housing arrangements • Pilot testing to determine how effective programs can be taken to large scale • Development of new types of modeling approaches for understanding how community factors operate as part of a system to influence dementia risk and the lived experience of dementia

REFERENCES

Adamsen, C., Manson, S.M., and Jiang, L. (2021). The association of cultural participation and social engagement with self-reported memory problems among American Indian and Alaska elders. *Journal of Aging Health*, 33(7–8_suppl), 60S–67S. https://doi.org/10.1177/08982643211014971

Administration for Community Living. (2021). *Area Agencies on Aging*. https://acl.gov/programs/aging-and-disability-networks/area-agencies-aging

Agrawal, Y., Platz, E.A., and Niparko, J.K. (2008). Prevalence of hearing loss and differences by demographic characteristics among U.S. adults: Data from the National Health and Nutrition Examination Survey, 1999-2004. *Archives of Internal Medicine*, 168(14), 1522–1530. https://doi.org/10.1001/archinte.168.14.1522

Ahn, J-A., Park, J., and Kim, C-J. (2018). Effects of an individualised nutritional education and support programme on dietary habits, nutritional knowledge and nutritional status of older adults living alone. *Journal of Clinical Nursing*, 27, 2142–2151.

Ailshire, J.A., and Clarke, P. (2015). Fine particulate matter air pollution and cognitive function among U.S. older adults. *Journals of Gerontology: Series B*, 70(2), 322–328. https://doi.org/10.1093/geronb/gbu064

Ailshire, J., and Crimmins, E.M. (2014). Fine particulate matter air pollution and cognitive function among older U.S. adults. *American Journal of Epidemiology*, 180(4), 359–366. https://doi.org/10.1093/aje/kwu155

Ailshire, J., Karraker, A., and Clarke, P. (2017). Neighborhood social stressors, fine particulate matter air pollution, and cognitive function among older U.S. adults. *Social Science and Medicine*, 172, 56–63. https://doi.org/10.1016/j.socscimed.2016.11.019

Alegría, M., Álvarez, K., and DiMarzio, K. (2017). Immigration and mental health. *Current Epidemiology Reports*, 4(2), 145–155. https://doi.org/10.1007/s40471-017-0111-2

Alzheimer's Association. (n.d.). *Community Environments*. https://www.alz.org/professionals/public-health/core-areas/community-environments

———. (2016). *Public Health Spotlight: Dementia-Friendly Communities*. https://www.alz.org/media/Documents/spotlight-dementia-friendly-communities.pdf

Alzheimer's Association and Centers for Disease Control and Prevention. (2019). *Healthy Brain Initiative: Road Map for Indian Country*. Chicago, IL: Alzheimer's Association. https://www.cdc.gov/aging/healthybrain/pdf/HBI-Road-Map-for-Indian-Country-508.pdf

Alzheimer's Australia. (2007). *Support Needs of People living with Dementia in Rural and Remote Australia*. https://www.dementia.org.au/sites/default/files/20070200_Nat_SUB_SuppNeedsPplLivDemRurRemAus.pdf

Bailey, Z.D., Krieger, N., Agénor, M., Graves, J., Linos, N., and Bassett, M.T. (2017). Structural racism and health inequities in the USA: Evidence and interventions. *Lancet*, 389(10077), 1453–1463. https://doi.org/10.1016/S0140-6736(17)30569-X

Balouch, S., Rifaat, W., Chen, H.L., and Tabet, N. (2019). Social networks and loneliness in people with Alzheimer's dementia. *International Journal of Geriatric Psychiatry*, 34(5). https://doi.org/10.1002/gps.5065

Barnes, L.L., and Bennett, D.A. (2014). Alzheimer's disease in African Americans: Risk factors and challenges for the future. *Health Affairs*, 33(4), 580–586.

Barnes, L.L., Lewis, T.T., Begeny, C.T., Yu, L., Bennett, D.A., and Wilson, R.S. (2012). Perceived discrimination and cognition in older African Americans. *Journal of the International Neuropsychological Society*, 18, 856–865.

Bolin, J.N., Bellamy, G.R., Ferdinand, A.O., Vuong, A.M., Kash, BA., Schulze, A., and Helduser, J.W. (2015). Rural healthy people 2020: New decade, same challenges. *Journal of Rural Health*, 31(3), 326–333. https://doi.org/10.1111/jrh.12116

Bravo, M.A., Anthopolos, R., Bell, M.L., and Miranda, M.L. (2016). Racial isolation and exposure to airborne particulate matter and ozone in understudied U.S. populations: Environmental justice applications of downscaled numerical model output. *Environment International*, 92–93, 247–255. https://doi.org/10.1016/j.envint.2016.04.008

Buckner, S., Mattocks, C., Rimmer, M., and Lafortune, L. (2018). An evaluation tool for age-friendly and dementia friendly communities. *Working With Older People*, 22(1). https://www.emerald.com/insight/content/doi/10.1108/WWOP-11-2017-0032/full/html

Buckner, S., Darlington, N., Woodward, M., Buswell, M., Mathie, E., Arthur, A., Lafortune, L., Killett, A., Mayrhofer, A., Thurman, J., and Goodman, C. (2019). Dementia friendly communities in England: A scoping study. *International Journal of Geriatric Psychiatry*, 34(5), 1235–1243. https://doi.org/10.1002/gps.5123

Cacciottolo, M., Wang, X., Driscoll, I., Woodward, N., Saffari, A., Reyes, J., Serre, M.L., Vizuete, W., Sioutas, C., Morgan, T.E., Gatz, M., Chui, H.C., Shumaker, S.A., Resnick, S.M., Espeland, M.A., Finch, C.E., and Chen, J.C. (2017). Particulate air pollutants, APOE alleles and their contributions to cognitive impairment in older women and to amyloidogenesis in experimental models. *Translational Psychiatry*, 7(1), e1022. https://doi.org/10.1038/tp.2016.280

Cagney, K.A., Browning, C.R., and Wen, M. (2005). Racial disparities in self-rated health at older ages: What difference does the neighborhood make? *The Journals of Gerontology: Series B*, 60(4), S181–S190. https://doi.org/10.1093/geronb/60.4.s181

Caldwell, J.T., Lee, H., and Cagney, K.A. (2019). Disablement in context: Neighborhood characteristics and their association with frailty onset among older adults. *Journals of Gerontology: Series B*, 74(7), e40–e49. https://doi.org/10.1093/geronb/gbx123

Calia, C., Johnson, H., and Cristea, M. (2019). Cross-cultural representations of dementia: An exploratory study. *Journal of Global Health*, 9(1), 011001. https://doi.org/10.7189/jogh.09.01101

Capital Region Collaborative. (2021). *The Village Movement*. https://crvillages.org/villages/the-village-movement

Casey, J.A., Morello-Frosch, R., Mennitt, D.J., Fristrup, K., Ogburn, E.L., and James, P. (2017). Race/ethnicity, socioeconomic status, residential segregation, and spatial variation in noise exposure in the contiguous United States. *Environmental Health Perspectives*, 125(7), 077017. https://doi.org/10.1289/EHP898

Choi, Y.J., and Matz-Costa, C. (2018). Perceived neighborhood safety, social cohesion, and psychological health of older adults. *Gerontologist, 58*(1), 196–206. https://doi.org/10.1093/geront/gnw187

Cipriani, G., and Borin, G. (2015). Understanding dementia in the sociocultural context: A review. *International Journal of Social Psychiatry, 61*(2), 198–204. https://doi.org/10.1177/0020764014560357

Clarke, P.J., Weuve, J., Barnes, L., Evans, D., and de Leon, C.M. (2015). Cognitive decline and the neighborhood environment. *Annals of Epidemiology, 25*(11), 849–854.

Clifford, A., Lang, L., Chen, R., Anstey, K.J., and Seaton, A. (2016). Exposure to air pollution and cognitive functioning across the life course—A systematic literature review. *Environmental Research, 147*, 383–398. https://doi.org/10.1016/j.envres.2016.01.018

Cohen-Mansfield, J., and Perach, R. (2015). Interventions for alleviating loneliness among older persons: A critical review. *American Journal of Health Promotion, 29*(3), e109–e125.

Dementia Friendly America. (2021). *What is DFA?*. https://www.dfamerica.org/what-is-dfa

Diez Roux, A.V., Mujahid, M.S., Hirsch, J.A., Moore, K., and Moore, L.V. (2016). The impact of neighborhoods on CV risk. *Global Heart, 11*(3), 353–363. https://doi.org/10.1016/j.gheart.2016.08.002

Dong, X., and Bergren, S. (2017). The associations and correlations between self-reported health and neighborhood cohesion and disorder in a community-dwelling U.S. Chinese population. *Gerontologist, 57*(4), 679–697. https://doi.org/10.1093/geront/gnw050

Downer, B., Garcia, M.A., Raji, M., and Markides, K.S. (2019). Cohort differences in cognitive impairment and cognitive decline among Mexican-Americans aged 75 years or older. *American Journal of Epidemiology, 188*(1), 119–129. https://doi.org/10.1093/aje/kwy196

Du Toit, S., Shen, X., and McGrath, M. (2019). Meaningful engagement and person-centered residential dementia care: A critical interpretive synthesis. *Scandinavian Journal of Occupational Therapy, 26*(5), 343–355. https://doi.org/10.1080/11038128.2018.1441323

Duncan, G.J., and Murnane, R.J., Eds. (2011). *Whither Opportunity? Rising Inequality, Schools, and Children's Life Chances.* New York: Russell Sage Foundation.

Dunkle, R., Harlow-Rosentraub, K., Pacce, G., and Coppard, L. (2019). Joining and remaining: Factors that contribute to membership in a village. *Innovation in Aging, 3*(Suppl 1), S277–S278. https://doi.org/10.1093/geroni/igz038.1028

Ellwardt, L., Aartsen, M., Deeg, D., and Steverink, N. (2013). Does loneliness mediate the relation between social support and cognitive functioning in later life? *Social Science & Medicine, 98,* 116–124. https://doi.org/10.1016/j.socscimed.2013.09.002

Eschbach, K., Ostir, G.V., Patel, K.V., Markides, K.S., and Goodwin, J.S. (2004). Neighborhood context and mortality among older Mexican Americans: Is there a barrio advantage? *American Journal of Public Health, 94*(10), 1807–1812. https://doi.org/10.2105/ajph.94.10.1807

Farina, M.P., Hayward, M.D., Kim, J.K., and Crimmins, E.M. (2020). Racial and educational disparities in dementia and dementia-free life expectancy. *Journals of Gerontology: Series B, 75*(7), e105–e112.

Fullilove, M.T., and Wallace, R. (2011). Serial forced displacement in American cities, 1916–2010. *Journal of Urban Health, 88*(3). https://doi.org/10.1007/s11524-011-9585-2

Gamoran, A. (2001). American schooling and educational inequality: A forecast for the 21st century. *Sociology of Education* (Extra Issue: Current of Thought: Sociology of Education at the Dawn of the 21st Century), 74, 135–153. https://doi.org/10.2307/2673258

Garcia, M.A., Saenz, J., Downer, B., and Wong, R. (2018). The role of education in the association between race/ethnicity/nativity, cognitive impairment, and dementia among older adults in the United States. *Demographic Research, 38,* 155–168. https://doi.org/10.4054/DemRes.2018.38.6

Gaugler, J.E., Bain, L.J., Mitchell, L., Finlay, J., Fazio, S., Jutkowitz, E., Banerjee, S., Butrum, K., Gaugler, J., Gitlin, L., Hodgson, N., Kallmyer, B., Le Meyer, O., Logsdon, R., Maslow, K., and Zimmerman, S. (2019). Reconsidering frameworks of Alzheimer's dementia when assessing psychosocial outcomes. *Alzheimer's and Dementia: Translational Research and Clinical Interventions, 5,* 388–397. https://doi.org/10.1016/j.trci.2019.02.008

Gitlin, L., Hodgson, N., Piersol, C.V., Hess, E., and Hauck, W. (2014). Correlates of quality of life for individuals with dementia living at home: The role of home environment, caregiver, and patient-related characteristics. *American Journal of Geriatric Psychiatry, 22*(6), 587–597. https://doi.org/10.1016/j.jagp.2012.11.005

Gobbens, R.J.J., and van Assen, M.A.L.M. (2018). Associations of environmental factors with quality of life in older adults. *Gerontologist, 58*(1), 101–110. https://doi.org/10.1093/geront/gnx051

Goins, R.T., Winchester, B., Jiang, L., Grau, L., Reid, M., Corrada, M., Manson, S.M., and O'Connell, J. (2021). Cardiometabolic conditions and all-cause dementia among American Indians and Alaska Native peoples. *Journal of Gerontology: Series A.* https://doi.org/10.1093/gerona/glab097

Graham, C., Scharlach, A.E., and Kurtovich, E. (2016). Do villages promote aging in place? Results of a longitudinal study. *Journal of Applied Gerontology, 37*(3), 310–331. https://doi.org/10.1177/0733464816672046

Graham, C.L., Scharlach, A.E., and Stark, B. (2017). Impact of the village model: Results of a national survey. *Journal of Gerontological Social Work, 60*(5), 335–354. https://doi.org/10.1080/01634372.2017.1330299

Greenfield, E.A., Scharlach, A., Lehning, A., and Davitt, J. (2012). A conceptual framework for examining the promise of the NORC program and village models to promote aging in place. *Journal of Aging Studies, 26*(3), 273–284.

Grenier, A., Lloyd, L., and Phillipson, C. (2017). Precarity in late life: Rethinking dementia as a 'frailed' old age. *Sociology of Health & Illness, 39*(2), 318–330. https://doi.org/10.1111/1467-9566.12476

Guo, Y., Chan, C.H., Chang, Q., Liu, T., and Yip, P. (2019). Neighborhood environment and cognitive function in older adults: A multilevel analysis in Hong Kong. *Health & Place, 58,* 102146. https://doi.org/10.1016/j.healthplace.2019.102146

Hayward, M.D., Farina, M.P., Zhang, Y.S., Kim, J.K., and Crimmins, E.M. (2021). The importance of improving educational attainment for dementia prevalence trends from 2000–2014, among non-Hispanic Black and White Americans. *Journals of Gerontology: Series B.* https://doi.org/10.1093/geronb/gbab015

Hill, T.D., Ross, C.E., and Angel, R.J. (2005). Neighborhood disorder, psychophysiological distress, and health. *Journal of Health and Social Behavior, 46*(2), 170–186. https://doi.org/10.1177/002214650504600204

Hultsch, D.F., Hertzog, C., Small, B.J., and Dixon, R.A. (1999). Use it or lose it: Engaged lifestyle as a buffer of cognitive decline in aging? *Psychology and Aging, 14*(2), 245–263.

James, P., Banay, R.F., Hart, J.E., and Laden, F. (2015). A review of the health benefits of greenness. *Current Epidemiology Reports, 2*(2), 131–142. https://doi.org/10.1007/s40471-015-0043-7

Jervis, L.L., Cullum, C.M, Cox, D., and Manson, S.M. (2018). Dementia assessment in American Indians. In G. Yeo, L.A. Gerdner, and D. Gallagher-Thompson (Eds.), *Ethnicity and the Dementias, 3rd edition* (pp. 108–123). New York: Routledge.

Joint Center for Housing Studies of Harvard University. (2019). *Housing America's Older Adults 2019.* https://www.jchs.harvard.edu/sites/default/files/reports/files/Harvard_JCHS_Housing_Americas_Older_Adults_2019.pdf

Jung, H., and Lee, J-E. (2017). The impact of community-based eHealth self-management intervention among elderly living alone with hypertension. *Journal of Telemedicine and Telecare*, 23, 167–173.

Kelly, M.E., Duff, H., Kelly, S., McHugh Power, J.E., Brennan, S., Lawlor, B.A., and Loughrey, D.G. (2017). The impact of social activities, social networks, social support and social relationships on the cognitive functioning of healthy older adults: A systematic review. *Systematic Reviews*, 6(1), 259. https://doi.org/10.1186/s13643-017-0632-2

Kind, A.J.H., and Buckingham, W.R. (2018). Making neighborhood-disadvantage metrics accessible—The neighborhood atlas. *New England Journal of Medicine*, 378(26), 2456–2458. https://doi.org10.1056/NEJMp1802313

Kitwood, T. (1998). Toward a theory of dementia care: Ethics and interaction. *Journal of Clinical Ethics*, 9, 23–34.

Kramer, B.J. (1996). Dementia and American Indian populations. In G. Yeo and D. Gallagher-Thompson (Eds.), *Ethnicity and the Dementias* (pp. 175–181). Washington, DC: Taylor & Francis.

Larson, E.B. (2010). Prospects for delaying the rising tide of worldwide, late-life dementias. *International Journal of Geriatric Psychiatry*, 22(8), 1196–1202.

Latham, K., and Clarke, P. (2016). Neighborhood disorder, perceived social cohesion, and social participation among older Americans: Findings from the National Health & Aging Trends Study. *Journal of Aging and Health*, 30(1). https://doi/org/10.1177/0898264316665933

Lawrence, E., Hummer, R.A., and Harris, K.M. (2017). The cardiovascular health of young adults: Disparities along the urban-rural continuum. *ANNALS of the American Academy of Political and Social Science*, 672(1), 257–281. https://doi.org/10.1177/0002716217711426

LeadingAge. (2019). *How Do Older Baby Boomers Envision Their Quality of Life If They Need Long-Term Care Services?* https://leadingage.org/sites/default/files/HOW%20DO%20OLDER%20BABY%20BOOMERS%20ENVISION_FINAL.pdf

Lepore, M., Ferrell, A., and Wiener, J. (2017). *Living Arrangements of People with Alzheimer's Disease and Related Dementias: Implications for Services and Supports.* https://aspe.hhs.gov/system/files/pdf/257966/LivingArran.pdf

Leventhal, T., and Brooks-Gunn, J. (2000). The neighborhoods they live in: The effects of neighborhood residence on child and adolescent outcomes. *Psychological Bulletin*, 126(2), 309–337. https://doi.org/10.1037/0033-2909.126.2.309

Levy, B.L., Phillips, N.E., and Sampson, R.J. (2020). Triple disadvantage: Neighborhood networks of everyday urban mobility and violence in U.S. cities. *American Sociological Review*, 85(6), 925–956. https://doi.org/10.1177/0003122420972323

Lewis, J.P., Manson, S.M., Jernigan, V., and Noonan, C. (2020). "Making sense of a disease that makes no sense": Understanding Alzheimer's disease and related disorders among caregivers and providers in Alaska. *Gerontologist*, 61(3), 363–373. https://doi.org/10.1093/geront/gnaa102

Liang, J., Aranda, M.P., and Lloyd, D.A. (2020). Association between role overload and sleep disturbance among dementia caregivers: The impact of social support and social engagement. *Journal of Aging and Health*, 32(10), 1345–1354. https://doi.org/10.1177/0898264320926062

Lin, S.Y. (2017). "Dementia-friendly communities" and being dementia friendly in healthcare settings. *Current Opinion in Psychiatry*, 30(2), 145–150. https://doi.org/10.1097/YCO.0000000000000304

McHugh Power, J.E., Lee, O., Aspell, N., McCormack, E., Loftus, M., Connolly, L., Lawlor, B., and Brennan, S. (2016). RelAte: Pilot study of the effects of a mealtime intervention on social cognitive factors and energy intake among older adults living alone. *British Journal of Nutrition*, 116, 1573–1581.

Millar, R.J. (2020). Neighborhood cohesion, disorder, and physical function in older adults: An examination of racial/ethnic differences. *Journal of Aging and Health*, *32*(9), 1133–1144. https://doi.org/10.1177/0898264319890944

Mulvaney-Day, N.E., Alegría, M., and Sribney, W. (2007). Social cohesion, social support, and health among Latinos in the United States. *Social Science & Medicine*, *64*(2), 477–495. https://doi.org/10.1016/j.socscimed.2006.08.030

Nardone, A., Rudolph, K.E., Morello-Frosch, R., and Casey, J.A. (2021). Redlines and greenspace: The relationship between historical redlining and 2010 greenspace across the United States. *Environmental Health Perspective*, *129*(1), 17006. https://doi.org/10.1289/EHP7495

NASEM (National Academies of Sciences, Engineering, and Medicine). (2017). *Communities in Action: Pathways to Health Equity*. Washington, DC: The National Academies Press. https://doi.org/10.17226/24624

———. (2019a). *Fostering Healthy Mental, Emotional, and Behavioral Development in Children and Youth: A National Agenda*. Washington, DC: The National Academies Press. https://doi.org/10.17226/25201

———. (2019b). *Investing in Interventions that Address Non-Medical, Health-Related Social Needs: Proceedings of a Workshop*. Washington, DC: The National Academies Press. https://doi.org/10.17226/25544

———. (2020). *Social Isolation and Loneliness in Older Adults: Opportunities for the Health Care System*. Washington, DC: The National Academies Press. https://doi.org/10.17226/25663

———. (2021). *Population Health in Rural America: Proceedings of a Workshop*. Washington, DC: The National Academies Press. https://doi.org/10.17226/25989

National Council on Aging. (2015). *Get the Facts on Senior Centers*. https://www.ncoa.org/article/get-the-facts-on-senior-centers#intraPageNav4

Ng, T.P., Nyunt, M., Shuvo, F.K., Eng, J.Y., Yap, K.B., Hee, L.M., Chan, S.P., and Scherer, S. (2018). The neighborhood built environment and cognitive function of older persons: Results from the Singapore Longitudinal Ageing Study. *Gerontology*, *64*(2), 149–156. https://doi.org/10.1159/000480080

Nieuwenhuijsen, M.J. (2018). Influence of urban and transport planning and the city environment on cardiovascular disease. *Nature Reviews Cardiology*, *15*(7), 432–438. https://doi.org/10.1038/s41569-018-0003-2

Office of the Assistant Secretary for Planning and Evaluation. (2019, October 21). *Expanding Access to LTSS through Caregiver Support*. https://aspe.hhs.gov/advisory-council-october-2019-meeting-presentation-expanding-access-ltss

Penninkilampi, R., Casey, A.N., Singh, M.F., and Brodaty, H. (2018). The association between social engagement, loneliness, and risk of dementia: A systematic review and meta-analysis. *Journal of Alzheimer's Disease*, *66*(4), 1619–1633. https://doi.org/10.3233/JAD-180439

Phillipson, L., Hall, D., Cridland, E., Fleming, R., Brennan-Horley, C., Guggisberg, N., Frost, D., and Hasan, H. (2019). Involvement of people with dementia in raising awareness and changing attitudes in a dementia friendly community pilot project. *Dementia (London, England)*, *18*(7-8), 2679–2694. https://doi.org/10.1177/1471301218754455

Powell, W.R., Buckingham, W.R., and Larson, J.L. (2020). Association of neighborhood-level disadvantage with Alzheimer Disease neuropathology. *JAMA Network Open*, *3*(6), e207559. https://doi.org/10.1001/jamanetworkopen.2020.7559

Power, M.C., Adar, S.D., Yanosky, J.D., and Weuve, J. (2016). Exposure to air pollution as a potential contributor to cognitive function, cognitive decline, brain imaging, and dementia: A systematic review of epidemiologic research. *Neurotoxicology*, *56*, 235–253. https://doi.org/10.1016/j.neuro.2016.06.004

Probst, J., Eberth, J.M., and Crouch, E. (2019). Structural urbanism contributes to poorer health outcomes for rural America. *Health Affairs (Project Hope)*, 38(12), 1976–1984. https://doi.org/10.1377/hlthaff.2019.00914

Riley, A. (2018). Neighborhood disadvantage, residential segregation, and beyond—Lessons for studying structural racism and health. *Journal of Racial and Ethnic Health Disparities*, 5, 357–365. https://doi.org/10.1007/s40615-017-0378-5

Robertson, D., Killimannis, B., and Kenny, R. (2016). Negative perceptions of aging predict longitudinal decline in cognitive function. *Psychology and Aging*, 31(1), 71–81. https://doi.org/10.1037/pag0000061

Rodrigues, D.E., César, C.C., Xavier, C.C., Caiaffa, W.T., and Proietti, F.A. (2021). Exploring neighborhood socioeconomic disparity in self-rated health: A multiple mediation analysis. *Preventive Medicine*, 145, 106443. https://doi.org/10.1016/j.ypmed.2021.106443

Rote, S.M., Angel, J.L., and Markides, K. (2017). Neighborhood context, dementia severity, and Mexican American caregiver well-being. *Journal of Aging and Health*, 29(6), 1039–1055. https://doi.org/10.1177/0898264317707141

Saczynski, J.S., Pfeifer, L.A., Masaki, K., Korf, E.S., Laurin, D., White, L., and Launer, L.J. (2006). The effect of social engagement on incident dementia: The Honolulu-Asia Aging Study. *American Journal of Epidemiology*, 163(5), 433–440. https://doi.org/10.1093/aje/kwj061

Saenz, J.L., Wong, R., and Ailshire, J.A. (2018). Indoor air pollution and cognitive function among older Mexican adults. *Journal of Epidemiology and Community Health*, 72(1), 21–26. https://doi.org/10.1136/jech-2017-209704

Sanders, A., Smathers, K., Patterson, T., Stone, R., Kahn, J., Marshall, J., and Alecxih, L. (2015). *Service Availability in HUD-Assisted Senior Housing: Findings from a Survey on the Availability of Onsite Services in HUD-Assisted Senior Housing*. Washington, DC: LeadingAge. http://www.ltsscenter.org/resource-library/Service_Availability_in_HUD_Assisted_Senior_Housing.pdf

Sheffield, K.M., and Peek, M.K. (2009). Neighborhood context and cognitive decline in older Mexican Americans: Results from the Hispanic Established Populations for Epidemiologic Studies of the Elderly. *American Journal of Epidemiology*, 169(9), 1092–1101. https://doi.org/10.1093/aje/kwp005

Sherman, C. (2014). *Environmental Influence on the Developing Brain: A Report from the Fifth Annual Aspen Brain Forum*. Dana Foundation. https://dana.org/article/environmental-influence-on-the-developing-brain

Solomon, D., Maxwell, C., and Castro, A. (2019, August 7). *Systemic Inequality: Displacement, Exclusion, and Segregation*. Center for American Progress. https://www.americanprogress.org/issues/race/reports/2019/08/07/472617/systemic-inequality-displacement-exclusion-segregation

South, E.C., Kondo, M.C., Cheney, R.A., and Branas, C.C. (2015). Neighborhood blight, stress, and health: A walking trial of urban greening and ambulatory heart rate. *American Journal of Public Health*, 105(5), 909–913. https://doi.org/10.2105/AJPH.2014.302526

Sundström, A., Adolfsson, A.N., Nordin, M., and Adolfsson, R. (2020). Loneliness increases the risk of all-cause dementia and Alzheimer's disease. *Journals of Gerontology: Series B*, 75(5), 919–926.

Sutin, A.R., Stephan, Y., Luchetti, M., and Terracciano, A. (2020). Loneliness and risk of dementia. *Journals of Gerontology: Series B*, 75(7), 1414–1422.

Swarbrick, C.M., Doors, O., Scottish Dementia Working Group, Educate, Davis, K., and Keady, J. (2019). Visioning change: Co-producing a model of involvement and engagement in research (innovative practice). *Dementia*, 18(7–8), 3165–3172. https://doi.org/10.1177/1471301216674559

University of Southern California. (2020). *Contextual Data Resource for Aging Surveys.* https://gero.usc.edu/cbph/cdr

Victor, C.R., Rippon, I., Nelis, S.M., Martyr, A., Litherland, R., Pickett, J., Hart, N., Henley, J., Matthews, F., Clare, L., and IDEAL programme team. (2020). Prevalence and determinants of loneliness in people living with dementia: Findings from the IDEAL programme. *International Journal of Geriatric Psychiatry, 35*(8), 851–858. https://doi.org/10.1002/gps.5305

Warshaw, R. (2017, October 31). *Health Disparities Affect Millions in Rural U.S. Communities.* Association of American Medical Colleges. https://www.aamc.org/news-insights/health-disparities-affect-millions-rural-us-communities

Weuve, J., D'Souza, J., Beck, T., Evans, D.A., Kaufman, J.D., Rajan, K.B., de Leon, C., and Adar, S.D. (2020). Long-term community noise exposure in relation to dementia, cognition, and cognitive decline in older adults. *Alzheimer's & Dementia, 17*(2) 525–533. https://doi.org/10.1002/alz.12191

Williams, D.R., and Collins, C. (2001). Racial residential segregation: A fundamental cause of racial disparities in health. *Public Health Reports, 116*(5), 404–416. https://doi.org/10.1093/phr/116.5.404

Williams, D.R., and Earl, T.R. (2007). Commentary: Race and mental health—More questions than answers. *International Journal of Epidemiology, 36*, 758–760.

Wilson, R.S., Krueger, K.R., Arnold, S.E., Schneider, J.A., Kelly, J.F., Barnes, L.L., Tang, Y., and Bennett, D.A. (2007). Loneliness and risk of Alzheimer Disease. *Archives of General Psychiatry, 64*(2), 234–240.

Witten, D. (2019). *When Medicaid in Washington State Will Pay for a Nursing Home, Assisted Living, or Home Health Care.* Nolo. https://www.nolo.com/legal-encyclopedia/when-washington-state-medicaid-will-pay-for-long-term-care.html

Woo, B., Kravitz-Wirtz, N., Sass, V., Crowder, K., Teixeira, S., and Takeuchi, D.T. (2019). Residential segregation and racial/ethnic disparities in ambient air pollution. *Race and Social Problems, 11*(1), 60–67. https://doi.org/10.1007/s12552-018-9254-0

World Dementia Council. (2019). *Impacts of Dementia Friendly Initiatives: Presenting a Global Evidence Base for Dementia Friendly Initiatives.* https://worlddementiacouncil.org/sites/default/files/2020-12/DFIs%20-%20Paper%202_V15.pdf

Wu, Y.T., Prina, A.M., and Brayne, C. (2015a). The association between community environment and cognitive function: A systematic review. *Social Psychiatry and Psychiatric Epidemiology, 50*(3), 351–362. https://doi.org/10.1007/s00127-014-0945-6

Wu, Y.T., Prina, A.M., Jones, A.P., Barnes, L.E., Matthews, F.E., Brayne, C., and Medical Research Council Cognitive Function and Ageing Study. (2015b). Community environment, cognitive impairment and dementia in later life: Results from the Cognitive Function and Ageing Study. *Age and Ageing, 44*(6), 1005–1011. https://doi.org/10.1093/ageing/afv137

Wu, Y.T., Beiser, A.S., Breteler, M.M.B., Fratiglioni, L., Helmer, C., Hendrie, H.C., Honda, H., Ikram, M.A., Langa, K., Lobo, A., Matthews, F., Ohara, T., Pérès, K., Qiu, C., Seshadri, S., Sjölund, B., Skoog, I., and Brayne, C. (2017). The changing prevalence and incidence of dementia over time—Current evidence. *Nature Reviews Neurology, 13*(6), 327–339. https://doi.org10.1038/nrneurol.2017.63

Wurm, S., and Benyamini, Y. (2014). Optimism buffers the detrimental effect of negative self-perceptions of ageing on physical and mental health. *Journal of Psychological Health.* https://doi.org/10.1080/08870446.2014.891737

Yin, S., Yang, Q., Xiong, J., Li, T., and Zhu, X. (2020). Social support and the incidence of cognitive impairment among older adults in China: Findings from the Chinese Longitudinal Healthy Longevity Survey Study. *Frontiers in Psychiatry, 11*, 254. https://doi.org/10.3389/fpsyt.2020.00254

Zahodne, L.B., Manly, J.J., Smith, J., Seeman, T., and Lachman, M.E. (2017). Socioeconomic, health, and psychosocial mediators of racial disparities in cognition in early, middle, and late adulthood. *Psychology and Aging*, *32*(2), 118.

Zuckerman, I.H., Ryder, P.T., Simoni-Wastila, L., Shaffer, T., Sato, M., Zhao, L., and Stuart, B. (2008). Racial and ethnic disparities in the treatment of dementia among Medicare beneficiaries. *Journals of Gerontology: Series B*, *63*(5), S328–S333.

Zuelsdorff, M., Larson, J.L., Hunt, J.F.V., Kim, A.J., Koscik, R.L., Buckingham, W.R., Gleason, C.E., Johnson, S.C., Asthana, S., Rissman, R.A., Bendlin, B.B., and Kind, A.J.H. (2020). The Area Deprivation Index: A novel tool for harmonizable risk assessment in Alzheimer's disease research. *Alzheimer's & Dementia*, *6*(1), e12039. https://doi.org/10.1002/trc2.12039

6

Health Care, Long-Term Care, and End-of-Life Care

People living with dementia are most often diagnosed and treated by a primary care physician, but many are also treated by numerous other medical specialists, for both dementia and other conditions, as their diseases progress. They also are likely to interact with many different institutions that provide health care and social support as their dementia symptoms become more severe and they lose their ability to function independently. And many of those who become totally dependent upon others will spend time living in long-term care facilities and ultimately receive such care as hospice at the end of life.

Thus, people living with dementia have relationships with numerous professionals and institutions—often a great many, over time—including primary care providers; neurologists, psychiatrists, geriatricians, and nurse practitioners who specialize in dementia care; social workers; and public and private entities that provide residential and end-of-life care. Each interaction may be comforting and beneficial, or may fall short of that ideal. These interactions are shaped by the characteristics of the institutions that provide care, which are often large and complex, and the systems of which they are a part. These systems, in turn, are shaped by the policy environment and other contextual factors discussed in Chapter 1. Earlier chapters have also explained how differences in the quality and availability of all types of care and the way these services are funded have significant impacts on individuals and families. This chapter examines the functioning of the systems that provide health care, long-term care, and end-of-life care for people living with dementia, including how well they support those people and their families, as well as how they are funded.

The committee's aim for this chapter was to provide an overview of key issues for these fundamental supports for people living with dementia, but we were unable to address every issue of importance in detail. We note that the experiences individuals have with the institutions that provide these supports vary enormously depending on where they live, as well as their financial circumstances, level of educational attainment, access to care, assumptions about need, help-seeking behavior, and other factors: there is no "average" experience. Therefore, we focused on care delivery models that have been evaluated and described in the research literature, and looked for opportunities to improve care.

THE HEALTH CARE SYSTEM

People living with dementia need care for the disease that causes it, which is typically offered by a primary care provider. They also require routine health care, and individuals in this predominantly older population frequently have other serious medical conditions. Managing this care is a challenge for people living with dementia and their family caregivers. Questions about the quality of dementia care provided by nonspecialists and how patients fare when they have other significant medical conditions are key to reducing negative impacts. This section looks first at what is known about the quality of primary care and then at approaches to coordinating care.

Quality of Primary Care

Primary care providers, such as physicians and advanced practice providers (nurse practitioners, physician assistants, and clinical nurse specialists), provide first-line care for people with dementia. These practitioners often have long-term relationships with their patients, which can be an advantage for identifying and managing dementia. However, the training received by primary care physicians in internal and family medicine provides limited opportunities to learn about managing care for people living with dementia in an ambulatory care setting, although some may have had experience with patients in the later stages of dementia through working in nursing home settings. A lack of training and experience in caring for people with dementia can mean missed or delayed diagnosis and less-than-optimal management of care. A recent survey of primary care physicians showed that many feel they lack knowledge and confidence in their skills in this area, are uncertain about how to diagnose dementia, and find the condition challenging to manage (Lee et al., 2020). By one estimate, of the 730,026 physicians practicing in the United Sates in 2019, 228,936, or 31 percent, were primary care physicians (Willis et al., 2020), and in 2020, only 6,896 primary care physicians were geriatricians with specific training in providing care for patients with dementia (American Board of Medical Specialties, 2020).

There are guidelines for the care that people living with dementia should receive, such as the quality indicators shown in Box 6-1. However, related research indicates that many patients do not receive optimal care and that few of these indicators of quality are routinely met. By one estimate based on a series of observational studies, adherence to current standards averaged 44 percent across all dementia quality indicators (Jennings et al., 2016).

Unfortunately, little research is available to guide further development of policies and best practices related to the provision of primary care to persons living with dementia. For example, one might expect that a

---

BOX 6-1
Quality Indicators for Dementia Care

Domain: Assessment and Screening
- Annual assessment of cognition
- Staging of dementia
- Annual evaluation of function
- Labs performed
- Depression screening
- Annual screening for behavioral symptoms
- Annual medication review

Domain: Counseling
- Caregiver counseled in at least two of the following domains:
  - dementia diagnosis, prognosis, or behavioral symptoms
  - safety
  - community resources
- Counseled regarding driving
- Counseled about advance care planning or palliative care
- Identification of a surrogate decision maker

Domain: Treatment
- Discussion about acetylcholinesterase inhibitors
- Cerebrovascular accident or stroke prophylaxis, if indicated
- Treatment with behavioral interventions before or concurrently with medications
- Assessment of response to new medication for dementia or depression
- Risks/benefits discussion documented for new antipsychotics
- Medications discontinued or justified when associated with mental health status changes

SOURCE: Adapted from Jennings et al. (2016). Used with permission from John Wiley and Sons, *Journal of the American Geriatrics Society*.

multispecialty practice would be better able to manage the complex needs of persons with dementia, either because some primary care physicians could specialize in managing such patients or because centralized care management resources could be available to the entire practice. However, there is as yet no evidence pointing to specific ways to improve the quality and consistency of the dementia care provided by primary care practitioners in settings that do not include specific dementia care programs.

Fragmentation of Care Delivery

From the perspective of patients and families, what is most important is that they are aware of, understand, and are able to easily access the care and services they need. The current care delivery system offers little guidance to older adults, including those with dementia or mild cognitive impairment (MCI) and their families, in navigating and managing health care and long-term care systems. In practice, needs for care include medical issues, such as management of other conditions and coordination of prescriptions, as well as help with daily living, such as preventing falls, ensuring that prescriptions are taken correctly, and managing incontinence. Individuals living with dementia experience more frequent hospitalizations and longer stays relative to their peers without dementia, and these hospitalizations are a prime contributor both to high medical costs for this population and to morbidity (Lin, 2020).

The challenges of managing multiple conditions are exacerbated by cognitive impairment. Each progressive, chronic condition an individual develops may involve an additional specialist or clinic for a patient who is likely to be challenged by the need to manage that added complexity. While care coordination is very important for all older patients with complex chronic conditions, it is especially important for those living with dementia and their caregivers, who must navigate the complex transitions between care settings and health care providers. Many such care providers have limited experience with the needs of people with impaired cognition. There is evidence, for example, that dementia patients with other medical issues receive less consistent treatment and monitoring for such conditions as visual impairment and diabetes relative to those with similar conditions who do not have dementia (Bunn et al., 2014).

Comprehensive Dementia Care

Increasingly, health care delivery systems are responding both to the needs of their patients and to a movement for incentive-based changes in health care financing by exploring comprehensive approaches to providing care. For example, a program developed at the University of California,

Los Angeles, the UCLA Alzheimer's and Dementia Care Program, was designed to coordinate the care provided by diverse practitioners, with the goal of maximizing patients' functioning, independence, and dignity and decreasing strain on caregivers (Reuben et al., 2013). Another example is the Integrated Memory Care Clinic, a medical home designed to coordinate the care provided by geriatric nurses, social workers, and various medical specialists (Clevenger et al., 2018). Other models include home visits and telephone management by nonlicensed or licensed providers supported by clinical professionals (Haggerty et al., 2020). Programs designed to provide comprehensive care include such elements as

- continuous monitoring and assessment,
- development of a care plan,
- psychosocial interventions,
- providing the patient with self-management tools,
- caregiver support,
- medication management,
- treatment of related conditions, and
- coordination of care (Boustani et al., 2019).

Studies of such programs suggest benefits that include improvements in behavioral and emotional symptoms and reductions or delay in the need for admission to a long-term care facility (Reuben et al., 2019b; Jennings et al., 2019, 2020; see also Haggerty et al., 2020). A study of Medicare fee-for-service claims suggests that people with dementia who had access to some plan for ensuring continuity of care had lower rates of hospital admission and fewer emergency room visits relative to those who had less continuity of care (Amjad et al., 2016).

Although the committee that produced a recent National Academies' report recommended disseminating collaborative care models that use multidisciplinary teams, care of this kind is not yet readily available in most communities (National Academies of Sciences, Engineering, and Medicine [NASEM], 2021). Dissemination has stalled at least in part because these models are not financially viable under current reimbursement structures. Some comparative effectiveness research to test such comprehensive approaches is under way, but additional pragmatic trials and assessment of the impacts of reimbursement structure and other issues, will be important extensions of existing research.

A Model of Comprehensive Care at the Population Level

Researchers have explored ways to bring the benefits of evidence-based dementia care to larger populations. One proposed model is for health systems to design dementia care from a population perspective by planning for the types and intensity of medical and support services likely to be needed by different segments of the dementia population they serve (Reuben et al., 2019a). This model allows a health system to use estimates of the number of people it serves who currently have dementia, combined with assessments of the patient needs typical at different phases of the disease, to project the types of services likely to be needed. Figure 6-1 shows a model of the stages experienced by persons living with dementia (five stages identified in the tiers of the pyramid) and the severity of the symptoms associated with each (on the left side of the pyramid) (Reuben et al., 2019a). It identifies how many persons (among the 5,000 in the example) are likely to be at each stage at a given time and indicates the likely needs of individuals for health care system resources at each tier (on the right side of the pyramid). The information in the tiers indicates the intensity and resources associated with each stage of disease progression.

Figure 6-2 shows in more detail the issues at play in caring for individuals who progress through the stages of disease.

A comprehensive dementia care approach such as this may benefit patients and families, and also yield cost savings for both patients and the health care system. For example, this type of analysis could support improved planning to strengthen the resources in the home (allowing individuals to live at home longer), coordinate medical care, establish and maintain links to community resources, and provide support to caregivers—thus helping to delay the phase when patients need the highest levels of care (Jennings et al., 2019). For those with behavioral symptoms, behavioral health

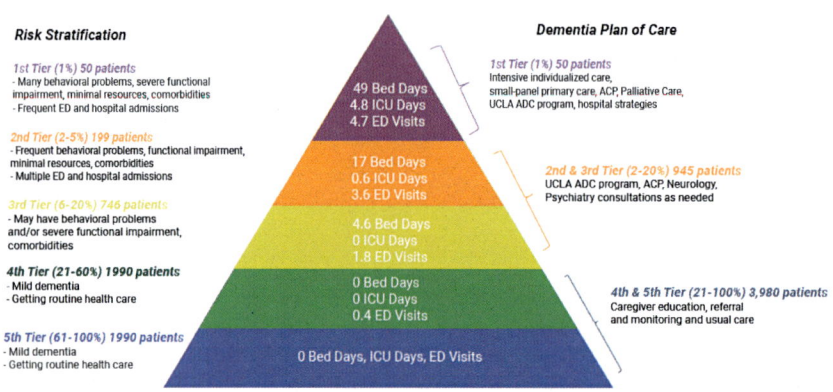

FIGURE 6-1 Stages of dementia and care needs.
SOURCE: Reuben et al. (2019a). Reprinted with permission from Project Hope/ *Health Affairs Journal.*

HEALTH CARE, LONG-TERM CARE, AND END-OF-LIFE CARE

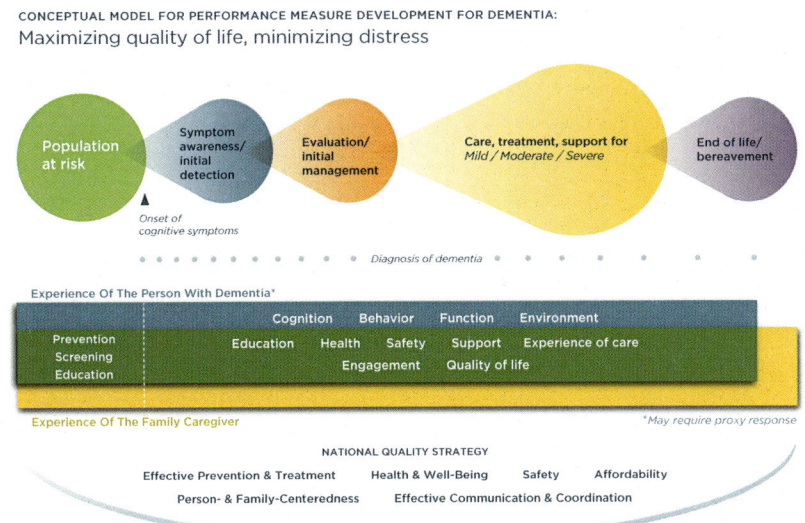

FIGURE 6-2 Conceptual model of disease progression and care.
SOURCE: National Quality Forum (2014). Reprinted with permission.

care providers may be helpful in reducing admissions to psychiatric units and long-term nursing home placement. We note that integrating mental health care with care for dementia symptoms and with the care provided in residential facilities is a challenge, as it is in other parts of the health care system, though a detailed exploration of these issues was beyond the scope of this report.

The potential benefits of a population-based approach can be considerable. For patients who enter the top tier shown in Figure 6-1, the costs of institutional care are extraordinarily high, and the benefits of such expenditures in terms of the duration or quality of life are uncertain. People at this stage frequently have patterns of recurrent or prolonged hospitalization, most often for infectious diseases or behavioral complications of dementia (e.g., agitation, aggression). Those admitted to a psychiatry unit because of behavioral problems often have prolonged stays (some more than 40 days) because it is usually very difficult to find nursing or assisted living facilities that will accept these patients (for reasons that include staff time needed and potential liability resulting from patient or staff injuries). Some patients require a legally authorized guardian (conservatorship) to make discharge decisions, and the legal system for establishing this arrangement is often slow. Palliative care or hospice (discussed below) is not a substitute for permanent nursing home placement, although among those with very advanced dementia, it can help prevent repeated hospital transfers that are distressing for the patient and result in little or no benefit.

Knowledge Gaps

The disease and health care needs model discussed above offers a valuable heuristic for assessing the progression of dementia and associated needs. However, population-based management of the disease trajectory of people living with dementia is realistic only in an integrated health system that cares for enough dementia patients to justify creating such programs. Many people living with dementia do not receive care in a health system but rely on a primary care physician who serves a wide array of patients, relatively few of whom have dementia. It is difficult for small or solo practices to provide the expertise and access to programs needed by dementia patients. In one study of dementia diagnoses and health care over the 5-year period following diagnosis, 85 percent of Medicare beneficiaries were diagnosed by a primary care or an internal medicine physician or other nondementia specialist physician. Five years later, only about one-third had received any care by a dementia specialist (Drabo et al., 2019). Among older fee-for-service Medicare beneficiaries with a dementia diagnosis, lower continuity of care is associated with higher rates of hospitalization, emergency department visits, testing, and health care spending (Amjad et al., 2016). It is not known what proportion of providers are embedded in an integrated delivery system, but it is reasonable to assume that access to such delivery systems varies by urban or rural location and by the patient's race, ethnicity, income, and education.

Additional information is needed to support widespread adoption of comprehensive care models. One challenge is the considerable variation in the clinical progression of the disease and the associated variability in the range and timing of health care utilization. To date, few empirical, population-based studies have systematically documented individuals' progression through the phases of dementia and the care needs and health care costs associated with a dementia diagnosis. One study that focused on Medicare fee-for-service beneficiaries used indicators of patients' use of services (e.g., diagnosis date, initial postacute care, nursing home placement) as a measure (Bentkover et al., 2012). However, this approach captured data only for individuals who use services that incur charges, excluding data for care provided by, for example, family members. Better empirical estimates of the rate of progression through the natural phases of the disease would be extremely helpful to the field in general but also to the many health care systems trying to plan for the needs of this population.

A second issue is that although a number of care models have been implemented and studied (e.g., Possin et al., 2019; Callahan et al., 2006), few of these studies have been replicated. Such studies have established that model programs can be efficacious under optimal conditions. However, more embedded pragmatic clinical trials are needed to identify how such models can be implemented in real-world circumstances. Some work is under way to pursue this goal. The National Institute on Aging has recently made a considerable investment in testing pilot projects that, once completed, can be launched as pragmatic clinical trials embedded in fully functioning health care systems. The **IM**bedded Pragmatic Alzheimer's disease (AD) and AD-Related Dementias (AD/ADRD) Clinical Trials (IMPACT) Collaboratory was established to solicit pilot applications of promising interventions for which there is evidence of efficacy and then to fund, support, and monitor them as part of an effort to build the evidence base for embedded pragmatic trials focused on improving care for persons living with dementia and their caregivers (Mitchell et al., 2020).

LONG-TERM AND END-OF-LIFE CARE

There are several ways to meet the needs of patients and families in the later stages of dementia, when they require more comprehensive daily support. While it is common for people entering the terminal stage of dementia to be admitted to a nursing home or the memory care unit of an assisted living facility, the duration of such placements varies considerably, and many of these individuals are cared for at home.

State policies and regulations have a significant impact on residential care such as assisted living and memory care. Aside from an infrequently used accreditation program, there are no national definitions, standards, enforcement mechanisms, financing programs, or regulations for these residential settings, although they serve nearly 1 million people across the states; 41.9 percent of individuals in residential care and 47.8 percent of nursing home residents (2016 data) are diagnosed with dementia (Harris-Kojetin et al., 2019).[1] Thus, it falls to states to regulate the safety of and care provided in these facilities. States also set Medicaid reimbursement rates for various services, including nursing home care, home care, and case management, and states have some flexibility with Medicaid eligibility. Reimbursement methods differ across states, and reimbursement rates vary substantially. State legislatures may also pursue unique policy goals. For instance, in 2019 Washington State became the first state to establish an entitlement to funding for long-term services and supports by enacting the Washington State Long-Term Care Trust Act, recognizing the impact of dementia and other functional impairments that lead to a need for paid help (Gleckman, 2019).

Options for providing the necessary care and support for patients in their own homes have been expanding, but payment for long-term care, which is extremely expensive, remains a challenge. This section considers issues associated with assisted living and memory units, nursing homes, alternatives to nursing homes, and palliative and hospice care.

---

[1] These data include only facilities that are regulated by states or the federal government.

Assisted Living and Memory Units

Assisted living and memory care or dementia units serve a small but significant percentage of dementia patients. The number of specialty care memory units, including those housed within a larger care system (e.g., part of an assisted living setting), has increased recently, from approximately 63,000 in 2013 to 98,000 in 2018 (Adler, 2018). Unlike nursing homes, which rely heavily on Medicaid financing, assisted living facilities are usually paid for privately, generally out of pocket, but occasionally through long-term care insurance.[2] These units often feature modified environments (e.g., exit controls, safety accommodations, and other designs that promote security and safety); offer dementia-related services, such as medication management; and have staff who have completed training in dementia. Such targeted dementia care has been associated with outcomes that include reduced rates of depression, improved medication adherence, and decreased emergency room use (Zimmerman et al., 2005). However, relatively little is known about the attributes of and regulatory requirements for this type of care that affect outcomes and quality of life for people with dementia, or the delivery, structure, quality, and financing of these facilities.

Nursing Homes

Dementia is the most common clinical diagnosis among persons residing in the approximately 15,600 nursing homes in the United States. Just under 70 percent of nursing homes are privately owned for-profit entities (Harris-Kojetin et al., 2019). Nursing homes serve two populations:

1. long-stay patients, for whom costs are often paid by Medicaid, predominantly at or below the actual cost of providing care; and
2. postacute residents, for whom fees are paid by Medicare or commercial insurers at a higher reimbursement rate generally exceeding care costs.

Postacute residents, who account for more than 90 percent of admissions to most nursing homes, come from hospitals to receive skilled, rehabilitative care following an acute care hospital episode, with the goal of being discharged to the community (Rahman et al., 2014; Tyler et al., 2013). Although the majority of nursing homes provide both long-stay and postacute care, many have sought to specialize in the latter, marketing their facilities to hospitals and Medicare Advantage plans to increase admissions

---

[2]In 2014, 330,000 Medicaid beneficiaries received assisted living services (U.S. Government Accountability Office, 2018a, 2018b).

of such patients and competing to build preferred relationships with local hospitals to maintain their referral base (Mor et al., 2016; Rahman et al., 2013). While most postacute nursing home patients return home, persons living with dementia are more likely to "get stuck" and become permanent nursing home residents. A recent study found that those admitted with a secondary diagnosis of dementia were substantially less likely to return home and also remained longer in the nursing home (Bardenheier et al., 2020).

Medicaid is the primary payer for long-stay nursing home care. Thus, it is important to note that the care financed by Medicaid has long been plagued by quality and safety problems, ranging from inadequate staffing to high rates of infection and hospitalization (Institute of Medicine, 1986, 2001; Mor et al., 2004).[3] While major regulatory policies, including the Nursing Home Reform Act of 1987 and subsequent revisions, have attempted to address these deficiencies in the quality of care, concerns remain. One is that the current oversight system, implemented by individual states, produces inconsistent outcomes and emphasizes punishment rather than quality improvement (Angelelli et al., 2003). On the other hand, recent efforts to increase the transparency of nursing home quality and tie it directly to payment have also produced only modest quality improvements (Werner et al., 2009, 2012, 2013, 2016).

The COVID-19 pandemic has highlighted the shortcomings of the current system of long-term care. Nursing home residents and staff in the United States were hit particularly hard by the virus, which caused extremely high rates of infection and death in nursing homes and other congregate care settings (35–40% of COVID-19 deaths as of fall 2020 [Soucheray, 2020]; see Chapter 1). Although the primary determinant of an outbreak of COVID-19 is the prevalence of the virus in the adjacent area, most nursing homes lacked the resources necessary to contain an outbreak, including tests and personal protective equipment (Altman, 2020; Gorges and Konetzka, 2020; Chatterjee et al., 2020; White et al., 2020; Abrams et al., 2020; Panagiotou et al., 2021; Ouslander and Grabowski, 2020). Moreover, regulatory requirements were difficult to follow and subject to rapid change. New York State, for instance, at one point imposed stiff fines on nursing homes that refused to admit patients diagnosed with COVID but later rescinded this requirement under public pressure (Sapien and Sexton, 2020). Furthermore, nursing home staff are routinely underpaid and undertrained, and many work multiple jobs, which increased the risk of transmitting the virus across facilities (Chen et al., 2020; Van Houtven et al., 2020). The spread of the virus also was exacerbated by the use of

---

[3] A forthcoming National Academies' report will address nursing home quality issues in detail; see https://www.nationalacademies.org/our-work/the-quality-of-care-in-nursing-homes.

shared living quarters and communal spaces in nursing homes, as well as the intimate nature of the needed care, which makes social distancing or isolation difficult if not impossible.

Alternatives to Nursing Homes

Many Americans would prefer to avoid living in a nursing home, and the continuing quality problems discussed above have given rise to the development of numerous alternative residential settings specifically for dementia care. These alternatives include assisted living communities, independent or retirement communities, and memory care communities, and can encompass both institutional and residential care. Access to and payment for such settings vary, and states have significant discretion over what Medicaid will cover. For example, while Medicaid will not pay for the room and board portion of senior living fees, some states do have waivers that allow Medicaid to cover the portion associated with enriched services (e.g., care coordination, nurse practitioner clinics, meals, and transportation). Most states provide reimbursement for assisted living through Medicaid programs. However, all but a few states have imposed limits on the number of places that are paid by Medicaid, and they have capped daily reimbursement rates at well under the prevailing private pay rates. Lack of long-term care insurance and the limits of Medicaid mean that most people finance their senior living using personal savings, housing equity, or family out-of-pocket contributions. Unfortunately, the ways in which families in different populations finance care and the impact on their financial security have not been well studied.

As researchers and policy makers contemplate the future of long-term care after COVID-19, one intriguing approach is to reimagine the physical layout of nursing homes for long-stay residents. Emerging evidence suggests that smaller facilities serving approximately a dozen individuals and emphasizing a home-like environment, such as those developed by the Green House Project (see Box 6-2), are associated with superior quality of life (Grabowski and Mor, 2020; Werner et al., 2020; Zimmerman et al., 2016). However, current evidence on home-like residential care models is limited (Ausserhofer et al., 2016). In addition, models that involve replacing an existing physical plant or undertaking a comprehensive redesign require substantial capital outlay, and ongoing operating costs could be higher as well. The cost to government in terms of the number of inspectors visiting a large number of small facilities would be an additional consideration in contemplating such a transformation of the residential care system. Evaluation of such projects would provide a foundation for further innovation and the real-world application of these kinds of approaches.

It would also be useful to know more about patterns of use of alternatives to nursing homes. States are increasingly using Medicaid waivers for home and

> **BOX 6-2**
> **The Green House Project**
>
> The Green House Project[a] is a nonprofit organization that develops small-scale nursing homes to provide residential care for elders and dementia patients, with a focus on promoting self-sufficiency in a home-like environment. The Project began with the aim of building new homes designed to meet its objectives but has also developed the Cultural Transformation program to support traditional nursing home settings in rethinking their programs and facilities to provide care based on the Green House model. A key element of the Green House model is its Best Life dementia care approach, designed to emphasize the accomplishments of the residents, foster relationships, and establish the least restrictive environment possible. The Green House model may not work as well once residents progress to severe dementia, when higher staffing levels than the model can incorporate are needed; additional research clarifying this issue would be helpful.
>
> ---
> [a]https://www.thegreenhouseproject.org

community-based services to shift care out of nursing homes and into home settings, partly in response to a Supreme Court decision requiring Medicaid to pay for care in the least restrictive settings possible (*Olmsted v. L. C.*, 527 U.S. 581 [1999][4]). This shift may be beneficial for individuals. Surveys suggest that people want to live at home for as long as possible (Guo et al., 2014; Brown et al., 2012), and there is some evidence that helping people stay home reduces health care spending (Newcomer et al., 2016). There is also evidence that both fee-for-service and Medicare Advantage members (see below) increased their use of home health care between 2007 and 2010, for example, but that usage subsequently declined primarily because of reimbursement and regulatory changes (Li et al., 2018). Home health care is among the fastest-growing Medicare expenditures: in 2019 it grew faster than all other types of care.[5]

The effects of the COVID-19 pandemic on nursing home and alternative care settings are not yet fully understood, but it appears that many families are substituting home care for facility-based rehabilitative and recuperative care (Flynn et al., 2020). Some prior work has demonstrated that patients receiving home health care in place of institutional postacute care in a nursing home have worse outcomes (Werner et al., 2019), but the trade-off for people living with dementia is not known. Sources of risk for patients receiving home care include the complexity of adhering to postacute care instructions from multiple physicians and higher rates

---
[4]https://supreme.justia.com/cases/federal/us/527/581
[5]https://www.cms.gov/files/document/highlights.pdf

of rehospitalization (which can cause confusion and delirium in elderly patients, especially those with dementia).

Nursing homes were already one of the least desirable health care settings before the pandemic, but with the high COVID death rates and the accompanying forced isolation of residents, they are even more likely to become care settings of last resort. Research on the implications of greater reliance on home health, including the increased responsibilities assumed by families, as well as how health care systems can better coordinate the care provided by home health agencies with the medical treatment being managed by primary care physicians, is badly needed.

Palliative and Hospice Care

There is evidence that both palliative and hospice care improve the quality of life for people at the end of life, including dementia patients (Evans et al., 2019). Palliative care is designed to address the symptoms of a serious condition and preserve the patient's comfort and dignity, as opposed to curing the underlying condition, and is an option for any dementia patient.[6] It is a way of thinking about the nature of the care a patient chooses, and physicians may specialize in providing this type of care (Mor and Teno, 2016). Although palliative care can be offered along with curative care for patients who may recover or improve (e.g., some cancer patients), it is the term commonly used for cases in which patients have chosen, usually though an advance directive or their family caregiver proxy, to receive only care that alleviates discomfort. This option is particularly valuable to many people living with dementia who do not wish to receive aggressive medical treatments or be in a hospital setting at the end of life, although palliative care may be provided long before the end of life. Palliative care is relatively rarely available in nursing homes or on an outpatient basis. Medicare may cover palliative care costs as it would cover any physician or nurse practitioner visit, depending on the benefits the individual has and the specifics of the treatment plan (National Institute on Aging, 2016).

Hospice care, in the context of Medicare coverage, differs from palliative care primarily in that it is offered only close to the end of life and is for situations in which the attending physician believes the patient is not expected to live more than 6 additional months. Like palliative care, hospice care focuses on the patient's comfort, and it can be provided in an inpatient hospice facility, in another institution, or in the patient's home, but there are limits on the length of time patients can receive some hospice care benefits. Regardless of setting, patients receiving hospice care do not

---

[6]For more information on palliative and hospice care, see https://www.nia.nih.gov/health/what-are-palliative-care-and-hospice-care.

receive curative treatments (Centers for Medicare & Medicaid Services [CMS], 2021b).

Hospice care has become increasingly common since Medicare began including it as a benefit in 1983, and significant changes to the program were made in 1986, as discussed below. Medicare covers the costs of hospice care even if it is needed for longer than 6 months, as long as the hospice medical director or other hospice doctor recertifies that the patient is terminally ill (CMS, n.d.). While evidence indicates that hospice care improves quality of life, growing numbers of patients receiving the care for longer than 6 months have resulted in increased costs (Miller et al., 2002; Teno et al., 2014).

There are several questions to consider regarding palliative and hospice care for dementia patients. One is whether it would be beneficial to offer either of these services to people living with dementia earlier in their disease progression than is currently typical. Even though several randomized controlled trials suggest that earlier intervention can improve quality of life and perhaps even reduce health care costs, it is not yet clear whether these effects would be replicated in the real world of fee-for-service Medicare, particularly for persons living with dementia whose prognosis is much less well understood than is the care for those with cancer diagnoses (Temel et al., 2010; Mor et al., 2018).

Study of other issues could support improvements in the design of palliative and hospice care programs and policies regarding their use. For example, the length of stay under hospice care prior to dying has been relatively steady over several decades, with some 40 percent of patients experiencing less than 7 days of such care, even though advocates believe that allowing more time would increase the benefit of the care (Teno et al., 2013). Hospice length of stay tends to be longer among those with dementia relative to those with other diagnoses, but the reasons for this are not clear. It would also be useful to know more about how persons living with dementia use palliative and hospice care; the preferences of dementia patients, their caregivers, and providers; the care choices made on patients' behalf in the last months and weeks of life; and how advance care directives affect the use of these kinds of care.

PAYING FOR CARE: MEDICARE AND MEDICAID

A key factor in the quality of dementia care, the timeliness of dementia detection, and the quality of life for persons living with dementia is how their care is paid for. The federal government has a direct impact on the way health and long-term care services are structured, delivered, and financed through Medicare (the federal health insurance program for people 65 or older and certain younger people with disabilities) and

Medicaid (the federal and state-funded provider of health care coverage to low-income individuals of any age, including those with disabilities).[7] Medicare covers 95 percent of all persons with dementia, and approximately one-quarter of adults with dementia also receive Medicaid benefits (Garfield et al., 2015). Medicare is complex, however, and the coverage it offers for dementia care has limitations and gaps. Medicare has also undergone changes in the past few years that have differing implications for those who are enrolled in *traditional Medicare* (the original version of Medicare), which includes both hospital insurance (Part A) and outpatient medical insurance (Part B) on a fee-for-service basis, with optional Part D prescription insurance, and those enrolled in *Medicare Advantage*, in which Parts A and B, and usually also Part D prescription insurance, are bundled together; see Box 6-3.[8] This section examines two key challenges associated with how aspects of dementia care are covered and the current state of thinking about managed care.

Coverage

Two issues related to dementia-related coverage under Medicare and Medicaid are important to note. The first concerns cognitive assessments. Since 2011, Medicare has covered an annual wellness visit that must include a cognitive assessment, which could promote earlier detection of dementia (see Chapter 3). Although the type of assessment has not been specified, typically it is a brief screening that, if positive, needs to be followed by a more extensive diagnostic evaluation. The annual wellness visit is covered in full by Medicare, but subsequent follow-up evaluations must be billed according to other codes. Implementation of the annual wellness visit in practice has been slow: it is estimated that 5 years after it was instituted,

---

[7]The health insurance provisions of the Affordable Care Act had limited impact on older individuals because most of them already had coverage through Medicare. However, the law included a number of delivery system reforms that have consequences for those on Medicare and those who are dually eligible for both Medicare and Medicaid. Dually eligible individuals account for a disproportionate share of spending in both Medicare and Medicaid. In 2013, 15 percent of Medicaid enrollees were dually eligible, but they accounted for 32 percent of Medicaid spending; 20 percent of Medicare enrollees had dual eligibility, and they accounted for 34 percent of all Medicare spending (Medicaid and CHIP Payment and Access Commission, 2020). Among dually eligible individuals over age 65, 23 percent had a diagnosis of dementia (Medicare Payment Advisory Commission and Medicaid and CHIP Payment and Access Commission, 2018).

[8]For more information about the components of Medicare and the differences among plans, see https://www.medicare.gov/what-medicare-covers/your-medicare-coverage-choices/whats-medicare. Additional information can be found at https://www.kff.org/medicare/issue-brief/an-overview-of-medicare/?gclid=CjwKCAjw0On8BRAgEiwAincsHE3No4tHUSNvqb--BjbFQzoZHX93wQURevpzFM4_jRuh3F-M7hihCRoCWH8QAvD_BwE.

> **BOX 6-3**
> **Medicare Advantage**
>
> Medicare Advantage (MA) is the privately run and capitated segment of the Medicare program: medical providers receive a set fee for each enrolled patient rather than fees for each service provided. In 2019, 37 percent of all Medicare beneficiaries were enrolled in MA plans. MA insurers may each offer dozens of different plans that compete in an open market, but all must be actuarially comparable to the benefits offered beneficiaries under the traditional fee-for-service Medicare plan. MA plans also often include additional coverage, such as for vision, hearing, and dental care. MA as a share of the entire Medicare program has grown substantially since 2005 (CMS, 2020b).
>
> SOURCE: Adapted from CMS (2020a).

only one-quarter of eligible beneficiaries had received this cognitive assessment (Ganguli et al., 2017; Hu et al., 2015). Data about annual wellness visits and cognitive assessments are limited, but another study, based on a nationally representative sample of older Americans, showed that in 2019, only 30 percent had undergone a cognitive assessment in the primary care setting; rates were higher among persons enrolled in Medicare Advantage compared with those enrolled in traditional Medicare (Jacobson et al., 2020). The research also revealed that detection of cognitive impairment was no more common among those who had had annual wellness visits than among those who had not had such visits (see also Fowler et al., 2018). Results of one study suggest that up to two-thirds of those identified through screening as having cognitive impairment do not undergo a subsequent diagnostic assessment (Fowler et al., 2015). In 2021, CMS increased payment levels for these follow-up diagnostic assessments and care plan services, but it is not yet clear whether this payment increase will result in improved follow-up care (CMS, 2021a).

The other issue is that Medicare does not cover two classes of services that are critical for dementia patients: institutional long-term nursing home care and certain home and community-based services. After spending down their savings and existing financial resources, about 30 percent of persons with dementia are also covered by Medicaid, which covers some long-term services and supports not included in Medicare's benefit package (Mor et al., 2010). However, persons living with dementia who are eligible for both Medicare and Medicaid face fragmented financing, and the conflicting incentives for the two programs can lead to potentially unnecessary and intensive care. For instance, Medicaid typically pays nursing homes a daily custodial rate that covers room, board, and nursing care. When a resident becomes acutely ill, the nursing home has an incentive to transfer the patient to a hospital, thereby shifting the costs to the Medicare program, even though such a transfer may not be in the patient's interest (Unruh et al., 2013). The nursing home can also earn a higher per-day rate for providing Medicare-financed skilled nursing home care when the same patient returns to the nursing home after discharge. These incentives can lead to a "revolving door" between nursing homes and hospitals, with adverse consequences for cognitively impaired and frail elderly people (Mor et al., 2010; Goldfeld et al., 2013; Polniaszek et al., 2011).

The Federal Role in Innovation

CMS has taken significant steps to document, measure, and address fragmentation in the health and long-term care systems. Starting in the 1990s, CMS provided the first waivers for the Program of All-Inclusive Care for the Elderly, a program that provides comprehensive medical and social services to adults over age 55 who are dually enrolled in Medicare and Medicaid and are sufficiently frail to be categorized as "nursing home eligible" by their state's Medicaid program. The CMS Innovation Center (created under the Affordable Care Act) allows the Medicare and Medicaid programs to test models that improve care, lower costs, and better align payment systems with models that support patient-centered practices. Furthermore, Congress provided CMS the authority to expand the scope and duration of models being tested through rulemaking. Evaluating innovative payment and service delivery models to determine whether they are appropriate for expansion and which characteristics are associated with success is a key focus of the Innovation Center (Howell et al., 2015).

The Obama Administration set ambitious goals for the Innovation Center's study of the effects of payment and delivery reforms; however, the Trump Administration rolled back many of the initial efforts. According to a 2018 report from the U.S. Government Accountability Office, of the 37 models for delivering and paying for health care implemented by 2018, very few succeeded in maintaining or reducing health care cost savings while maintaining or enhancing quality (U.S. Government Accountability Office, 2018a). The Innovation Center has made investments in models that include postacute or long-term care, some of which addressed the needs of individuals with dementia. Still, the Center could be used to test new models for this population and to provide evidence to support congressional action on new models.

In addition, under the value-based insurance design (VBID) program, plans may apply to test innovative interventions and their benefit design, including cost-sharing reductions, additional supplemental benefits, and targeted benefits for enrollees with certain chronic conditions. The benefits typically offered are quite limited but include caregiver supports, meal delivery, and transportation for groceries. The goals of the VBID program are to test innovations designed to reduce Medicare spending, enhance quality of care for Medicare beneficiaries, and improve the coordination and efficiency of health care service delivery. Dementia was added explicitly to the list of seven chronic condition categories in 2018.

These flexibilities are new, untested, and as yet not widely utilized by plans. More research on such innovations is needed. While they hold promise, it will be essential for researchers to track their implementation closely; measure their outcomes and return on investment; and ascertain whether and how they reach those with significant, complex conditions such as dementia.

Managed Care

A key focus of innovation has been managed care, an approach to health care in which the financing and delivery of care are integrated, with the goal of improving quality and lowering costs and with potential advantages for the care of people living with dementia. Medicare was originally designed to finance acute hospitalizations, postacute skilled nursing, surgeries, and curative care in the outpatient setting, although its coverage has expanded since it was established in 1965. It generally pays providers on a per-service basis, and each service has a unique code. This approach has meant that definitions of codes and providers' interpretations of those definitions affect the services received by beneficiaries, as well as the diagnoses associated with each service rendered. In general, this coding system motivates providers to increase the volume and intensity of services rendered to a particular patient instead of striving to avert potentially unnecessary and costly care (Song et al., 2010). Managed care programs have different incentives, encouraging providers to use resources prudently while maximizing patient outcomes, which may permit them to provide better management of care for people living with dementia.[9]

One promising new opportunity is a set of developments allowing Medicare Advantage plans to deliver supplemental services as part of the Medicare benefit package. This opportunity holds promise for Medicare beneficiaries who need extensive care coordination and some long-term services and supports. The underlying theory is that providing some social supports and other nonmedical assistance can help the beneficiary while also minimizing overuse of costly hospital and nursing home services. One example of this approach is CMS's modification of the definition of what the nearly 3,000 Medicare Advantage plans nationwide could classify as "primarily health

---

[9] Medicare Advantage is Medicare's managed care program.

related services." The new interpretation includes such services as adult day care, home-based palliative care, in-home support, and memory fitness.

How Managed Care Works

Conceptually, the managed care approach to care delivery and outcomes is driven by three underlying factors: incentives, competition, and organizational capabilities.

In a managed care approach, a health insurance plan bears the risk of paying for covered services for a defined population; payments can be adjusted for patients' risk and expected health care expenditures so the plan will have less reason to avoid higher-risk patients. With this approach, the plan has an incentive to coordinate care for persons with dementia to reduce unnecessary service use, thus keeping overall costs down. For decades, Medicare Advantage plans were able to attract Medicare beneficiaries who were healthier than the average fee-for-service patient, although the past several years have seen a substantial increase in the number of beneficiaries enrolling in Medicare Advantage plans who have disabilities or are otherwise eligible for both Medicare and Medicaid (Park et al., 2020). Such enrollments may increase as a result of the introduction of dementia into the calculation of codes that determine reimbursement, which took place in 2020.

Competition plays a role in managed care because the presence of managed care plans in a market generates competitive pressure for plans to attract more enrollees through lower premiums, more generous benefits, or better quality of care. Finally, managed care plans have specific organizational capabilities absent from the original Medicare program. Specifically, Medicare providers reimbursed solely through fee-for-service are not part of an organizational structure that is accountable for both care quality and financing. In contrast, organizations providing care through Medicare Advantage have the capacity to manage supply by restricting the providers their members can use and employing other cost-containment approaches, such as utilization review or prior authorization policies. Plans may also influence provider behavior by altering the payment method or profiling providers' treatment patterns. Or they may contract selectively with more efficient providers and/or attempt to steer enrollees to receive care from such providers by forming restricted provider networks. Finally, plans can engage directly with enrollees to implement preventive health, case management, disease management, or other related interventions.

Medicare Advantage and Dementia Care

How might managed care improve outcomes for dementia patients? First, in contrast to traditional Medicare, Medicare Advantage plans have the flexibility to cover services or alter payment policies in ways that avert preventable spending on hospital care or improve quality of care. For instance, while traditional Medicare will pay for skilled nursing care only for patients who have first experienced a 3-day hospital stay, most Medicare Advantage plans waive this requirement to facilitate direct admission for subacute care in a nursing home (Zissimopoulos et al., 2014; White et al., 2019; Yang et al., 2012; Grebla et al., 2015). Unlike traditional Medicare, moreover, Medicare Advantage plans can elect to cover case management by social workers, adult day care services, respite for caregivers, in-home meal delivery, and other long-term services and supports should the plans decide that these interventions make it possible to avert other medical spending or improve outcomes (White et al., 2019; Yang et al., 2012; Thomas et al., 2019; Durfey et al., 2021).

A few examples illustrate this point. A care consultation service (using the managed care approach) for people living with dementia implemented by a Medicare Advantage plan in Ohio, together with the Cleveland Alzheimer's Association, achieved lower service utilization, improved patient and family satisfaction, and decreased caregiver strain (Fishman et al., 2019). A case management and quality improvement program implemented by a Medicare Advantage plan in Los Angeles also produced significant improvements in caregiver satisfaction and greater adherence to guideline-based quality measures, including routine assessments of cognition, activities of daily living, decision-making capacity, and wandering risk (Kuo et al., 2008).

Managed care plans may also use health-risk assessments to identify enrollees with cognitive impairment and provide them with intensive case management, which is an important benefit because of the problem with underdiagnosis discussed in Chapter 3 (Lin et al., 2016; Hudomiet et al., 2019; Albert et al., 2002; Eaker et al., 2002; Gaugler et al., 2013; Geldmacher et al., 2013; Suehs et al., 2013; Zhu et al., 2015; Lin et al., 2010; Bynum et al., 2004; Hill et al., 2002; Carter and Porell, 2005). Finally, managed care organizations can contract selectively with home health and nursing home providers that achieve better outcomes, such as lower readmissions and hospitalization rates for functionally impaired older adults (Albert et al., 2002). Thus, in principle, managed care may help patients live longer in the community and prevent unnecessary hospitalizations.

Risks Despite its benefits, managed care may also compromise outcomes for people living with dementia. The capitated payment structure (in which physicians are paid a preset monthly amount for each patient) may give Medicare plans an incentive to attract and retain healthier enrollees and to promote the disenrollment of patients with complex health care needs.

There is evidence that Medicare Advantage patients who use short- or long-term nursing home care have high rates of switching to traditional Medicare in the following year (Meyers et al., 2021). This may indicate that Medicare Advantage plans are attempting to "cream-skim" healthy patients so that traditional Medicare will bear the cost when patients enter a period of increased health care needs. Indeed, recent research on disenrollment in Medicare Advantage plans shows that once Medicare beneficiaries receive a dementia diagnosis, they are much more likely to switch back to traditional Medicare or switch to another Medicare Advantage plan relative to Medicare Advantage members without a new dementia diagnosis. This finding is consistent with other research indicating that Medicare Advantage members who have chronic conditions and are users of nursing home or home health services are more likely to disenroll from their plan in the year in which they have these utilization experiences than in other years (Jung et al., 2018; Goldberg et al., 2017, 2018).

Plans may also restrict access to some high-cost services, particularly for frail patients. For example, in a sample of several hundred managed care patients in four California skilled nursing facilities, managed care patients had substantially shorter stays and received less therapy compared with fee-for-service patients, even after adjusting for an extensive set of demographic and clinical variables and site of care (Eaker et al., 2002). Similarly, a study comparing the experiences of Medicare Advantage and fee-for-service patients with hip fracture discharged from a hospital to a skilled nursing facility found, after propensity score matching, that Medicare Advantage patients spent 5 fewer days in the skilled nursing facility but were less likely to be rehospitalized and more likely to remain home (Kumar et al., 2018). In a population-based sample of frail Medicare beneficiaries in San Diego, managed care enrollees received 71 percent fewer home visits compared with fee-for-service participants, independent of health and sociodemographic characteristics (Gaugler et al., 2013). In this same sample, the odds of preventable rehospitalization were 3.51 times higher for Medicare Advantage enrollees than for Medicare fee-for-service participants. A recent national study demonstrated that Medicare Advantage members used less home health care and skilled nursing care and had fewer hospital days compared with Medicare fee-for-service beneficiaries, controlling for demographic, regional, and clinical factors (Li et al., 2018). These studies support the notion that the practices managed care plans may adopt to limit the use of services may have significant unintended consequences at later points along the continuum of care.

Knowledge gaps Theoretically, Medicare Advantage plans may be able to manage the care needs of people living with dementia better than the fee-for-service system can precisely because they have an incentive to manage and coordinate care so as to reduce unnecessary utilization while improving the quality of the care and care partners' satisfaction with care. Under optimal conditions, Medicare Advantage plans focused on managing their patients' care could achieve the same sorts of positive outcomes observed in studies of integrated health care delivery systems that provide the full range of inpatient, outpatient, and community-based services.

Unfortunately, there is limited empirical evidence to support this proposition. On the one hand, Medicare Advantage special needs plans are available to some persons living with dementia.[10] These plans are tailored to meet needs associated with specific conditions, provide targeted care (e.g., dementia care specialists), and cover drugs typically prescribed for the covered conditions, and they often include a care coordinator. Special needs plans increase the use of primary care and improve the management of such chronic conditions as diabetes (Cohen et al., 2012). However, these plans are now growing rapidly, and further research on their effects would be valuable.

Another relatively new development in the realm of Medicare Advantage plans pertains to the growth of institutional as well as disability-based special needs plans. These plans have begun to draw an increasingly large population of persons who are dually eligible for Medicare and Medicaid. Disability-based special needs plans that cover permanent residents of nursing homes combine the per diem payment for nursing home care from Medicaid with the highest level of Medicare monthly payment for those patients with the most complex mix of diagnoses.

Although there is ample evidence that enrollees in Medicare Advantage plans have lower rates of hospitalization and readmission relative to those enrolled in traditional Medicare, after risk adjustment, whether these broad differences are applicable to people living with dementia is unknown (Cohen et al., 2012). Furthermore, like other populations with high needs and costs, those with dementia appear to be particularly likely to disenroll from Medicare Advantage. It is not known, however, whether these disenrollment choices are made by the person with dementia or a caregiver, or whether they reflect subtle pushes from the Medicare Advantage plan itself. It will be important to determine whether disenrollment reflects patients' dissatisfaction with access to care and care coordination or has some other cause.

Several recent policy changes have increased the flexibility of Medicare Advantage plans in meeting the needs of people living with dementia. In 2019, for example, the list of Medicare Advantage plan benefits was expanded to include adult day care, in-home personal care attendants,

---

[10]For more information, see https://www.medicare.gov/sign-up-change-plans/types-of-medicare-health-plans/special-needs-plans-snp.

home safety, and assistive devices. In 2020, plans were allowed to offer supplemental benefits, including home-delivered meals, help with daily activities, and nonmedical transportation, to chronically ill beneficiaries. While some of these services were available to some people living with dementia before these policy changes, access to them was constrained by income limits, as well as local availability. The recent changes make it possible for Medicare Advantage plans to offer services that directly address some of the social needs that are significant determinants of health outcomes for frail and chronically ill beneficiaries such as people living with dementia.

Because these changes are recent, however, there is little empirical evidence about how Medicare Advantage plans are organizing such services and making them available, or whether the services are effective in improving quality of life. It will be important to study how Medicare Advantage plans contract with and arrange for these services for their chronically ill members. Indeed, because Medicare Advantage plans are serving more individuals living with dementia and an increasingly impaired population, research on how different types of Medicare Advantage plans can affect the care and outcomes experienced by persons living with dementia is critical. The structure of emerging special needs plans varies, so it will be important to examine whether any of these structures are more effective than the others in improving the outcomes of persons with dementia living in nursing homes (Meyers et al., 2020). New alternative payment models (e.g., accountable care organizations, primary care first, direct contracting) also allow the flexibility to provide greater benefits for people living with dementia. Whether these models will also provide augmented payment to cover services for people living with dementia remains to be determined.

RESEARCH DIRECTIONS

The committee identified numerous gaps in the available research on the capacity of the health care system and long-term and end-of-life care to meet the needs of people living with dementia and their families. With respect to health care, we point to the need for observational research using existing data (e.g., electronic health records, administrative claims data) to develop more detailed understanding of patients' needs as they move through the stages of dementia and related questions. Research on new models of care is also needed. In addition to intervention development research, further evaluation research is needed as well, including

- traditional clinical trials;
- pragmatic trials; and
- quasi-experimental designs (e.g., stepped wedge) (Hemming et al., 2015), as well as hybrid designs that include a summative

evaluation of the impact of an intervention, treatment, or practice and formative evaluation of the implementation process itself (Curran et al., 2012).

To date, moreover, there has been minimal research on how to accelerate the implementation and dissemination of successful models, which will be necessary if the products of intervention research are to reach large numbers of persons with dementia.

The committee also identified gaps in research on residential and community-based long-term care. Cluster randomized and quasi-experimental studies are needed to define the critical elements of assisted living facilities, including those with dementia/memory care programs, and their effectiveness in real-world settings. The COVID-19 pandemic has underscored the need for study of the current structure and processes of nursing homes, and studies examining the failures and successes of nursing homes during the pandemic may provide insights for nursing home reform. Study of alternatives to the current nursing home structure (e.g., smaller facilities serving fewer than 20 individuals that emphasize a home-like environment) is needed to determine what influences patients' and families' choices and how to disseminate and finance preferred options. Research also is needed on how and when to implement palliative and hospice care to provide the optimal benefit for persons living with dementia; these questions could be addressed through Medicare demonstration projects, such as those included under Medicare Advantage.

Study of the barriers to financing new, effective approaches to dementia care, particularly in fee-for-service settings, is also needed. Research evaluating new payment models, including managed care plans, and their outcomes and the potential to use their flexibility to provide additional services that improve dementia care would provide evidence as to whether the potential of these plans is being fulfilled. Research on the structures of different dementia services offered by health plans and, in turn, their effects on quality of care and outcomes among Medicare Advantage beneficiaries could provide insight into how policies and regulations pertaining to dementia care can best be revised. Such research conducted over the next decade could support the development of policy and the delivery of more effective, more efficient care.

The committee identified priority areas for additional research on how persons living with dementia and their caregivers interact with and are served by the health and social service systems in the domains of the quality and structure of health care, the quality and structure of long-term and end-of-life care, and financing of dementia care. These research needs are summarized in Conclusions 6-1, 6-2, and 6-3 and detailed in Tables 6-1, 6-2, and 6-3, respectively.

CONCLUSION 6-1: Research in the following areas has the potential to substantially strengthen the quality and structure of the health care provided to people living with dementia:
- Documentation of the diagnosis and care management received by persons living with dementia from their primary care providers.
- Clarification of disease trajectories to help health systems plan care for persons living with dementia.
- Identification of effective methods for providing dementia-related services (e.g., screening and detection, diagnosis, care management and planning, transition management) for individuals living with dementia throughout the disease trajectory.
- Development and evaluation of standardized systems of coordinated care for comprehensively managing multiple comorbidities for persons with dementia.
- Identification of effective approaches for integrating care services across health care delivery and community-based organizations.

TABLE 6-1 Detailed Research Needs

1: Documentation of Care Received from Primary Care Providers	• Documentation of existing practices and experiences of diagnosis and subsequent care management; how those practices and experiences are associated with stages of disease and symptom progression, and how they vary across type of dementia as well as racial, ethnic, and socioeconomic groups and geography • Assessment of the effectiveness of patient and caregiver support and management systems embedded in health care systems, and system capacity for mounting comprehensive, multifaceted interventions • Assessment of the effectiveness of population health management systems designed to identify and care for persons living with dementia and their caregivers as implemented by health plans and accountable care organizations • Identification of care gaps and unmet needs of persons living with dementia and caregiver support • Identification of gaps in current standardized systems of coordinated care, including management of multiple comorbidities • Identification of effective care practices that can be disseminated
2: Clarification of Disease Trajectories	• Observational studies examining how persons with dementia progress clinically and in their use of services, including behavioral health care, long-term care, and end-of life care, and how these trajectories vary across type of dementia; racial, ethnic, and socioeconomic groups; and geography, as well as among those with comorbidities

TABLE 6-1 Continued

3: Identification of Effective Methods for Providing Dementia Care Services	• Studies that optimize how screening is conducted and results are communicated • Studies of the impact of strategies for integrating dementia-focused interventions into the workflow of primary care practices • Clinical trials to test the effectiveness of promising strategies for providing persons living with dementia with diagnostic and longitudinal care for all their health care needs, including care for behavioral problems and comorbid conditions, in various settings • Studies of the impact of advance care planning at all stages of dementia and assessment of preferences, including patients' preferences regarding palliative, hospice, and end-of-life care • Development and evaluation of systems for comprehensive care at the population level, including study of the use of existing and emerging models
4 and 5: Standardized Systems of Coordinated Care and Integrated Care Services	• Studies of the application of principles of design, implementation, and diffusion that integrate science and engineering (e.g., agile management) to promote dissemination of care innovations for people living with dementia • Studies of the application of network science tools and processes in the dissemination of innovations • Investigation of strategies for disseminating evidence-based models of dementia care in rural areas and demographically diverse populations • Development and evaluation of comprehensive care models that span health care and community-based organizations • Studies of the use of electronic health record systems for integration across platforms and providers, including caregivers, to promote more efficient transactions between care facilities and community-based partners and track the effects of interventions • Creation and evaluation of innovative financing structures that support persons with dementia and caregivers receiving both health care and social services

CONCLUSION 6-2: Research in the following areas has the potential to substantially strengthen the quality and structure of long-term and end-of-life care provided to people living with dementia:
- Identification of future long-term and end-of-life needs and available care for persons living with dementia.
- Description and monitoring of factors that contribute to problems with nursing home quality, particularly in light of the acceleration

of those problems caused by the COVID-19 pandemic, to provide evidence for ongoing changes to the long-term care system.
- Development and evaluation of alternatives to traditional nursing home facilities, including home care options and innovative facility designs.
- Improved understanding of how and when patients use palliative and hospice care options and variation in the end-of-life care available across regions and populations.

TABLE 6-2 Detailed Research Needs

1: Long-Term and End-of-Life Patient Needs and Available Care	• Studies that produce demographic projections, including dementia-specific microsimulation models, based on the anticipated family structure of households in the United States and the availability of family caregivers able and willing to undertake the task of providing care for persons living with late-stage dementia • Studies of how patients and families are informed about their options and how decisions are made, including use of advance directives
2: Improved Nursing Home Quality	• Effects of changes (or differences) in Medicaid payment models on the quality of nursing home and community-based services
3: Development and Evaluation of Alternative Long-Term Care Options	• Studies of the implications for patients and families of greater reliance on home care • Analysis of how innovative alternatives may function in varied settings (e.g., low-income, urban, rural) • Analysis of how alternative staffing models function with patients at different stages of impairment • Comparison of effects of alternative sites and modes of care (e.g., home, assisted living facilities, small residential facilities) on caregivers and clinical outcomes for persons with dementia, as well as on utilization of facilities and services and costs
4: Use of and Variation in End-of-Life Care	• Effects of different types of dementia care programs and payment structures on the timing of hospice referrals • Evaluation of the feasibility of a palliative/home care benefit for patients and families willing to forgo aggressive, life-prolonging services and treatments

CONCLUSION 6-3: Research in the following areas has the potential to substantially strengthen the arrangements through which most dementia care is funded—traditional Medicare, Medicare Advantage, alternative payment models, and Medicaid:
- Comparison of the effects of different financing structures on the quality of care and clinical outcomes for persons living with dementia, as well as effects on their caregivers.
- Examination of ways to modify incentives in reimbursement models to optimize care and reduce unnecessary hospitalizations and other negative outcomes for people living with dementia.
- Development and testing of approaches to integrated financing of medical and social services.

Finally, we note that persistent challenges affect the workforces in both health care and the direct care system. Issues that go well beyond the context of dementia care have been documented. These include, to name a few, shortages of qualified workers, limitations in the quality and availability of training and education for both prospective workers and those developing their careers, as well as multiple factors specific to domains within these sectors. The aging of the U.S. population is likely to exacerbate the stress on these workforces, as the ratio of working-age people to older people shifts. The issues are likely to be most acute for the direct care workforce because of financial disincentives such as low pay and poor benefits, as well as limited opportunities for career advancement.

TABLE 6-3 Detailed Research Needs

1: Comparative Effectiveness of Financing Structure	• Comparison of the quality of care, clinical and quality-of-life outcomes, and costs experienced by Medicare beneficiaries living with dementia versus those in managed care plans • Comparison of the outcomes of persons living with advanced dementia being cared for and managed under various specialized managed care programs and alternative payment models, such as special needs plans, accountable care organizations, and Program of All-Inclusive Care for the Elderly programs
2: Ways to Modify Incentives	• Studies of how Medicare Advantage plans and alternative payment models best provide incentives to implement active care management for people living with dementia
3: Evaluation of Approaches to Integrated Financing	• Identification of optimal means of financing and paying for individual services across health care delivery and community-based organizations provided to individual persons with dementia and their caregivers

Many of the challenges that affect the supply of qualified individuals to care for people living with dementia are broad workforce issues for the entire health care system and the providers of direct care for the elderly and people with disabilities. These include, for example, national-level health care policies affecting payment and insurance as well as workforce trends and policies affecting lower-income workers. Little of the potentially pertinent research is structured by the diagnosis of persons being cared for. It was beyond the scope of this study to conduct a review of the state of the research in each of the relevant areas that was detailed enough to support specific conclusions about the research direction that should be given highest priority. Nevertheless, we regard emerging knowledge about workforce issues as a vital complement to the research directions described here.

REFERENCES

Abrams, H.R., Loomer, L., Gandhi, A., and Grabowski, D.C. (2020). Characteristics of U.S. Nursing Homes with COVID-19 Cases. *Journal of the American Geriatrics Society*, 68(8), 1653–1656. https://doi.org/10.1111/jgs.16661

Adler, J. (2018, June 4). *Investors Rethink Memory Care*. Seniors Housing Business. https://seniorshousingbusiness.com/investors-rethink-memory-care

Albert, S.M., Glied, S., Andrews, H., Stern, Y., and Mayeux, R. (2002). Primary care expenditures before the onset of Alzheimer's disease. *Neurology*, 59(4), 573–578. https://doi.org/10.1212/wnl.59.4.573

Altman, D. (2020, July 21). Hotspot states see more COVID cases in nursing homes. *Axios*. https://www.axios.com/coronavirus-cases-infections-nursing-homes-b5260d20-47f2-4a56-9574-e63e9dafd012.html

American Board of Medical Specialties. (2020). *ABMS Board Certification Report 2019–2020*. https://www.abms.org/wp-content/uploads/2020/11/ABMS-Board-Certification-Report-2019-2020.pdf

Amjad, H., Carmichael, D., Austin, A.M., Chang, C.-H., and Bynum, J.P.W. (2016). Continuity of care and healthcare utilization in older adults with dementia in fee-for-service Medicare. *JAMA Internal Medicine*, 176(9), 1371–1378. https://doi.org/10.1001/jamainternmed.2016.3553

Angelelli, J., Mor, V., Intrator, O., Feng, Z., and Zinn, J. (2003). Oversight of nursing homes: Pruning the tree or just spotting bad apples? *Gerontologist*, 43(suppl 2), 67–75. https://doi.org/10.1093/geront/43.suppl_2.67

Ausserhofer, D., Deschodt, M., De Geest, S., van Achterberg, T., Meyer, G., Verbeek, H., Sjetne, I.S., Malinowska-Lipień, I., Griffiths, P., Schlüter, W., Ellen, M., and Engberg, S. (2016). "There's no place like home": A scoping review on the impact of homelike residential care models on resident-, family-, and staff-related outcomes. *Journal of the American Medical Directors Association*, 17(8), 685–693. https://doi.org/10.1016/j.jamda.2016.03.009

Bardenheier, B.H., Rahman, M., Kosar, C., Werner, R.M., and Mor, V. (2020). Successful discharge to community gap of FFS Medicare beneficiaries with and without ADRD narrowed. *Journal of the American Geriatrics Society*, 69(4), 972–978. https://doi.org/10.1111/jgs.16965

Bentkover, J., Cai, S., Makineni, R., Mucha, L., Treglia, M., and Mor, V. (2012). Road to the nursing home: Costs and disease progression among Medicare beneficiaries with ADRD. *America Journal of Alzheimer's Disease and Other Dementias*, 27(2), 90–99. https://doi.org/10.1177/1533317512440494

Boustani, M., Alder, C.A., Solid, C.A., and Reuben, D. (2019). An alternative payment model to support widespread use of collaborative dementia care models. *Health Affairs, 38*(1), 54–59. https://doi.org/doi:10.1377/hlthaff.2018.05154

Brown, J.R., Goda, G.S., and McGarry, K. (2012). Long-term care insurance demand limited by beliefs about needs, concerns about insurers, and care available from family. *Health Affairs (Project Hope), 31*(6), 1294–1302. https://doi.org/10.1377/hlthaff.2011.1307

Bunn, F., Burn, A-M., Goodman, C., Rait, G., Norton, S., Robinson, L., Schoeman, J., and Brayne, C. (2014). Comorbidity and dementia: A scoping review of the literature. *BMC Medicine, 12*, 192. https://doi.org/10.1186/s12916-014-0192-4

Bynum, J.P., Rabins, P.V., Weller, W., Niefeld, M., Anderson, G.F., and Wu, A.W. (2004). The relationship between a dementia diagnosis, chronic illness, Medicare expenditures, and hospital use. *Journal of the American Geriatrics Society, 52*(2), 187–194. https://doi.org/10.1111/j.1532-5415.2004.52054.x

Callahan, C.M., Boustani, M.A., Unverzagt, F.W., Austrom, M.G., Damush, T.M., Perkins, A.J., Fultz, B.A., Hui, S.L., Counsell, S.R., and Hendrie, H.C. (2006). Effectiveness of collaborative care for older adults with Alzheimer disease in primary care: A randomized controlled trial. *Journal of the American Medical Association, 295*(18), 2148–2157.

Carter, M.W., and Porell, F.W. (2005). Vulnerable populations at risk of potentially avoidable hospitalizations: The case of nursing home residents with Alzheimer's disease. *American Journal of Alzheimer's Disease and Other Dementias, 20*, 349–358.

Chatterjee, P., Kelly, S., Qi, M., and Werner, R.M. (2020). Characteristics and quality of U.S. nursing homes reporting cases of coronavirus disease 2019 (COVID-19). *JAMA Network Open, 3*(7), e2016930. https://doi.org/10.1001/jamanetworkopen.2020.16930

Chen, M.K, Chevalier, J.A., and Long, E.F. (2020). *Nursing Home Staff Networks and COVID-19*. NBER Working Paper 27608. Cambridge, MA: National Bureau of Economic Research. https://doi.org/10.3386/w27608

Clevenger, C.K., Cellar, J., Kovaleva, M., Medders, L., and Hepburn, K. (2018). Integrated memory care clinic: Design, implementation, and initial results. *Journal of the American Geriatrics Society, 66*(12), 2401–2407. https://doi.org/10.1111/jgs.15528

CMS (Centers for Medicare & Medicaid Services). (n.d.). *Medicare Hospice Benefits*. https://www.medicare.gov/Pubs/pdf/02154-medicare-hospice-benefits.pdf

———. (2020a). *Medicare Enrollment Dashboard*. https://www.cms.gov/Research-Statistics-Data-and-Systems/Statistics-Trends-and-Reports/CMSProgramStatistics/Dashboard

———. (2020b). *Total Medicare Enrollment: Total, Original Medicare, and Medicare Advantage and Other Health Plan Enrollment, Calendar Years 2014-2019*. https://www.cms.gov/files/document/2019cpsmdcrenrollab1.pdf

———. (2021a). *Cognitive Assessment and Care Plan Services*. https://www.cms.gov/cognitive

———. (2021b). *Hospice*. https://www.cms.gov/Medicare/Medicare-Fee-for-Service-Payment/Hospice

Cohen, R., Lemieux, J., Schenborn, J., and Mulligan, T. (2012). Medicare Advantage chronic special needs plan boosted primary care, reduced hospital use among diabetes patients. *Health Affairs, 31*(1), 110–119. https://doi.org/10.1377/hlthaff.2011.0998

Curran, G.M., Bauer, M., Mittman, B., Pyne, J.M., and Stetler, C. (2012). Effectiveness-implementation hybrid designs: Combining elements of clinical effectiveness and implementation research to enhance public health impact. *Medical Care, 50*(3), 217–226. https://doi.org/10.1097/MLR.0b013e3182408812

Drabo, E., Barthold, D., Joyce, G., Ferido, P., Chui, H., and Zissimopoulos, J. (2019). Longitudinal analysis of dementia diagnosis and specialty care among racially diverse Medicare beneficiaries. *Alzheimer's & Dementia, 15*(11), 1402–1411. https://doi.org/10.1016/j.jalz.2019.07.005

Durfey, S., Gadbois, E.A., Meyers, D.J., Brazier, J.F., Wetle, T., and Thomas, K.S. (2021). Health care and community-based organization partnerships to address social needs: Medicare Advantage Plan representatives' perspectives. *Medical Care Research and Review*. Advance online publication. https://doi.org/10.1177/10775587211009723

Eaker, E.D., Mickel, S.F., Chyou, P.H., Mueller-Rizner, N.J., and Slusser, J.P. (2002). Alzheimer's disease or other dementia and medical care utilization. *Annals of Epidemiology*, 12, 39–45. https://doi.org/10.1016/s1047-2797(01)00244-7

Evans, C.J., Ison, L., Ellis-Smith, C., Nicholson, C., Costa, A., Oluyase, A.O., Namisango, E., Bone, A.E., Brighton, L.J., Yi, D., Combes, S., Bajwah, S., Gao, W., Harding, R., Ong, P., Higginson, I.J., and Maddocks, M. (2019). Service delivery models to maximize quality of life for older people at the end of life: A rapid review. *Milbank Quarterly*, 97(1), 113–175. https://doi.org/10.1111/1468-0009.12373

Fishman, P., Coe, N.B., White, L., Crane, P.K., Park, S., Ingraham, B., and Larson, E.B. (2019). Cost of dementia in Medicare managed care: A systematic literature review. *American Journal of Managed Care*, 25(8), e247–e253.

Flynn, H., Morley, M., and Bentley, F. (2020, September 8). Hospital discharges to home health rebounding, but SNF volumes lag. *Avalere*. https://avalere.com/press-releases/hospital-discharges-to-home-health-rebound-while-snf-volumes-lag

Fowler, N.R., Frame, A., Perkins, A.J., Gao, S., Watson, D.P., Monahan, P., and Boustani, M.A. (2015). Traits of patients who screen positive for dementia and refuse diagnostic assessment. *Alzheimer's & Dementia (Amsterdam, Netherlands)*, 1(2), 236–241. https://doi.org/10.1016/j.dadm.2015.01.002

Fowler, N.R., Campbell, N.L., Pohl, G.M., Munsie, L.M., Kirson, N.Y., Desai, U., Trieschman, E.J., Meiselbach, M.K., Andrews, J.S., and Boustani, M.A. (2018). One-year effect of the Medicare annual wellness visit on detection of cognitive impairment: A cohort study. *Journal of the American Geriatrics Society*, 66(5), 969–975. https://doi.org/10.1111/jgs.15330

Ganguli, I., Souza, J., McWilliams, J.M., and Mehrotra, A. (2017). Trends in use of the U.S. Medicare annual wellness visit, 2011-2014. *Journal of the American Medical Association*, 317(21), 2233–2235. https://doi.org/10.1001/jama.2017.4342

Garfield, R., Musumeci, M.B., and Reaves, E.L. (2015). Medicaid's role for people with dementia. *Kaiser Family Foundation*. https://www.kff.org/medicaid/issue-brief/medicaids-role-for-people-with-dementia

Gaugler, J.E., Hovater, M., Roth, D.L., Johnston, J.A., Kane, R.L., and Sarsour, K. (2013). Analysis of cognitive, functional, health service use, and cost trajectories prior to and following memory loss. *Journals of Gerontology: Series B*, 68(4), 562–567. https://doi.org/10.1093/geronb/gbs078

Geldmacher, D.S., Kirson, N.Y., Birnbaum, H.G., Eapen, S., Kantor, E., Cummings, A.K., and Joish, V.N. (2013). Pre-diagnosis excess acute care costs in Alzheimer's patients among a U.S. Medicaid population. *Applied Health Economics and Health Policy*, 11, 407–413.

Gleckman, H. (2019, May 15). What you need to know about Washington State's public long-term care insurance program. *Forbes*. https://www.forbes.com/sites/howardgleckman/2019/05/15/what-you-need-to-know-about-washington-states-public-long-term-care-insurance-program/?sh=493dcc982cdc

Goldberg, E.M., Trivedi, A.N., Mor, V., Jung, H.Y., and Rahman, M. (2017). Favorable risk selection in Medicare Advantage: Trends in mortality and plan exits among nursing home beneficiaries. *Medical Care Research and Review*, 74(6), 736–749. https://doi.org/10.1177/1077558716662565

Goldberg, E.M., Keohane, L.M., Mor, V., Trivedi, A.N., Jung, H.Y., and Rahman, M. (2018). Preferred provider relationships between Medicare Advantage plans and skilled nursing facilities reduce switching out of plans: An observational analysis. *Inquiry*, 55. https://doi.org/10.1177/0046958018797412

Goldfeld, K.S., Hamel, M.B., and Mitchell, S.L. (2013). The cost-effectiveness of the decision to hospitalize nursing home residents with advanced dementia. *Journal of Pain and Symptom Management, 46*(5), 640–651. https://doi.org/10.1016/j.jpainsymman.2012.11.007

Gorges, R.J., and Konetzka, R.T. (2020). Staffing levels and COVID-19 cases and outbreaks in U.S. nursing homes. *Journal of the American Geriatrics Society, 68*(11), 2462–2466. https://doi.org/10.1111/jgs.16787

Grabowski, D.C., and Mor, V. (2020). Nursing home care in crisis in the wake of COVID-19. *Journal of the American Medical Association, 324*(1), 23–24. https://doi.org/10.1001/jama.2020.8524

Grebla, R.C., Keohane, L., Lee, Y., Lipsitz, L.A., Rahman, M., and Trivedi, A.N. (2015). Waiving the three-day rule: Admissions and length-of-stay at hospitals and skilled nursing facilities did not increase. *Health Affairs, 34*(8), 1324–1330. https://doi.org/10.1377/hlthaff.2015.0054

Guo, J., Konetzka, R.T., and Dale, W. (2014). Using time trade-off methods to assess preferences over health care delivery options: A feasibility study. *Value in Health, 17*(2), 302–305. https://doi.org/10.1016/j.jval.2013.11.010

Haggerty, K.L., Epstein-Lubow, G., Spragens, L.H., Stoeckle, R.J., Evertson, L.C., Jennings, L.A., and Reuben, D.B. (2020). Recommendations to improve payment policies for comprehensive dementia care. *Journal of the American Geriatrics Society, 68*(11), 2478–2485. https://doi.org/10.1111/jgs.16807

Harris-Kojetin, L., Sengupta, M., Lendon, J.P., Rome, V., Valverde, R., and Caffrey, C. (2019). Long-term care providers and services users in the United States, 2015–2016. *Vital and Health Statistics, 3*(43). National Center for Health Statistics. https://www.cdc.gov/nchs/data/series/sr_03/sr03_43-508.pdf

Hemming, K., Haines, T.P., Chilton, P.J., Girling, A.J., and Lilford, R.J. (2015). The stepped wedge cluster randomised trial: Rationale, design, analysis, and reporting. *BMJ (Clinical Research Ed.), 350*, h391. https://doi.org/10.1136/bmj.h391

Hill, J.W., Futterman, R., Duttagupta, S., Mastey, V., Lloyd, J.R., and Fillit, H. (2002). Alzheimer's disease and related dementias increase costs of comorbidities in managed Medicare. *Neurology, 58*(1), 62–70. https://doi.org/10.1212/wnl.58.1.62

Howell, B.L., Conway, P.H., and Rajkumar, R. (2015). Guiding principles for Center for Medicare & Medicaid Innovation model evaluations. *Journal of the American Medical Association, 313*(23), 2317–2318. https://doi.org/10.1001/jama.2015.2902

Hu, J., Jensen, G.A., Nerenz, D., and Tarraf, W. (2015). Medicare's annual wellness visit in a large health care organization: Who is using it? *Annals of Internal Medicine, 163*(7), 567–568. https://doi.org/10.7326/L15-5145

Hudomiet, P., Hurd, M.D., and Rohwedder, S. (2019). The relationship between lifetime out-of-pocket medical expenditures, dementia, and socioeconomic status in the U.S. *Journal of the Economics of Ageing, 14*. https://doi.org/10.1016/j.jeoa.2018.11.006

Institute of Medicine. (1986). *The Quality of Care in Nursing Homes*. Washington, DC: The National Academies Press. https://www.nap.edu/catalog/646/improving-the-quality-of-care-in-nursing-homes

———. (2001). *Improving the Quality of Long-Term Care*. Washington, DC: The National Academies Press. https://www.nap.edu/catalog/9611/improving-the-quality-of-long-term-care

Jacobson, M., Thunell, J., and Zissimopoulos, J. (2020). Structured cognitive assessment at Medicare's annual wellness visit among beneficiaries in fee-for-service and Medicare Advantage plans. *Health Affairs, 39*(11), 1935–1942. https://doi.org/10.1377/hlthaff.2019.01795

Jennings, L.A., Tan, Z., Wenger, N.S., Cook, E.A., Han, W., McCreath, H.E., Serrano, K.S., Roth, C.P., and Reuben, D.B. (2016). Quality of care provided by a comprehensive dementia care comanagement program. *Journal of the American Geriatrics Society, 64*(8), 1724–1730. https://doi.org/10.1111/jgs.14251

Jennings, L.A., Laffan, A.M, Schlissel, A.C., Colligan, E., Tan, Z., Wenger, N.S., and Reuben, D.B. (2019). Health care utilization and cost outcomes of a comprehensive dementia care program for Medicare beneficiaries. *JAMA Internal Medicine, 179*(2), 161–166. https://doi.org/10.1001/jamainternmed.2018.5579

Jennings, L.A., Hollands, S., Keeler, E., Wenger, N.S., and Reuben, D.B. (2020). The effects of dementia care co-management on acute care, hospice, and long-term care utilization. *Journal of the American Geriatrics Society, 68*(11), 2500–2507. https://doi.org/10.1111/jgs.16667

Jung, H.Y., Li, Q., Rahman, M., and Mor, V. (2018). Medicare Advantage enrollees' use of nursing homes: Trends and nursing home characteristics. *American Journal of Managed Care, 24*(8), e249–e256.

Kumar, A., Rahman, M., Trivedi, A.N., Resnik, L., Gozalo, P., and Mor, V. (2018). Comparing post-acute rehabilitation use, length of stay, and outcomes experienced by Medicare fee-for-service and Medicare Advantage beneficiaries with hip fracture in the United States: A secondary analysis of administrative data. *PLoS Medicine, 15*(6), e1002592. https://doi.org/10.1371/journal.pmed.1002592

Kuo, T.C., Zhao, Y., Weir, S., Kramer, M.S., and Ash, A.S. (2008). Implications of comorbidity on costs for patients with Alzheimer disease. *Medical Care, 46*(8), 839–846. https://doi.org/10.1097/MLR.0b013e318178940b

Lee, L., Hillier, L., Patel, T., Weston, W. (2020). A decade of dementia care training: Learning needs of primary care clinicians, *Journal of Continuing Education in the Health Professions, 40(2)*, 131-140. doi: 10.1097/CEH.0000000000000288

Li, Q., Rahman, M., Gozalo, P., Keohane, L.M., Gold, M.R., and Trivedi, A.N. (2018). Regional variations: The use of hospitals, home health, and skilled nursing in traditional Medicare and Medicare Advantage. *Health Affairs, 37*(8), 1274–1281. https://doi.org/10.1377/hlthaff.2018.0147

Lin, P. (2020). *Commissioned Paper on AD/ADRD Health Economics and Public Policy.* Paper prepared for the National Academies of Sciences, Engineering, and Medicine, Decadal Survey of Behavioral and Social Science Research on Alzheimer's Disease and Alzheimer's Disease-Related Dementias. https://www.nationalacademies.org/event/10-17-2019/meeting-2-decadal-survey-of-behavioral-and-social-science-research-on-alzheimers-disease-and-alzheimers-disease-related-dementias

Lin, P.J., Kaufer, D.I., Maciejewski, M.L., Ganguly, R., Paul, J.E., and Biddle, A.K. (2010). An examination of Alzheimer's disease case definitions using Medicare claims and survey data. *Alzheimer's & Dementia, 6*(4), 334–341. https://doi.org/10.1016/j.jalz.2009.09.001

Lin, P.J., Zhong, Y., Fillit, H.M., Chen, E., and Neumann, P.J. (2016). Medicare expenditures of individuals with Alzheimer's disease and related dementias or mild cognitive impairment before and after diagnosis. *Journal of the American Geriatrics Society, 64*(8), 1549–1557. https://doi.org/10.1111/jgs.14227

Medicaid and CHIP Payment and Access Commission. (2020). *Report to Congress on Medicaid and CHIP*. https://www.macpac.gov/wp-content/uploads/2020/06/June-2020-Report-to-Congress-on-Medicaid-and-CHIP.pdf

Medicare Payment Advisory Commission and Medicaid and CHIP Payment and Access Commission. (2018). *Data Book: Beneficiaries Dually Eligible for Medicare and Medicaid*. http://medpac.gov/docs/default-source/data-book/jan18_medpac_macpac_dualsdatabook_sec.pdf?sfvrsn=0

Meyers, D.J., Gadbois, E.A., Brazier, J., Tucher, E., and Thomas, K.S. (2020). Medicare plans' adoption of special supplemental benefits for the chronically ill for enrollees with social needs. *JAMA Network Open, 3*(5), e204690. https://doi.org/10.1001/jamanetworkopen.2020.4690

Meyers, D.J., Rahman, M., Rivera-Hernandez, M., Trivedi, A.N., and Mor, V. (2021). Plan switching among Medicare Advantage beneficiaries with Alzheimer's disease and other dementias. *Alzheimer's & Dementia*, 7(1), e12150. https://doi.org/10.1002/trc2.12150

Miller, S.C., Mor, V., Wu, N., Gozalo, P., and Lapane, K. (2002). Does receipt of hospice care in nursing homes improve the management of pain at the end of life? *Journal of the American Geriatrics Society*, 50(3), 507–515. https://doi.org/10.1046/j.1532-5415.2002.50118.x

Mitchell, S.L., Mor, V., Harrison, J., and McCarthy, E.P. (2020). Embedded pragmatic trials in dementia care: Realizing the vision of the NIA IMPACT Collaboratory. *Journal of the American Geriatrics Society*, 68(Suppl 2), S1–S7. https://doi.org/10.1111/jgs.16621

Mor, V., and Teno, J.M. (2016). Regulating and paying for hospice and palliative care: Reflections on the Medicare hospice benefit. *Journal of Health Politics, Policy, and Law*, 41(4), 697–716. https://doi.org/10.1215/03616878-362089

Mor, V., Zinn, J., Angelelli, J., Teno, J.M., and Miller, S.C. (2004). Driven to tiers: Socioeconomic and racial disparities in the quality of nursing home care. *Milbank Quarterly*, 82(2), 227–256. https://doi.org/10.1111/j.0887-378X.2004.00309.x

Mor, V., Intrator, O., Feng, Z., and Grabowski, D.C. (2010). The revolving door of rehospitalization from skilled nursing facilities. *Health Affairs*, 29(1), 57–64. https://doi.org/10.1377/hlthaff.2009.0629

Mor, V., Rahman, M., and McHugh, J. (2016). Accountability of hospitals for Medicare beneficiaries' postacute care discharge disposition. *JAMA Internal Medicine*, 176(1), 19–21. https://doi.org/10.1001/jamainternmed.2015.6508

Mor, V., Thomas, K.S., and Rahman, M. (2018). Defining and measuring nursing home placement. *Journal of the American Geriatric Society*, 66(10), 1866-1868.

NASEM (National Academies of Sciences, Engineering, and Medicine). (2021). *Meeting the Challenge of Caring for Persons Living with Dementia and Their Care Partners and Caregivers: A Way Forward*. Washington, DC: The National Academies Press. https://doi.org/10.17226/26026

National Institute on Aging. (2016). *End of Life: Helping with Comfort and Care*. https://order.nia.nih.gov/sites/default/files/2017-07/End_of_Life_508.pdf

National Quality Forum. (2014). *Priority Setting for Healthcare Performance Measurement: Addressing Performance Measure Gaps for Dementia, Including Alzheimer's Disease*. https://www.qualityforum.org/priority_setting_for_healthcare_performance_measurement_alzheimers_disease.aspx

Newcomer, R.J., Ko, M., Kang, T., Harrington, C., Hulett, D., and Bindman, A.B. (2016). Health care expenditures after initiating long-term services and supports in the community versus in a nursing facility. *Medical Care*, 54(3), 221–228. https://doi.org/10.1097/MLR.0000000000000491

Ouslander, J.G., and Grabowski, D.C. (2020). COVID-19 in nursing homes: Calming the perfect storm. *Journal of the American Geriatrics Society*, 68(10), 2153–2162. https://doi.org/10.1111/jgs.16784

Panagiotou, O.A., Kosar, C.M., White, E.M., Bantis, L.E., Yang, X., Santostefano, C.M., Feifer, R.A., Blackman, C., Rudolph, J.L., Gravenstein, S., and Mor, V. (2021). Risk factors associated with all-cause 30-day mortality in nursing home residents with COVID-19. *JAMA Internal Medicine*, 181(4), 439–448. https://doi.org/10.1001/jamainternmed.2020.7968

Park, S., White, L., Fishman, P., Larson, E.B., and Coe, N.B. (2020). Health care utilization, care satisfaction, and health status for Medicare Advantage and traditional Medicare beneficiaries with and without Alzheimer disease and related dementias. *JAMA Network Open*, 3(3), e201809. https://doi.org/10.1001/jamanetworkopen.2020.1809

Polniaszek, S., Walsh, E.G., and Wiener, J.M. (2011). *Hospitalizations of Nursing Home Residents: Background and Options.* Washington, DC: Office of the Assistant Secretary for Planning and Evaluation, U.S. Department of Health and Human Services. https://aspe.hhs.gov/system/files/pdf/76296/NHResHosp.pdf

Possin, K.L., Merrilees, J.J., Dulaney, S., Bonasera, S.J., Chiong, W., Lee, K., Hooper, S.M., Allen, I.E., Braley, T., Bernstein, A., Rosa, T.D., Harrison, K., Begert-Hellings, H., Kornak, J., Kahn, J.G., Naasan, G., Lanata, S., Clark, A.M., Chodos, A., Gearhart, R., Ritchie, C., and Miller, B.L. (2019). Effect of collaborative dementia care via telephone and internet on quality of life, caregiver well-being, and health care use: The care ecosystem randomized clinical trial. *JAMA Internal Medicine,* 179(12), 1658–1667. https://doi.org/10.1001/jamainternmed.2019.4101

Rahman, M., Foster, A.D., Grabowski, D.C., Zinn, J.S., and Mor, V. (2013). Effect of hospital-SNF referral linkages on rehospitalization. *Health Services Research,* 48(6pt1), 1898–1919. https://doi.org/10.1111/1475-6773.12112

Rahman, M., Gozalo, P., Tyler, D., Grabowski, D.C., Trivedi, A., and Mor, V. (2014). Dual eligibility, selection of skilled nursing facility, and length of Medicare paid postacute stay. *Medical Care Research and Review,* 71(4), 384–401. https://doi.org/10.1177/1077558714533824

Reuben, D.B., Evertson, L.C., Wenger, N.S., Serrano, K., Chodosh, J., Ercoli, L., and Tan, Z.S. (2013). The University of California at Los Angeles Alzheimer's and Dementia Care Program for comprehensive, coordinated, patient-centered care: Preliminary data. *Journal of the American Geriatrics Society,* 61(12), 2214–2218. https://doi.org/10.1111/jgs.12562

Reuben, D.B., Gupta, R., and Skootsky, S. (2019a). How a population-based approach can improve dementia care. *Health Affairs Blog.* https://doi.org/10.1377/hblog20190506.543619

Reuben, D.B., Tan, Z.S., Romero, T., Wenger, N.S., Keeler, E., and Jennings, L.A. (2019b). Patient and caregiver benefit from a comprehensive dementia care program: 1-Year results from the UCLA Alzheimer's and Dementia Care Program. *Journal of the American Geriatrics Society,* 67(11), 2267–2273. https://doi.org/10.1111/jgs.16085

Sapien, J., and Sexton, J. (2020, June 16). "Fire through dry grass": Andrew Cuomo saw COVID-19's threat to nursing homes. Then he risked adding to it. *Pro Publica.* https://www.propublica.org/article/fire-through-dry-grass-andrew-cuomo-saw-covid-19-threat-to-nursing-homes-then-he-risked-adding-to-it

Song, Y., Skinner, J., Bynum, J., Sutherland, J., Wennberg, J.E., and Fisher, E.S. (2010). Regional variations in diagnostic practices. *New England Journal of Medicine,* 363(1), 45–53. https://doi.org/10.1056/NEJMsa0910881

Soucheray, S. (2020, June 16). *Nursing Homes Might Account for 40% of U.S. COVID-19 Deaths.* Center for Infectious Disease Research and Policy, University of Minnesota. https://www.cidrap.umn.edu/news-perspective/2020/06/nursing-homes-might-account-40-us-covid-19-deaths

Suehs, B.T., Davis, C.D., Alvir, J., van Amerongen, D., Pharmd, N.C., Joshi, A.V., Faison, W.E., and Shah, S.N. (2013). The clinical and economic burden of newly diagnosed Alzheimer's disease in a Medicare Advantage population. *American Journal of Alzheimer's Disease and Other Dementias,* 28(4), 384–392. https://doi.org/10.1177/1533317513488911

Temel, J.S., Greer, J.A., Muzikansky, A., Gallagher, E.R., Admane, S., Jackson, V.A., Dahlin, C.M., Blinderman, C.D., Jacobsen, J., Pirl, W.F., Billings, J.A., and Lynch, T.J. (2010). Early palliative care for patients with metastatic non-small-cell lung cancer. *New England Journal of Medicine,* 363(8), 733–742. https://doi.org/10.1056/NEJMoa1000678

Teno, J.M., Gozalo, P.L., Bynum, J.P., Leland, N.E., Miller, S.C., Morden, N.E., Scupp, T., Goodman, D.C., and Mor, V. (2013). Change in end-of-life care for Medicare beneficiaries: Site of death, place of care, and health care transitions in 2000, 2005, and 2009. *Journal of the American Medical Association,* 309(5), 470–477. https://doi.org/10.1001/jama.2012.207624

Teno, J.M., Plotzke, M., Gozalo, P., and Mor, V. (2014). A national study of live discharges from hospice. *Journal of Palliative Medicine, 17*(10), 1121–1127. https://doi.org/10.1089/jpm.2013.0595

Thomas, K.S., Durfey, S., Gadbois, E.A., Meyers, D.J., Brazier, J.F., McCreedy, E.M., Fashaw, S., and Wetle, T. (2019). Perspectives of Medicare Advantage plan representatives on addressing social determinants of health in response to the CHRONIC Care Act. *JAMA Network Open, 2*(7), e196923. https://doi.org/10.1001/jamanetworkopen.2019.6923

Tyler, D.A., Feng, Z., Leland, N.E., Gozalo, P., Intrator, O., and Mor, V. (2013). Trends in postacute care and staffing in US nursing homes, 2001–2010. *Journal of the American Medical Directors Association, 14*(11), 817–820. https://doi.org/10.1016/j.jamda.2013.05.013

Unruh, M.A., Grabowski, D.C., Travedi, A.N., and Mor, V. (2013). Medicaid bed-hold policies and hospitalization of long-stay nursing home residents. *Health Services Research, 48*(5), 1617–1633. https://doi.org/10.1111/1475-6773.12054

U.S. Government Accountability Office. (2018a). *CMS Innovation Center: Model Implementation and Center Performance*. https://www.gao.gov/assets/gao-18-302.pdf

———. (2018b). *Medicaid Assisted Living Services: Improved Federal Oversight of Beneficiary Health and Welfare Is Needed*. https://www.gao.gov/assets/gao-18-179.pdf

Van Houtven, C.H., DePasquale, N., and Coe, N.B. (2020). Essential long-term care workers commonly hold second jobs and double- or triple-duty caregiving roles. *Journal of the American Geriatrics Society, 68*(8), 1657–1660. https://doi.org/10.1111/jgs.16509

Werner, R.M., Konetzka, R.T., Stuart, E.A., Norton, E.C., Polsky, D., and Park, J. (2009). Impact of public reporting on quality of postacute care. *Health Services Research, 44*(4), 1169–1187. https://doi.org/10.1111/j.1475-6773.2009.00967.x

Werner, R.M., Norton, E.C., Konetzka, R.T., and Polsky, D. (2012). Do consumers respond to publicly reported quality information? Evidence from nursing homes. *Journal of Health Economics, 31*(1), 50–61. https://doi.org/10.1016/j.jhealeco.2012.01.001

Werner, R.M., Konetzka, R.T., and Polsky, D. (2013). The effect of pay-for-performance in nursing homes: Evidence from state Medicaid programs. *Health Services Research, 48*(4), 1393–1414. https://doi.org/10.1111/1475-6773.12035

———. (2016). Changes in consumer demand following public reporting of summary quality ratings: An evaluation in nursing homes. *Health Services Research, 51*(Suppl 2), 1291–1309. https://doi.org/10.1111/1475-6773.12459

Werner, R.M., Coe, N.B., Qi, M., and Konetzka, R.T. (2019). Patient outcomes after hospital discharge to home with home health care vs to a skilled nursing facility. *JAMA Internal Medicine, 179*(5), 617–623. https://doi.org/10.1001/jamainternmed.2018.7998

Werner, R.M., Hoffman, A.K., and Coe, N.B. (2020). Long-term care policy after COVID-19: Solving the nursing home crisis. *Faculty Scholarship at Penn Law, 2215*. https://scholarship.law.upenn.edu/faculty_scholarship/2215

White, L., Fishman, P., Basu, A., Crane, P.K., Larson, E.B., and Coe, N.B. (2019). Medicare expenditures attributable to dementia. *Health Services Research, 54*(4), 773–781. https://doi.org/10.1111/1475-6773.13134

White, E.M., Kosar, C.M., Feifer, R.A., Blackman, C., Gravenstein, S., Ouslander, J., and Mor, V. (2020). Variation in SARS CoV 2 prevalence in U.S. skilled nursing facilities. *Journal of the American Geriatrics Society, 68*(10), 2167–2173. https://doi.org/10.1111/jgs.16752

Willis, J., Antono, B., Bazemore, A., Jetty, A., Petterson, S., George, J., Rosario, B.L., Scheufele, E., Rajmane, A., Dankwa-Mullan, I., and Rhee, K. (2020). *The State of Primary Care in the United States: A Chartbook of Facts and Statistics*. Robert Graham Center. https://www.graham-center.org/content/dam/rgc/documents/publications-reports/reports/PrimaryCareChartbook2021.pdf

Yang, Z., Zhang, K., Lin, P.J., Clevenger, C., and Atherly, A. (2012). A longitudinal analysis of the lifetime cost of dementia. *Health Services Research, 47,* 1660–1678.

Zhu, C.W., Cosentino, S., Ornstein, K., Gu, Y., Scarmeas, N., Andrews, H., and Stern, Y. (2015). Medicare utilization and expenditures around incident dementia in a multiethnic cohort. *Journals of Gerontology: Series A, 70*(11), 1448–1453. https://doi.org/10.1093/gerona/glv124

Zimmerman, S., Sloane, P.D., Williams, C.S., Reed, P.S., Preisser, J.S., Eckert, J.K., Boustani, M., and Dobbs, D. (2005). Dementia care and quality of life in assisted living and nursing homes. *Gerontologist, 45*(suppl_1), 133–146. https://doi.org/10.1093/geront/45.suppl_1.133

Zimmerman, S., Bowers, B.J., Cohen, L.W., Grabowski, D.C., Horn, S.D., Kemper, P., and THRIVE Research Collaborative. (2016). New evidence on the Green House Model of Nursing Home Care: Synthesis of findings and implications for policy, practice, and research. *Health Services Research, 51*(Suppl 1), 475–496. https://doi.org/10.1111/1475-6773.12430

Zissimopoulos, J., Crimmins, E., and St. Clair, P. (2014). The value of delaying Alzheimer's disease onset. *Forum for Health Economics & Policy, 18,* 25–39.

7

Economic Costs of Dementia

As the numbers of cases of dementia grow in the United States, the economic costs to individuals and to society are likely to increase as well. Yet developing an understanding of the full extent of the economic impacts of dementia—and how to reduce them—is not a straightforward challenge. The economic costs for persons living with the disease, their caregivers and families, and society are described in multiple studies, but important questions remain. How do costs vary across diverse populations, disease types, disease severity, and trajectory of disease? What is the value of improvements in health and well-being or effective prevention measures? How do policy and practice in the health care and long-term care sectors affect costs? What are the economic impacts of innovations in prevention, diagnosis, and treatment? Answers to these and other questions can point to opportunities to reduce both the economic costs of dementia overall and disparities in who bears those costs, and to implement changes effectively.

There are two broad ways to decrease the negative economic impacts of dementia: reducing unnecessary costs and increasing value, that is, achieving significant improvements in health, quality of life, and other outcomes that justify their costs. This chapter reviews what is known about the economic costs of dementia and explores both the drivers of these costs and the potential economic impacts of innovations in treatment and care, policies, and programs. It identifies directions for research that would support the goals of reducing costs and distributing them more equitably. The committee recognizes that while research in economics makes a valuable contribution to reducing the negative impacts of dementia, it does not address the multiple noneconomic losses endured by persons living with dementia and their families.

MAGNITUDE OF ECONOMIC COSTS

The primary economic costs of dementia to persons living with dementia and their families are (1) medical and long-term care costs, and (2) the value of unpaid caregiving provided by family (most commonly) and friends. Most estimates of these costs in the literature draw on such nationally representative data sources as the Health and Retirement Study, the Medicare Current Beneficiary Survey, and Medicare claims data. An estimate of annual per-person costs for 2019, which includes health care and the value of unpaid care provided to persons with Alzheimer's disease, is approximately $81,000 ($31,000 is the value of the unpaid care) (Zissimopoulos et al., 2014). This estimate is about four times higher than the costs of the same care provided to similarly aged persons without the disease. Other estimates of annual costs are lower, with a range of $41,000–$56,000; estimates of the cost of unpaid care are less variable (Hurd et al., 2013; Moore et al., 2001). Cost estimates vary for reasons including, but not limited to, the methodology used for valuing the time spent by unpaid caregivers (e.g., replacement rate or opportunity cost of time); how medical care costs associated specifically with a dementia diagnosis are distinguished from the costs associated with other conditions; and the time frame over which costs are being evaluated (i.e., whether they include pre-diagnosis costs or end-of-life care).

Residential care is very expensive. Estimates of the typical costs of long-term care range from $52,624 per year for a home health aide to $90,000 for a semiprivate room in a nursing home and up to $102,000 for a private room (Genworth Financial, 2020). Medicaid, which covers long-term care for low-income individuals and those who become poor as a result of paying for health care and long-term care, is the largest public payer for long-term care, covering 62 percent of nursing home residents (Kaiser Family Foundation, 2017), and one-quarter of adults with dementia who live in the community are covered by Medicaid over the course of a year (Garfield et al., 2015). Recently, attention has turned to the "forgotten middle"—those who neither qualify for Medicaid nor have the resources to pay for long-term care (Pearson et al., 2019).

Additional insight into the economic costs of dementia can be gained by considering costs aggregated over a specific period of time. For example, one study calaculates the costs, including rest-of-lifetime medical care, unpaid caregiving, and long-term care, for a 70-year-old who develops dementia (Zissimopoulos et al., 2014). This estimate—more than $700,000—is three times higher than estimated lifetime health care costs for a 70-year-old who dies without developing dementia. Another study estimates that lifetime out-of-pocket medical costs for a person living with dementia are about $38,000 higher than the costs for a similar person without dementia (Hudomiet et al., 2019). An estimate of 5-year incremental costs to the traditional Medicare program for each dementia diagnosis (additional costs associated with the diagnosis for the 5-year period) is approximately $15,700 per patient, with nearly half of these costs incurred in the first year after diagnosis (White et al., 2019). A systematic review of nine studies provides ranges for costs attributable to both prevalent and incident dementia in private Medicare managed care plans. For prevalent cases, the estimates range from $3,700 to $8,700. The variation is wider—$8,900 to $38,800—for incident cases (based on first-year postdiagnosis costs) (Fishman et al., 2019).

Despite the methodological differences that yield varied estimates, the high costs of dementia are well documented. When aggregated to the U.S. population, the costs are estimated to have exceeded $500 billion in 2019 and are projected to increase to about $1.5 trillion by 2050 (Alzheimer's Association, 2021; Zissimopoulos et al., 2014).

Unaccounted for in these estimates are other economic costs, such as the impact on caregivers' wages and future employability; when included, these costs increase estimates of unpaid caregiver costs by as much as 20 percent (Coe et al., 2018). Moreover, these costs may be underestimated because the physical and mental strain associated with unpaid caregiving likely translates to other costs, such as for caregivers' own health care (Chen et al., 2020; Watson et al., 2019; Goren et al., 2016). Also not included in the estimates reported above are costs to employers, such as the costs of absenteeism, productivity losses, and turnover associated with employees' need to provide care for loved ones. Other costs unaccounted for include financial harm to persons living with dementia and their families. Cognitive impairment may lead to financial decision-making errors, including payment delinquency and susceptibility to financial exploitation, starting years before diagnosis (Nicholas et al., 2020). Financial harm to individuals living with dementia may also have long-term implications for the surviving spouse.

Poorly documented as well are disparities in who bears the costs of dementia, such as differences across racial and ethnic lines (Cantarero-Prieto et al., 2019). Estimated annual medical care and caregiving costs associated with dementia, based on data from the Health and Retirement Study, are about $20,000 higher for Hispanic and Black individuals than for their White counterparts (Alzheimer's Association, 2016). Other studies have found lower medical expenditures that may reflect differential access to care and preferences for types of care (Park and Chen, 2020). Questions about how persons living with dementia and their families finance the high costs of dementia are urgent and will grow more so if not addressed as dementia cases increase.

The financing and delivery of long-term care represent a challenge that policy makers have yet to address. The nation's long-term services and supports system is fragmented and inadequate (see Chapter 6).[1] The Congressional Budget Office has estimated that unpaid (informal) care accounted for 55 percent of the economic value of long-term care for older adults in 2019; institutional care accounted for about 39 percent and home and community-based care for the remaining 14 percent (Congressional Budget Office, 2013). Private long-term care insurance has not filled the gap, with only 8 percent of Americans having such coverage. This insurance is costly and has been deemed a failed product by many experts: the number of companies offering it declined from 125 in 2000 to 15 in 2014 (National Association of Insurance Commissioners and the Center for Insurance Policy and Research, 2016).

State legislatures have begun exploring options for filling the financing gap. Washington became the first state to enact an entitlement for all residents with a sufficient work history through a minimal payroll deduction of 0.58 percent for every working person in the state. This measure will go into effect in 2022, and eligible inidividuals will receive a benefit of up to $36,500. Additional research on the long-term sustainability of various financing options, as well as on the trade-offs among different spending priorities and implications for those who will bear the costs, is needed to support state and federal policy makers as they consider and implement long-term care programs.

Among the many questions whose answers may point to opportunities for reducing economic burden are how the costs of dementia affect generations of family members and contribute to the intergenerational transmission of inequality; how the costs are distributed among public sources, individuals, and families; how policy changes related to dementia care benefits affect costs; how reimbursement for dementia care and long-term care insurance affect the costs of dementia; and how to finance long-term care for persons living with dementia.

DRIVERS OF COSTS

Many factors affect the high costs of the care needed by people living with dementia. People living with these diseases are more likely to be hospitalized and have longer stays and utilize more postacute skilled nursing in facilities and home health care relative to otherwise similar older adults without dementia (White et al., 2019; Leibson et al., 2015; Lin et al., 2016).

---

[1] Medicare pays for time-limited care after a hospital stay or acute episode and is beginning to cover a small amount of supplemental services (typically a few days per year) but does not cover true long-term care.

High rates of comorbid conditions and complicated management of those conditions make a key contribution to the excess health care costs incurred by individuals with dementia (Lin et al., 2013). Coordination of care across multiple conditions may therefore provide opportunities to improve outcomes and increase the efficiency of care (see Chapter 6) (Zulman et al., 2015; Boyd et al., 2005).

Systematic reviews of cost drivers have identified consistent findings that costs increase as dementia progresses from the mild or early stage to the severe or late stage (Schaller et al., 2015). The last year of life is typically the most expensive for people living with dementia because of the amount and nature of care they need (see Chapers 3 and 6) (Kelley et al., 2015). The heterogeneity of costs within disease stages, however, is less well understood. Several new models for comprehensive dementia care have shown promise not only for improving care and outcomes but also for reducing costs (see Chapter 6 for discussion of comprehensive dementia care) (Haggerty et al., 2020). Although similar in aims, such programs differ in many ways, including scope of services and cost and effectiveness; the rigor of the studies that have evaluated them also varies (Boustani et al., 2019). Dissemination of such care models has thus far been limited. Traditional Medicare and Medicare Advantage plans do not cover all components of comprehensive care, and the health care systems that would implement those services often lack the infrastructure needed to deliver them. Further research on the cost-effectiveness and value of different programs and how payment structures can be modified to deliver better and lower-cost dementia care would support the achievement of value in care.

The cost and reimbursement structures of traditional Medicare and Medicare Advantage plans also play a key role in the overall cost picture. Newer Medicare benefits, such as the annual wellness visit with its required cognitive screening, may increase early detection, but the effects on costs are as yet unknown (Jacobson et al., 2020). The factors driving differences in costs across the types of Medicare plans (see Chapter 6) are not well understood, but differences in benefits are likely a factor. For example, Medicare Advantage special needs plans (coverage for defined disabilities; see Chapter 6) are available to persons with dementia and provide targeted care (e.g., dementia care specialists) and drug formularies designed for these beneficiaries; they often also cover the cost of a care coordinator. These special needs plans increase use of primary care and improve management of such chronic conditions as diabetes; however, whether this is the case for persons living with dementia and with what implications for costs are not well understood (Cohen et al., 2012).

While there is ample evidence that participants in Medicare Advantage plans have lower rates of hospitalization and readmission compared with participants in traditional Medicare, after risk adjustment, whether these broad differences persist for persons living with dementia is unknown (Cohen et al., 2012). Beginning in 2020, Medicare Advantage risk adjustment includes dementia, which will increase payments to Medicare Advantage plans for medical care for persons living with dementia. The adjustment provides incentives for better detection of dementia and improved care, with unknown impacts on costs. Further research is needed to explore how the organization of health care and reimbursement and payment systems affect costs and their distribution across payers.

THE ECONOMICS OF INNOVATION

Several types of innovation have the potential to provide value through their impact on costs (cost savings) and by extending life-years and the quality of those life-years. Innovations may reduce direct medical costs and may also reduce the costs associated with caregiving or long-term care. Improvements in quality of life may not be easily measurable but have value beyond reduction in costs. The potential benefits of models for comprehensive care have already been discussed in Chapter 6, but there are other possibilities.

First, more than 130 innovative treatments for Alzheimer's disease and related dementias are being investigated in clinical trials, and some may turn out to slow or halt disease progression and reduce costs (Cummings et al., 2019). A simulation study found that a hypothetical treatment innovation that delayed the onset of Alzheimer's disease by 5 years would reduce the population with the disease by 41 percent in 2050, which would reduce annual costs by $640 billion (Zissimopoulos et al., 2014). However, novel treatments, which would likely have high prices, could exacerbate the overall economic impact of the disease. Such treatments would also likely be less available to disadvantaged populations and in underserved regions, which could increase disparities in outcomes (Jervis et al., 2007). Furthermore, the potential treatments currently under study, even if successful, are mostly designed to prevent or delay progression from mild cognitive impairment (MCI) or mild dementia, and would not likely improve outcomes for the millions of Americans who already meet criteria for moderate to severe dementia.

Innovations may extend life or bring a greater number of years with improved quality of life. Using a measure known as a quality-adjusted life-year, researchers can estimate the diverse costs of disease and the value of innovation. Uncertainty about the innovation's long-term effectiveness will pose challenges for value assessment, however. Novel treatments targeting younger patients (i.e., under age 65) present incentive challenges regarding coverage and reimbursement for health care payers. For example, biomarkers for Alzheimer's disease that are currently available or will soon be available (see Chapter 3) could identify large groups at risk for the disease, many of whom would never go on to develop clinical symptoms. Everyone in such a group might be eligible to take a novel medication that was approved, but a far smaller portion would actually benefit. Thus, the costs for these expensive medications could be quite large relative to the number of people they would benefit. If drugs are targeted to those with MCI or mild dementia, most recipients would be Medicare beneficiaries, so that program would bear the brunt of these new costs.

Research on alternative payment mechanisms, such as performance-based installment payments, may aid in aligning incentives and produce improved coverage and value outcomes. The clinical, economic, and social implications of innovations in diagnostics, such as the introduction of the Precivity blood test for Alzheimer's disease, are uncertain. Whether earlier and more accurate diagnostics would improve care, reduce avoidable hospitalizations, improve patient financial planning, and spur innovation in treatment is as yet unknown, although these new diagnostics would almost certainly increase costs associated with follow-up health care utilization.

Nonpharmacologic innovations may also have cost impacts warranting study. For example, innovations in housing (see Chapter 5) and in long-term care (see Chapter 6) are designed to allow individuals living with dementia to retain independence longer and avoid more expensive institutional placements. Although these innovations have their own costs, it will be valuable to understand the implications. Similarly, the use of technology to offset some labor costs could have varied implications, including allowing higher wages for direct care workers and reducing the need for highly paid care in certain settings.

APPLYING BEHAVIORAL ECONOMICS

Behavioral economics, an interdisciplinary field that draws on research in both psychology and economics, offers a valuable approach to identifying opportunities to reduce costs or add value to costly services. This approach breaks with the usual assumption of economists that individuals act purely according to rational self-interest. Behavioral economists acknowledge the role of reason but also take into account the influence of other factors that have traditionally been the province of psychology, such as limited cognition, biases, and social motivations (see, e.g., Thaler and Sunstein, 2008). Interventions designed by behavioral economists are intended to influence actions to encourage particular outcomes through subtle modifications of the choice environment, such as altering the way options are presented, how many are offered, or how incentives are conveyed or emphasized (Fox et al., 2020).

This approach has been applied to many aspects of health and health policy, leading to improvements in health and health behaviors (Meeker et al., 2016; Doctor et al., 2018; Halpern et al., 2013). In this context, behavioral economists have posited that individuals may not act in their own best interest for varied reasons, including incomplete information about an issue, heuristics (or rules of thumb) they use in making decisions, and the like (Rice, 2013). However, this approach has not been widely applied to challenges associated with dementia, and it could be of significant value in the design of interventions to, for example, support conversations about advance care planning among patients, caregivers, and clinicians; align nonfinancial incentives, such as by discouraging the inappropriate use of antipsychotics; or encourage health care providers to offer screening for cognitive impairment. Such tools as "nudges" that influence choices below the conscious level, and changes in features of the physical and social environments to change health-related behavior (choice architecture), may be more effective than investment in education or awareness campaigns.

A WORD ABOUT THE COSTS OF ADUCANUMAB

The recent approval by the U.S. Food and Drug Administration (FDA) of the first new drug in decades that is intended to treat Alzheimer's disease, aducanumab, is likely to have substantial impact on the cost picture (we discuss other issues related to this approval in Chapter 9). The economic costs of aducanumab or any other anti-amyloid drugs with similar pricing, administration, monitoring requirements, and possible adverse effects are considerable. These costs include the purchase price of the drug and the costs of the intravenous infusion, MRI scans (baseline and twice in the first year for aducanumab), and assessment and treatment of adverse effects. In addition, two tests used in the clinical trials cited in the FDA application suggest the possibility of additional costs: amyloid PET scans were used to determine patients' eligibility, and testing for certain genes linked with Alzheimer's disease was used to determine maximum dosing, because those with a particular genotype were more likely to develop the principal adverse effect of this medication. At present, neither of these tests is covered by Medicare, but these would either be substantial out-of-pocket expenses to patients or would further increase the cost to Medicare of covering the new drug.

The manufacturer of aducanumab initially estimated that 1 to 2 million persons would currently be eligible to receive the medication, although that number may change depending on eligibility guidelines. Using the manufacturer's estimated cost of $56,000 per patient per year, the total cost just for the drug could range from $56 billion to as much as $112 billion. Whatever number of people ultimately receive the drug, such estimates do not include the costs of infusion, monitoring and treating adverse effects, and additional pre-administration testing. The magnitude of ancillary costs is not yet established, but observers have suggested that they could add tens of thousands in costs per eligible patient (*New York Times*, Cubanski and Neuman, 2021). To put the cost of the drug alone into perspective, the total 2021 National Institutes of Health budget is $43 billion and the total 2021 Medicare budget is $688 billion.

Crucially, the out-of-pocket costs to patients may be substantial. Generally, Medicare covers 80 percent of the cost of drugs included under Part B, and beneficiaries pay the remaining 20 percent. For aducanumab treatment, that means a cost of roughly $11,500 each year, or nearly 40 percent of the $29,650 median annual income for Medicare beneficiaries in 2019 (Cubanski and Neuman, 2021). If private insurers and Medicare grant coverage of the drug, the distribution of out-of-pocket costs across individuals and families will depend on insurance type. There will be variation in the coverage provided by the private plans that younger persons not eligible for Medicare rely on. For those covered by traditional Medicare, out-of-pocket costs will depend on supplemental coverage, while for beneficiaries in Medicare Advantage costs will depend on plan type. Variation in out-of-pocket costs will contribute to inequities in drug access and financial impact across families. Since aducanumab would be covered under Part B, rather than Part D, the prescription drug plan, it is not clear that states' Medicaid programs would necessarily cover the treatment, and it is likely that few state Medicaid plans would cover the required copayment.

Apart from questions about the medical benefits of aducanumab, discussed in Chapter 9, an assessment of the value of it or similar treatments will depend on their impact on costs, both direct costs associated with treatment and associated medical care and indirect costs such as impacts on long-term care costs. Another aspect to be considered is social value, that is, the value of any extended life-years and how the treatment alters the quality of those life-years. Aducanumab and similar treatments may be valuable to individuals and their families, but improved means of measuring value are needed to make such assessments. A standard cost-effectiveness analysis has limitations in the context of serious illnesses such as Alzheimer's disease. For example, standard approaches typically do not allow value benchmarks (e.g., $100,000 per quality-adjusted life-year) to increase with disease severity, so they generally over-value treatments for less severe illnesses, relative to severe illnesses. Additionally, the difference between what sick people would pay to treat illness and what healthy people would pay to insure against illness may be larger for severe diseases such as Alzheimer's disease (Lakdawalla and Phelps, 2020). Valuation of aducanumab will require consideration of uncertainty and variability in treatment outcomes and how these may change over time as evidence is collected. Moreover, a true assessment of value would also take equity into account.

RESEARCH DIRECTIONS

Research in economics can aid in identifying and implementing opportunities to reduce the economic costs of dementia overall and disparities in who bears those costs. Social scientists from across disciplines can contribute understanding about the costs of dementia and their totality; the heterogeneity of costs across diverse populations, disease types, disease severity, and life course of disease; how policies regarding health and long-term care affect costs; and the economic impacts of innovations in prevention, diagnostics, and treatment. The committee identified high-priority research needs in the domain of the economic impact of dementia and how those costs can be reduced. These research needs are summarized in Conclusion 7-1 and detailed in Table 7-1.

> CONCLUSION 7-1: Research in the following areas is needed to improve understanding of the economic impact of dementia and identify ways to reduce those costs:
> - Assessment and quantification of the total economic impact of dementia for individuals and families, including current and future national costs.
> - Improved understanding of drivers of dementia-related costs.
> - Estimation of the value to individuals, families, and society of innovations in prevention; diagnostics; and treatment, including pharmacologic treatments.

TABLE 7-1 Detailed Research Needs

1: Total Economic Impact	• Quantifying of dementia-related costs not currently measured, including but not limited to caregivers' physical and mental health care use, current and future wages, employability, financial exploitation, harms related to dementia, and impacts across generations of family members • Quantifying and analysis of long-term financial impacts of dementia on a spouse and family members and the intergenerational transfer of inequality related to dementia care costs • Assessment of distribution of costs: how costs and types of costs vary across racial/ethnic populations and other vulnerable groups, etiological type of dementia, age at dementia onset, life course of disease, and type of health care system serving persons living with dementia • Assessment of how costs are distributed across payers • Analysis of innovations in long-term care financing • Assessment of factors, including methods utilized, that drive differences in cost estimates

TABLE 7-1 Continued

	• Improved means of estimating the impacts of new treatments, including new drugs, on Medicare, on patients and families, and on relevant policies
2: Drivers of Costs	• Identification of the multiple individual, familial, community, and societal drivers of costs, using rigorous methods for quantifying the costs attributable to dementia • Analysis of how health care institutions and organizations affect costs through policies and practices
3: Value of Innovations	• Analysis of the value of innovations in dementia prevention, diagnosis, treatment, and care models, considering both direct and indirect costs and the value of extended life-years and quality of years (social value) • Use of rigorous tools, including but not limited to dynamic microsimulation models, for analyzing and quantifying the cost and health implications of innovations in diagnostics and treatments for dementia • Application of the tools of behavioral economics to identify opportunities to reduce the economic impact of dementia

REFERENCES

Alzheimer's Association. (2016). 2016 Alzheimer's disease facts and figures. *Alzheimer's & Dementia, 12*(4), 459–509. https://doi.org/10.1016/j.jalz.2016.03.001

———. (2021). *2021 Alzheimer's Disease Facts and Figures.* https://www.alz.org/media/Documents/alzheimers-facts-and-figures.pdf

Belluck, P., & Robbins, R. (2021). Alzheimer's drug poses a dilemma for the F.D.A. New York Times (Online), *New York: New York Times Company.* Jun 5, 2021.

Boustani, M., Alder, C.A., Solid, C.A., and Reuben, D. (2019). An alternative payment model to support widespread use of collaborative dementia care models. *Health Affairs (Millwood), 38*(1), 54–59. https://doi.org/10.1377/hlthaff.2018.05154

Boyd, C.M., Darer, J., Boult, C., Fried, L.P., Boult, L., and Wu, A.W. (2005). Clinical practice guidelines and quality of care for older patients with multiple comorbid diseases: Implications for pay for performance. *Journal of the American Medical Association, 294*(6), 716–724. https://doi.org/10.1001/jama.294.6.716

Cantarero-Prieto, D., Leon, P.L., Blazquez-Fernandez, C., Juan, P.S., and Cobo, C.S. (2019). The economic cost of dementia: A systematic review. *Dementia, 19*(8), 2637–2657. https://doi.org/10.1177/1471301219837776

Chen, C., Thunell, J., and Zissimopoulos, J.C. (2020). Changes in physical and mental health of Black, Hispanic, and White caregivers and non-caregivers associated with onset of spousal dementia. *Alzheimer's & Dementia, 6*(1), e12082. https://doi.org/10.1002/trc2.12082

Coe, N.B., Skira, M.M., and Larson, E.B. (2018). A comprehensive measure of the costs of caring for a parent: Differences according to functional status. *Journal of the American Geriatrics Society, 66,* 2003–2008. https://doi.org/10.1111/jgs.15552

Cohen, R., Lemieux, J., Schoenborn, J., and Mulligan, T. (2012). Medicare Advantage Chronic Special Needs Plan boosted primary care, reduced hospital use among diabetes patients. *Health Affairs, 31*(1), 110–119.

Congressional Budget Office. (2013). *Rising Demand for Long-Term Services and Supports for Elderly People.* https://www.cbo.gov/sites/default/files/cbofiles/attachments/44363-LTC.pdf

Cubanski, J., and Neuman, T. (2021, June 10). PFA's approval of Biogen's new Alzheimer's drug has huge cost implications for Medicare beneficiaries. Kaiser Family Foundation. https://www.kff.org/medicare/issue-brief/fdas-approval-of-biogens-new-alzheimers-drug-has-huge-cost-implications-for-medicare-and-beneficiaries/

Cummings, J., Lee, G., Ritter, A., Sabbagh, M., and Zhong, K. (2019). Alzheimer's disease drug development pipeline: 2019. *Alzheimer's & Dementia, 5*(1), 272–293. https://doi.org/10.1016/j.trci.2019.05.008

Doctor, J.N., Nguyen, A., Lev, R., Lucas, J., Knight, T., Zhao, H., and Menchine, M. (2018). Opioid prescribing decreases after learning of a patient's fatal overdose. *Science, 361*(6402), 588–590.

Fishman, P., Coe, N.B., White, L., Crane, P., Park, S., Ingrahamm, B., and Larson, E. (2019). Cost of dementia in Medicare managed care: A systematic literature review. *American Journal of Managed Care, 25*(8), e247–e253. https://pubmed.ncbi.nlm.nih.gov/31419102

Fox, C.R., Doctor, J.N., Goldstein, N.J., Meeker, D., Persell, S.D., and Linder, J.A. (2020). Details matter: Predicting when nudging clinicians will succeed or fail. *British Medical Journal, 370*, m3256. https://doi.org/10.1136/bmj.m3256

Garfield, R., Mesumeci, M.B., Reaves, E., and Damico, A. (2015). *Medicaid's Role for People with Dementia.* Kaiser Family Foundation. https://www.kff.org/medicaid/issue-brief/medicaids-role-for-people-with-dementia

Genworth Financial. (2020). *Cost of Care Survey.* https://www.genworth.com/aging-and-you/finances/cost-of-care.html

Goren, A., Montgomery, W., Kahle-Wrobleski, K., Nakamura, T., and Ueda, K. (2016). Impact of caring for persons with Alzheimer's disease or dementia on caregivers' health outcomes: Findings from a community based survey in Japan. *BMC Geriatrics, 16*, 122. https://doi.org/10.1186/s12877-016-0298-y

Haggerty, K.L., Epstein-Lubow, G., Spragens, L., Stoeckel, R., Evertson, L., Jennings, L., and Reuben, D. (2020). Recommendations to improve payment policies for comprehensive dementia care. *Journal of the American Geriatrics Society, 68*(11), 2478–2485. https://doi.org/10.1111/jgs.16807jgs.16807

Halpern, S.D., Loewenstein, G., and Volpp, K.G. (2013). Default options in advance directives influence how patients set goals for end-of-life care. *Health Affairs, 32*(2), 408–417. https://doi.org/10.1377/hlthaff.2012.0895

Hudomiet, P., Hurd, M.D., and Rohwedder, S. (2019). The relationship between lifetime out-of-pocket medical expenditures, dementia, and socioeconomic status in the U.S. *Journal of the Economics of Ageing, 14*, 100181. https://doi.org/10.1016/j.jeoa.2018.11.006

Hurd, M.D., Martorell, P., Delavande, A., Mullen, K.J., and Langa, K.M. (2013). Monetary costs of dementia in the United States. *New England Journal of Medicine, 368*, 1326–1334. https://doi.org/10.1056/NEJMsa1204629

Jacobson, M., Thunell, J., and Zissimopoulos, J. (2020). Structured cognitive assessment at Medicare's annual wellness visit among beneficiaries in fee-for-service and Medicare Advantage plans. *Health Affairs, 39*(11), 1935–1942. https://doi.org/10.1377/hlthaff.2019.01795

Jervis, L.L., Shore, J., Hutt, E., and Manson, S.M. (2007). Suboptimal pharmacotherapy in a tribal nursing home. *Journal of the American Medical Directors Association, 8*(1), 1–7. https://doi.org/10.1016/j.jamda.2006.03.010

Kaiser Family Foundation. (2017). *Medicaid's Role in Nursing Home Care.* https://www.kff.org/infographic/medicaids-role-in-nursing-home-care

Kelley, A.S., McGarry, K., Gorges, R., and Skinner, J.S. (2015). The burden of health care costs for patients with dementia in the last 5 years of life. *Annals of Internal Medicine, 163*(10), 729–736. https://doi.org/10.7326/M15-0381

Lakdawalla, D.N., and Phelps, C.E. (2020). Health technology assessment with risk aversion in health. *Journal of Health Economics, 72,* 102346. https://doi.org/10.1016/j.jhealeco.2020.102346

Leibson, C.L., Long, K.H., Ransom, J.E., Roberts, R.O., Hass, S., Duhig, A., Smith, C., Emerson, J., Pankratz, V.S., and Petersen, R. (2015). Direct medical costs and source of cost differences across the spectrum of cognitive decline: A population-based study. *Alzheimer's & Dementia, 11*(8), 917–932. https://doi.org/10.1016/j.jalz.2015.01.007

Lin, P.J., Fillit, H.M., Cohen, J.T., and Neumann, P.J. (2013). Potentially avoidable hospitalizations among Medicare beneficiaries with Alzheimer's disease and related disorders. *Alzheimer's & Dementia, 9*(1), 30–38. https://doi.org/10.1016/j.jalz.2012.11.002

Lin, P.J., Zhong, Y., Fillit, H.M., Chen, E., and Neumann, P.J. (2016). Medicare expenditures of individuals with Alzheimer's disease and related dementias or mild cognitive impairment before and after diagnosis. *Journal of the American Geriatric Society, 64*(8), 1549–1557. https://doi.org/10.1111/jgs.14227

Meeker, D., Linder, J.A., Fox, C.R., Friedberg, M.W., Persell, S.D., Goldstein, N.J., Knight, T.K., Hay, J.W., and Doctor, J.N. (2016). Effect of behavioral interventions on inappropriate antibiotic prescribing among primary care practices: A randomized clinical trial. *Journal of the American Medical Association, 315*(6), 562–570.

Moore, M.J., Zhu, C.W., and Clipp, E.C. (2001). Informal costs of dementia care: Estimates from the National Longitudinal Caregiver Study. *Journals of Gerontology: Series B, 56*(4), S219–S228. https://doi.org/10.1093/geronb/56.4.s219

National Association of Insurance Commissioners and the Center for Insurance Policy and Research. (2016). *The State of Long-Term Care Insurance: The Market, Challenges and Future Innovations.* https://www.naic.org/documents/cipr_current_study_160519_ltc_insurance.pdf

Nicholas, L.H., Langa, K., and Bynum, J. (2020). Financial presentation of Alzheimer Disease and related dementias. *JAMA Internal Medicine, 181*(2), 220–227. https://doi.org/10.1001/jamainternmed.2020.6432

Park, S., and Chen, J. (2020). Racial and ethnic patterns and differences in health care expenditures among Medicare beneficiaries with and without cognitive deficits or Alzheimer's disease and related dementias. *BMC Geriatrics, 20*(482). https://doi.org/10.1186/s12877-020-01888-y

Pearson, C.F., Quinn, C.C., Loganathan, S., Datta, A.R., Mace, B.B., and Grabowski, D.C. (2019). The forgotten middle: Many middle-income seniors will have insufficient resources for housing and health care. *Health Affairs (Project Hope), 38*(5). https://doi.org/10.1377/hlthaff.2018.05233

Rice, T. (2013). The behavioral economics of health and health care. *Annual Review of Public Health, 34*(1), 431–447. https://doi.org/10.1146/annurev-publhealth-031912-114353

Schaller, S., Mauskopf, J., Kriza, C., Wahlster, P., and Kolominsky-Rabas, P.L. (2015). The main cost drivers in dementia: A systematic review. *International Journal of Geriatric Psychiatry, 30*(2), 111–129. https://doi.org/10.1002/gps.4198

Thaler, R.H., and Sunstein, C.R. (2008). *Nudge: Improving Decisions about Health, Wealth, and Happiness.* New Haven, CT: Yale University Press.

Watson, B., Tatangelo, G., and McCabe, M. (2019). Depression and anxiety among partner and offspring carers of people with dementia: A systematic review. *Gerontologist, 59*(5), e597–e610.

White, L., Fishman, P., Basu, A., Crane, P.K., Larson, E.B., and Coe, N.B. (2019). Medicare expenditures attributable to dementia. *Health Services Research*, *54*(4), 773–781. https://doi.org/10.1111/1475-6773.13134

Zissimopoulos, J., Crimmins, E., and St. Clair, P. (2014). The value of delaying Alzheimer's disease onset. *Forum for Health Economics & Policy*, *18*(1), 25–39. https://doi.org/10.1515/fhep-2014-0013

Zulman, D.M., Pal Chee, C., Wagner, T.H., Yoon, J., Cohen, D.M., Holmes, T., Ritchie, C., and Asch, S. (2015). Multimorbidity and healthcare utilisation among high-cost patients in the US Veterans Affairs health care system. *BMJ Open*, *5*, e007771. http://dx.doi.org/10.1136/bmjopen-2015-007771

8

Strengthening Data Collection and Research Methodology

Chapters 2 through 7 describe many priorities for social and behavioral research with the potential to reduce the negative impacts of dementia. In nearly every domain discussed, however, there are challenges related to data infrastructure and research methodology that could hamper the realization of these opportunities. New data and methodological developments shape social and behavioral research just as advances in genetic sequencing or DNA manipulation accelerate bench science. The committee has highlighted many specific evidence gaps and methodological challenges in prior chapters. In this chapter, we focus on issues of quantitative methodology because they present particular opportunities and challenges in the context of dementia research. Qualitative methods remain essential tools in social and behavioral research on dementia, especially when integrated with other approaches, but it is primarily in the quantitative domain that we see specific opportunities for notable theoretical and technical advances in the next decade.

Innovations and improvements in research methodology to address the challenges associated with quantitative dementia research could significantly increase the potential for research to reduce the negative impacts of dementia in the coming decade. This chapter reviews those challenges and then explores opportunities and challenges in four areas: data infrastructure, measurement, study design, and integration of evidence from varied sources to yield stronger conclusions (meta-research). The chapter closes with discussion of the importance of investing in human capital and research capacity, and directions for research.

CHALLENGES OF QUANTITATIVE RESEARCH ON DEMENTIA

Dementia research presents unique challenges for quantitative researchers (Weuve et al., 2015). For example, the relevant risk factors and outcomes are difficult to measure. The data sources often underrepresent or exclude the most relevant populations, such as racial/ethnic groups disproportionately affected by dementia or the caregivers and families of people living with dementia. And many of the data sources for which there are high-quality outcome measures are not large or diverse enough to support research on differences across diverse subgroups. Some of these difficulties arise in other fields as well, but in the context of dementia they have hindered progress in identifying effective preventive measures, managing disease, improving quality of life for people with dementia and their families, and even fully quantifying dementia's social impact.

One issue in dementia research is that the analytic approaches and study designs applied have been predominantly observational, sometimes longitudinal—designs that draw on covariate-controlled regression models. In other words, they seek to estimate causal effects by identifying and fully adjusting for all factors that may influence both the exposure and outcome under consideration (Matthay et al., 2020). This approach is likely to be biased in the study of dementia, a disease that develops and progresses slowly and has symptoms that are subtle, particularly in early stages.

The subtle early cognitive changes seen in dementia may induce changes in the constructs researchers seek to evaluate in their study of risk factors (see Chapter 2), such as social experiences, behaviors, health care utilization, emotions, or even physiology (e.g., body mass index). Establishing temporal order is foundational for establishing causality, but the long, slow development of dementia makes it difficult to pinpoint when someone does or does not have the disease. Thus, it is difficult to disentangle factors that increase the risk of developing dementia from factors that are influenced by incipient dementia. The slowly progressing nature of dementia in many patients necessitates long follow-up periods to detect changes using standard clinical measurements. Because its symptoms include diminishing capacity and because the disease is ultimately fatal, follow-up and longitudinal studies present particular challenges. As the disease progresses, patients are less able to communicate and require more help and input from their caregivers, which exacerbates measurement challenges and biases. The impact of these measurement biases depends on inclusion criteria, the prevalence of other risk factors in the population, and the outcomes that are selected for study, creating extreme difficulties in interpreting observational results.

These problems are even more acute because of the challenges of diagnosing and measuring dementia. As discussed in Chapters 1 and 3, diagnosis of dementia is not straightforward. The clinical tools and criteria for tracking and assessing cognitive changes have evolved over time (see Jack et al., 2018; Glymour et al., 2018; McCleery et al., 2019), and as researchers develop improved tools, patients will be better served. However, such changes make conducting long-term cohort studies or evaluating temporal trends more difficult. Ambiguity in diagnosis also makes it difficult to anticipate the likely benefits of proposed interventions, since the individuals in any specific group of patients will be at different disease stages. Based on differing social, demographic, and economic considerations, moreover, patients may receive care in heterogeneous settings. Similarly, the lack of data about family members and friends who provide care or are otherwise affected by dementia hampers research on interventions to support them. Because no one dataset encompasses all these kinds of information as well as clinical and patient-reported outcomes, it is impossible to identify the effectiveness of interventions in general or across different populations.

FOUR OPPORTUNITIES FOR IMPROVEMENTS IN METHODOLOGY

There are four broad areas in which significant advances can be made to address these challenges. These areas correspond to four primary domains of emerging, priority opportunities for research methodology development (see Figure 8-1).

Progress in any one of these areas will be relevant for one or more of the others. For example, research is constrained by the data sources available and the exposure and outcome measures that can be extracted from those sources. Novel data sources and linkages can both expand the measures available for dementia research and support the inclusion of populations

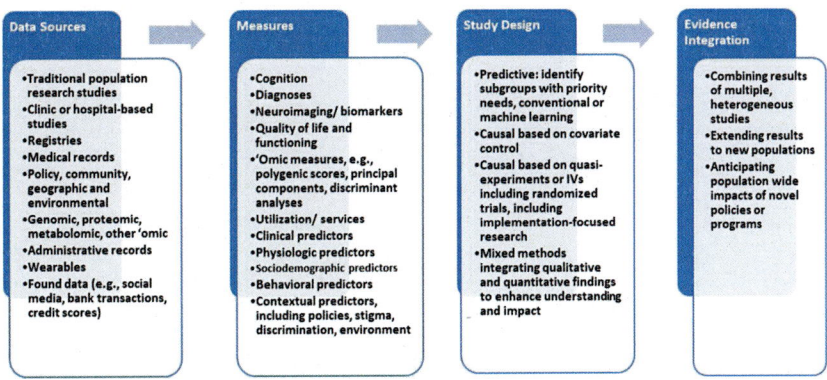

FIGURE 8-1 Domains for enhancing research methodology.

that have been underrepresented in dementia research (including specific racial/ethnic, socioeconomic, and geographically defined groups). Similarly, new data infrastructure can support novel study designs to improve identification, and more rigorous study designs to estimate biases and heterogeneity across populations will support stronger population effect estimates.

Data Sources

The availability of data fundamentally shapes the types of research that are conducted, so decisions about investments in data infrastructure have substantial influence. The strengths and weaknesses must be considered based on the goal of a particular research project. The discussion below considers data sources used in research to examine such topics as

- which treatments or exposures influence risk;
- the effectiveness of interventions to improve survival, functioning, and quality of life of people with dementia and their caregivers; and
- ways to identify individuals with incipient dementia and predict who will develop the disease.

Researchers studying aspects of dementia have relied heavily on a handful of sources. For example, analyses of community-based cohort studies, which often reflect a limited number of communities, are a primary source for prevention research (Fried et al., 1991; White et al., 1996; Bild et al., 2002). Outcomes research is often based on cohorts recruited through specialized memory clinics or Alzheimer's disease centers. Research based on billing records or more comprehensive electronic health record data has been informative in many cases because studies of such large size offer diversity and easy linkage with information on comorbidities, medications, or laboratory tests. Electronic health record data also have many weaknesses that have limited their usefulness (Beekly et al., 2004; Haneuse and Daniels, 2016; Jutkowitz et al., 2020). These include inconsistencies in how dementia is diagnosed, and selection biases based on when records were created (at what point in the disease trajectory individuals entered the system) and who is covered by the record system.

The available data sources shape who is included in studies, what risk factors or outcomes are measured, and what opportunities exist for estimating causal effects. One significant problem with current sources of data for dementia research is underrepresentation of population groups. Because of limitations in available data sources, non-Hispanic White individuals are particularly overrepresented in existing research; individuals from other racial/ethnic groups or multiracial individuals are underrepresented

(Wilkinson et al., 2018; Dahl et al., 2007; Brewster et al., 2019; Bynum et al., 2020). Recent estimates indicate, for example, that fewer than 200 American Indians are represented in the data on more than 40,000 individuals housed in the National Alzheimer's Coordinating Center's Uniform Data Set (NACC, 2021). These gaps are especially troubling because of dementia's disproportionate impact, with respect to incidence, caregiving needs, and economic consequences, on non-White individuals and families, as discussed in earlier chapters.

Individuals with less education and those from geographically underserved communities (e.g., rural towns far from tertiary care centers) are also underrepresented in datasets. Much research includes volunteers who are not only more likely to identify as White but also have high levels of education and convenient access to study centers. Data from the large UK Biobank cohort indicate that study participants not only are of higher socioeconomic status, more likely to be White, and healthier relative to average Britons, but also are of taller stature (likely indicating advantages during early-life growth periods) (Fry et al., 2017).

We review four paths forward for addressing these limitations: developing new data sources and adding items to existing sources, linking existing data sources in new ways, improving recruitment, and improving measuring exposures and outcomes.

Developing New Data Sources and Adding Items to Existing Sources

New data sources with potential relevance to dementia are rapidly emerging. These include "found" data, such as digital health data, phone records, and social media, as well as increasingly well-documented administrative sources, such as comprehensive electronic health records, claims records for health service billing, and the Minimum Data Set reported by nursing homes (Nicholas et al., 2021). While these data may offer powerful new research tools, however, their strengths and limitations and potential applications are as yet not well understood. Use of these sources to produce sound conclusions will require understanding of, for example, selection processes (who is represented and what data elements are present), the measurement limitations of the tool and individual data elements, and statistical considerations involved in analyzing the data.

Some of these data sources will be useful for dementia research only after transformation or screening with various algorithms (e.g., natural language processing algorithms to identify dementia cases based on language use or algorithms to identify stressful experiences). Innovations in machine learning offer promise for improving case identification but also introduce potential major problems because of algorithmic bias (Obermeyer et al., 2019). Without consistent and careful evaluation, existing biases or stereotypes can be built into new algorithms, or algorithms can be trained to recognize the experiences of the most well-represented groups. One study, for example, showed that a widely used algorithm intended to identify patients most in need of additional resources was based on health service utilization as a proxy for health (Obermeyer et al., 2019). Because barriers to access reduced utilization among Black patients, the algorithm systematically underestimated the degree of health need among Black patients and inappropriately deprioritized them for the additional resources.

Other challenges call for special consideration in dementia research. Respecting privacy while also fostering the use of new data sources is one. Dementia researchers also must grapple with identifying the most relevant data sources and needed data infrastructure. These determinations will be important for research investigating such emerging questions as how physical isolation affects people (e.g., whether electronic tools can partially or fully replace in-person interactions).

Disease registries, such as the Surveillance, Epidemiology, and End Results (SEER) registries for cancer, have been invaluable resources for the study of some diseases. No national registry is available to document and support the development of strategies for addressing dementia, but there have been some efforts to address this gap. One such effort is the Alzheimer's Disease Research Centers supported by the National Institute on Aging. These centers, housed in medical institutions that conduct a wide range of research activities, use a common study protocol and store data in a central repository, but are limited by variable sampling and follow-up priorities across the centers and over time, and lack of generalizability; there are particular concerns about race, socioeconomic status, and family history (NACC, 2021; Beekley et al., 2004; Besser et al., 2018; Weintraub et al., 2009, 2018). Registry efforts are also under way in a handful of states, including South Carolina, Georgia, West Virginia, and New York (Krysinska et al., 2017). However, access for research purposes is limited, and issues that have arisen regarding consent and reporting point to challenges for a national registry effort. Nonetheless, a national registry or improved coordination among existing registries with links to other data sources could provide improved resources for researchers.

The use of rich individual-level data presents ethical and legal challenges. Securing the consent of participants for the sharing and use of data about their health can be challenging when language barriers or limited education may hamper understanding of the issues at stake, and such issues are particularly challenging when participants have diminished decision-making capacity. Recommendations from a multidisciplinary team may provide best practices for consent in data-intensive dementia research and can support harmonization of consent practices across institutions and countries while facilitating data sharing (Thorogood et al., 2018).

Another way to create "new" data sources is to improve the dementia-relevant measures in available data sources. For example, the Health and Retirement Study used a comprehensive set of cognitive assessments in a small substudy (Langa et al., 2005), an important investment in validating the brief core assessments currently used (Plassman et al., 2008).[1] Substantial effort has gone into creating a crosswalk with clinical diagnoses, such as those in Medicare data (i.e., a mapping between the measures used in the Aging, Demographics, and Memory Study component of the Health and Retirement Study[2] and clinical diagnoses).

These findings frequently indicate that sources differ notably in their classifications at the individual level (although their performance may be acceptable at the population level if most people are cognitively normal). These variations indicate that one or all sources are fraught with substantial misclassification. For some purposes, this misclassification will not introduce bias or reflect authentic ambiguity as individuals progress through early stages of disease development. For many research questions, however, the misclassification is quite problematic, especially because it is likely to be differential across racial/ethnic groups, education levels, or other social indicators (Gianattasio et al., 2019, 2020; Power et al., 2020; Berkman, 1986).

Similar efforts to weave simple and more complex cognitive measures into other datasets are under way. In 2017, for example, the Panel Study of Income Dynamics added the AD8 dementia screen into the national household study. The National Longitudinal Study of Youth is adding cognitive measures that match those used in the Health and Retirement Study, and the National Longitudinal Study of Adolescent to Adult Health has incorporated various cognitive measures over the years and is adding more detailed neurocognitive assessments in planned future waves. Since 2006, the National Longitudinal Survey of Youth has administered a cognition module. Investments in these types of data enhancements pay off disproportionately, but research is needed to foster such additions and make it easier to establish links among relatively small studies.

Linking Existing Data Sources in New Ways

Linking different data sources can create powerful research opportunities. For example, establishing connections between self-reported

---

[1] More recently, the standard core assessments have been expanded to include the Harmonized Cognitive Assessment Protocol, which is integrated into many international sister studies, such as the Longitudinal Aging Study in India, the Health and Aging in Africa: A Longitudinal Study of an INDEPTH Community in South Africa Study, and the English Longitudinal Study of Aging.

[2] https://hrs.isr.umich.edu/publications/biblio/5761

quality-of-life outcomes and environmental or policy data from administrative records can allow researchers to examine many of the critical questions identified in Chapters 2 through 7. Linkages may be at the individual level (e.g., linkage of the 1940 detailed census data with data from participants in the Health and Retirement Study) or at a geographic level (e.g., linkage of state or county school policy changes with individual cognitive outcomes). The Health and Retirement Study's contextual data resource series links respondents to a variety of resources for data on crime, health care, and state policies.[3] Probabilistic linkages based on combinations of covariates (e.g., eligibility for social resources) or other units (e.g., schools, hospitals) are also possible.[4]

Further work on these methods is needed to expand and validate their applications. One challenge is building linkage opportunities into existing datasets. For example, collecting data on place of residence across the life course in cohorts for which detailed outcome data are available would make it possible to analyze age-specific place-level exposures to such variables as policies, pollution, and social context. However, few datasets include such life-course geographic data.

Another priority, alluded to above, is balancing the essential importance of data privacy with the goals of fostering data linkage. While many existing data security policies hamper research, alternative approaches that facilitate research while ensuring privacy have not been clearly established. Privacy is both an ethical concern (e.g., defining an acceptable probability of reidentification) and a technical concern (e.g., how to ensure adequate encryption when using cloud computing). Efforts to reduce cost and administrative barriers other than those strictly necessary to ensure privacy would accelerate research and help the field avoid the problem of researching only the most easily measured, most accessible risk factors. Data merges will not necessarily prevent "looking under the lamppost" (seeing only what happens to be easy to see or what is conveniently measured), but they effectively build more lampposts.

Data merges also need conceptual attention. Theories about the most important determinants of dementia have likely been constrained by limits on what it has been possible to measure. An example of an innovative approach that can open up new research opportunities is linking sources

---

[3] https://hrs.isr.umich.edu/data-products/restricted-data/available-products

[4] In the basic sciences, this type of linkage is also creating powerful study designs, such as two-sample Mendelian randomization analyses (in which genetic variants established in one sample as influencing a phenotype of interest are used as instrumental variables to estimate the effect of that phenotype on an outcome in a second sample) or research on gene expression profiles (in which information on genetic variants is scored based on tissue-specific data about how each variant relates to RNA or protein levels).

of data about exposures that may predict or increase dementia risk with data on cognitive or dementia-related outcomes. Recent work linking credit histories to cognitive status highlights the potential value of this type of innovation. Credit histories may reveal cognitive risk years before a dementia diagnosis, with implications for research design, public policy, and clinical care. For example, linking data from the Federal Reserve Bank of New York/Equifax Consumer Credit Panel with Medicare outcomes data made it possible to identify this connection and quantify how early it was detectable. This innovative work also illustrates the challenges involved: the link was based on census block, birth year, and zip code history and thus was not conducted at the individual level (Nicholas et al., 2021). Other valuable opportunities would come from linking health data with data from other sectors, such as data on labor experiences, trauma/violence exposures, income and social safety net protections, and educational resources.

Numerous relatively small or localized studies have used such approaches. To date, however, there has been little effort to synthesize those studies, compare their findings with national patterns, or even consider preferred settings for new proposed studies. A linked data resource tying together data from multiple sources—such as existing or newly reconstructed surveys and population-based, longitudinal population and health services data—could serve as the basis for a reference database. Such a reference database could in turn provide a comparator with more detailed localized databases that could be used, for example, to test the extent of representativeness of small trials or transfer results from small localized studies to new settings, or to guide design and settings for proposed new observational or intervention studies.

Creating such a database would require identifying studies with harmonizable measures; evaluating how each of those studies relates to a larger population (i.e., whether they are representative or approximately so); harmonizing the measures, which may entail creating latent variables if different instruments are used for the same construct; combining the datasets; developing recommended strategies for handling inconsistent measure availability (e.g., when multiple imputation is appropriate); and possibly creating weights to apply to the overall sample based on the intended reference population. Each of these tasks is technically difficult, but the payoff could be great.

Improved understanding of potential biases in selection and data collection is necessary to make new data linkage opportunities possible. No dataset is perfect. More systematic evaluation of selection biases and the differential effects of the data that are missing would strengthen research using both new and old data sources. Bias can be an issue with almost any existing data source, but this is an understudied topic that will become ever more urgent as new "big data" sources become popular.

Improving Recruitment

Although better leveraging of existing datasets will be valuable, improving recruitment is critical. The lack of racial/ethnic, socioeconomic, and geographic diversity in many major studies of dementia is well documented (e.g., Brewster et al., 2019). Lack of diversity in dementia research is now broadly recognized as a critical barrier to scientific progress and the achievement of health equity, and it is exacerbated in studies with intensive measurement protocols, such as neuroimaging. The lack of representation of many groups in dementia research has cascading effects that limit the relevance of scientific findings and in some cases may directly exacerbate health disparities that have adversely affected communities of color, individuals from disadvantaged socioeconomic backgrounds, and people living in certain geographic regions (see Chapters 2 and 5).

Developers of new data sources, such as the All of Us research program, have made impressive commitments to achieving racial/ethnic diversity (as of this writing, the 316,760 All of Us participants include 21% Black-, 17% Hispanic-, and 3% Asian-identified participants [National Institutes of Health, 2021]). An important challenge for All of Us will be ensuring that participants who provide more detailed measures, such as from wearables or linked data, are also diverse. Because All of Us is not based on a probability sample, opportunities for crosswalks between All of Us and representative samples will be important, for example, to reweight to U.S. population distributions. Although such reweighting is often based on only a handful of characteristics (e.g., age, sex, and race), it may fail to represent heterogeneity within these groups and paint very misleading pictures of population patterns (see below).

Nevertheless, although the importance of increased inclusion of underrepresented groups is widely recognized, efforts to this end are often isolated or cursory, or they occur too late in the scientific development process to be effective. In some cases, they may exacerbate bias by creating completely different recruitment paths for different groups (e.g., recruiting most White study participants from memory impairment clinics but most Black participants from church congregations).

The field needs insights from behavioral economics, social networks theory, or communications to create a toolbox of effective recruitment strategies. Researchers currently lack a coherent, comprehensive scientific framework for the inclusion of diverse groups (Dankwa-Mullan et al., 2021). Indeed, the definition of "diversity" is continually evolving, and ways to include people from varied racial/ethnic groups, geographic areas, sexual and gender minorities, cultural identities, and socioeconomic circumstances will need to evolve as well. The issue may require different remedies depending on the study focus: studies of dementia prevention, brain pathology, and quality of life among individuals living with dementia, for example, may each present different representation challenges. But regardless, a rigorous systematic framework that can be evaluated, challenged, modified, and adapted for varied research contexts is needed (Gilmore-Bykovskyi et al., 2021).

Measurement

Measurement of both exposures and outcomes presents another set of challenges for dementia researchers. The controversies about measurement of dementia will become even more salient as new data sources become available and as currently underrepresented groups are included more effectively in research. Selection and measurement of relevant exposures for dementia prevention and for improvement of quality of life for people living with dementia and caregivers are similarly critical and evolving. Social and behavioral researchers will need to be fully engaged to challenge narrow conceptualizations of relevant risk factors and consider the implications of alternative measurement approaches.

The challenge of measuring biologically meaningful and patient- and family-centered outcomes in dementia research is relevant to nearly every topic addressed in this report, but one example will illustrate the issues involved. The relatively modest correspondence between neuroimaging markers of pathophysiology and clinical or functional manifestations of disease has disappointed researchers who had hoped it would spur progress in research on both prevention and therapeutic responses (see Chapter 3). Some of the discrepancy may be the result of inadequacies in the measures used in neuropsychological assessments, including random noise, insensitivity to subtle early cognitive changes, or insensitivity to cultural context or test-taking artifacts. On the other hand, the discrepancy is at least in part a sign that the biomarkers are only modestly related to functional outcomes, either because meaningful cognitive reserve or resilience can counteract the damage indicated by the biomarkers or because researchers have not accurately measured or identified the relevant biological factors.

Another need is for evidence from cognitive assessments that are better able to capture the symptoms of dementia compared with most current measures.[5] Sensory, motor, and mood changes common in old age complicate the assessment of cognition, and assessments may conflate changes in capacity to participate in the assessment (e.g., to hear words read out loud

---

[5] Such properties include equal interval scaling, lack of ceilings/floors, absence of differential item functioning across sociodemographic groups, and adaptive test design to reduce participant burden. Differential item functioning is a special concern for evaluating the impact of many important social risk factors, which are very plausible sources of measurement bias.

from a verbal memory test) with changes in cognition. Substantial progress has recently been made in implementing advanced psychometric methods, but most commonly used measures still have important limitations in reliability and validity across linguistic background, educational attainment, and cultural identity.

To the extent that these limitations intersect with critical predictors or outcomes, they can also lead to significantly biased results. Cultural differences may relate to comfort level with the examiner (as well as other characteristics, such as pitch and enunciation) and may also intersect with other important predictors (Gershon et al., 2020; Kobayashi et al., 2020; Mukherjee et al., 2020; Gross et al., 2020; Walter et al., 2019). In addition, there are significant differences by mode of assessment (in person, video, phone) that contribute to variable results (particularly during the COVID-19 pandemic). Many of these challenges will require qualitative work to understand how people from different communities interpret and respond to the phrasing of specific assessments and the cultural norms or expectations that shape their responses. Passive cognitive measures (discussed below) may be helpful with respect to equivalence across groups and would support the collection of data from large samples, thus facilitating rigorous study designs.

Advances in two areas—measuring exposures and identifying valid early predictors of cognitive outcomes—show particular promise for improving measurement in the context of dementia research.

Measuring Exposures

Given the constrained set of measures available in datasets used in dementia research, research on risk factors has focused primarily on those that can be identified relatively late in life, which are most easily self-reported or documented in electronic health records. Researchers have been much less likely to evaluate life-course measures; contextual factors; social network variables, such as size, density, position of the respondent in the network, strength of ties, or support delivered by different ties; or other difficult-to-measure variables. This is an important limitation, especially when one is considering opportunities to prevent dementia. Earlier chapters have pointed to many early or midlife exposures that are likely to be profoundly important for dementia. Factors driven by structural racism contributing to disparities, structures and processes related to gender across the life course, and paid and unpaid work experiences, for example, have received short shrift because of the measurement challenges. Research on the progression and impacts of dementia could be especially enhanced by better access to measures of the social networks of individuals living with dementia, yet such measures are difficult to access. New technologies and other measurement innovations may help address this gap.

Concerns about establishing consent for people living with cognitive impairment is another serious issue for researchers. Some researchers avoid engaging people with dementia to circumvent this problem, which also emerges in longitudinal studies when people deteriorate. Evaluations of this issue are inconsistent across institutional review boards, so standardized guidance and best practices for establishing capacity to consent would be invaluable.

Novel insights will emerge from novel measures. Building out older datasets with risk information from earlier in the life course for individuals who are now older adults is another approach to help address the problem of measuring exposure (e.g., by following up old studies to incorporate late-life cognitive assessments). Since many of these datasets are unformatted, investments would be required to convert them to electronic format or machine learning or natural language processing tools so that relevant, analyzable data could be extracted. Funding to support this conversion and documentation for these sources would therefore be an important part of the larger data infrastructure buildout efforts. Linking of data sources (as discussed above) would also support this type of innovation, but would require methodological work on how to collect linking variables and how to complete probabilistic linkages.

Identifying Valid Early Predictors of Cognitive Outcomes

Dementia and the underlying pathological conditions that contribute to the disease develop and progress over decades, far beyond the time scale of typical research studies. Thus, substantial benefits could be realized with the development of methods for identifying outcomes that could serve as proxies for long-term outcomes but be accessible within the relatively short time frame of most research. Innovative research designs to identify the early manifestations of disease—for example, leveraging genetic factors to identify leading indicators of cognitive change—could help pinpoint the most sensitive markers. Such research will, however, require validation of proxies, perhaps through retrospective analyses of existing data, as well as tools for easily capturing such data.

Multiple efforts are under way to improve the sensitivity of cognitive tests for early recognition of cognitive loss while addressing some of the major deficits of existing cognitive assessment tools. Some new, more challenging, measures are designed to be more engaging (some are based on games, for example) as a means of improving participation and limiting educational bias. Some can be administered repeatedly to address significant reliability concerns related to such factors as illness, mood, and other fluctuations not related to underlying cognitive change. Some extract additional data from digital tasks to improve the reliability and granularity of measurement.

Strategies for extracting cognitive information from incidental data sources—such as metadata[6] from surveys, phone or other device usage, social network site activities, financial transactions, or writing samples—could provide longer timelines for cognitive assessments, better ways to control for early-life cognition, and a wide range of outcome measures. People reveal cognitive function or cognitive deterioration through such common daily activities as phone usage, bill paying, completion of routine forms, or travel outside the home. However, despite a handful of innovative efforts, no simple ways of routinely incorporating this information into research studies or clinical assessments currently exist (James et al., 2011; Nicholas et al., 2021). Protocols for extracting, calculating, and calibrating such assessments are therefore needed. Innovative work using survey metadata is promising, especially if it could be applied to extract comparable cognitive information across time from waves of survey assessments before the cohort had undergone formal cognitive assessment. In some cases, metadata from existing surveys may also reveal cognitive information.

New data sources are transforming many areas of research, but researchers with both data science skills and substantive knowledge of dementia research will be needed to take advantage of these possibilities (Salganik, 2019). Moreover, most cognitive measures assess proxies for cognitive functioning, such as processing speed, and more work is needed to identify their relationship to the capacities that decline with dementia. Measurement strategies spanning the entire spectrum of dementia, from the very subtle incipient changes through late-stage disease, are needed. To describe the full range of patient experience, it will be necessary to connect the various measures—not just cognitive measures but also measures that reflect individual priorities for a meaningful life, such as social connections, autonomy, dignity, and freedom from pain—to show the individual's disease trajectory.

Defining outcomes related to quality of life for people living with dementia, their caregivers, and other loved ones is another key goal for dementia researchers. In some cases, imperfect measurement is inevitable, but it is possible to use statistical tools to quantify the measures and correct for bias. Possible approaches include both contemporary quantitative psychometric methods and qualitative research methods.

---

[6]Metadata are data about the administration and completion of a survey rather than the survey responses specifically. Potentially useful metadata would include the time respondents needed to complete sections of the survey, which participants were interviewed by the same interviewers, the number of contacts before a participant agreed to taking part in the survey, and the date or time of survey completion.

Study Design

Although prediction and early identification have received extensive attention in recent dementia research, the ultimate goal is to identify interventions to prevent dementia, improve the well-being of individuals living with dementia and their loved ones, and ameliorate the potential adverse societal impact of expenses related to these diseases. Identifying such interventions—including both pharmacologic and behavioral approaches, resource programs, systems changes, social and health policies, and other strategies—will require methods for anticipating their causal effects. However, researchers in social and behavioral disciplines are far from having established standard methods for causal research, and indeed this challenge is the source of profound disagreements (Matthay et al., 2020) This state of affairs obscures the fact that researchers across these divides share goals and are developing new data sources and measures that may support the development of consensus on how to leverage the most relevant study design in any given setting. This section highlights a number of opportunities for supporting advances in study design.

Broadening the Repertoire of Tools

The challenge of disentangling causal determinants of dementia or dementia progression from noncausal correlates pervades nearly all dementia literature. Randomized controlled trials (RCTs) of nonpharmacologic interventions are often difficult and slow, and sometimes simply infeasible. Pragmatic trials can be more feasible, and their importance is likely to grow in the future as data options improve. However, the predominant methodologies to date have been based on observational cohort studies, often with diagnostic time-to-event outcomes, in which the causal identification strategy is based on measuring and controlling for all factors that might influence both exposure and outcome (Pearl, 2009). Alternative methodologies applied to observational data, such as difference-in-difference, interrupted time series, regression discontinuity, or instrumental variables methods, are much less commonly used, possibly because these methods must be modified or adapted for dementia outcomes.

These methods have various names but are based on the idea that some of the exposures individuals experience vary as a result of arguably random events or characteristics that would otherwise have no association with their health outcomes. For example, the date when a state adopts legalization of recreational marijuana may have nothing to do with the quality of life of people in the state, but if marijuana use influences quality of life, it would be reasonable to expect a change in quality of life to occur in that state after that date. The timing of the policy adoption introduces a quasi-random source of variation in the exposure to marijuana use. Put simply, most quantitative methods rely either on experimental (exogenous) variation in the treatment or on controlling for all common causes of treatment and outcome. Machine learning analytic approaches can be applied in either setting and may be useful, for example, in identifying and optimizing statistical control for potential confounders.

Quasi-experimental methods (including instrumental variables methods, regression discontinuity, and others noted above) can be powerful complements to conventional observational analyses because they often depend on entirely different assumptions. In many settings, the key assumptions for conventional analyses (e.g., no confounding of the exposure–outcome association) are clearly implausible. For example, it is not credible that there are no confounders of the association between engagement in cognitively demanding tasks in late life and subsequent dementia risk. In this situation, quasi-experimental and related methods can be invaluable. Policy changes and other sources of exogenous variation in important exposures have long been used for causal research in economics (Matthay et al., 2020).

Work is needed to improve causal methodologies for dementia-related outcomes: accommodating the slow and insidious development of dementia and distinguishing those changes from the physiologic changes related to age. New data sources would improve the feasibility of approaches based on instrumental variables, both because new potential instruments may be embedded in the new data and because these methods need very large samples to be informative. Some approaches that were promising but not quite workable in the past may be viable and informative as large administrative datasets become available. Research to identify, evaluate, and apply instrument-based approaches and compare their findings with those from conventional, covariate-control approaches is needed.

Likewise, methods for dealing with time-varying confounder mediators have been rapidly adopted in some domains of epidemiology but remain rare in dementia (Hernán et al., 2000; Robins et al., 2000), Time-varying confounder mediators are common in dementia research because the exposures of interest change over time, influencing mediators that in turn also influence future values of exposure. Leisure-time cognitive activities are an example: leisure-time cognitive engagement may preserve cognitive function, and preserved cognitive function may in turn lead older individuals to continue to engage in cognitively demanding activities (McDonald et al., 2003). Time-varying confounder mediators affect both prevention research and research on strategies for maintaining quality of life for people living with dementia. Specialized statistical tools are available for evaluating complex longitudinal exposures that may have different effects based on timing or duration of exposure. These tools are also helpful for quantifying and correcting bias attributable to selective mortality and selective attrition

(Hernán et al., 2004), both of which are common in dementia research. These methods remain challenging and underutilized, however.

Many argue that analyses of observational data should be structured to mirror RCTs; that is, they should have a defined moment of "randomization," no control for postrandomization variables, and clearly defined follow-up rules (Hernán and Robins, 2016; Labrecque and Swanson, 2017). This approach gained traction when it was found that the discrepancy between observational studies of postmenopausal hormone replacement and RCTs of the same medications could be almost fully accounted for by differences in the analytic approach. When the observational data were analyzed as an RCT, results were very similar to those from actual RCTs (Hernán et al., 2008). Emulated trial designs are seeing rapid uptake because of their conceptual clarity and natural alignment with the goal of developing actual RCTs based on observational studies (Caniglia et al., 2020; Rojas-Saunero, 2021).

Creating Opportunities for Quasi-Experimental Discovery, Including Leveraging Instrumental Variables Analyses

In many cases, major programs or interventions are rolled out with limited understanding of their likely impacts. Resource limitations or feasibility issues result in some individuals receiving the intervention while others do not, so in theory, it would be possible to learn about the intervention's effects. Yet it is rare for such roll-outs to be organized intentionally to create opportunities for rigorous program evaluation. Such methods as stepped wedge designs (in which a new treatment is introduced to a population in a staggered fashion with randomly selected units or clusters chosen for treatment initiation at successive time points across the follow-up) are powerful tools for enhancing what can be learned about interventions (Bärnighausen et al., 2017; Oldenburg et al., 2016; Handley et al., 2018), and many related designs could be introduced to take advantage of settings where there is true uncertainty or disagreement about the best treatments or the merits of a program. Researchers need to understand better why health care system administrators may not randomly allocate the units or settings where clinical innovations are to be implemented so that the results can be rigorously evaluated. Furthermore, study of ethical issues inherent in doing this kind of research is needed, as is methodologic work to optimize design and demonstrate most rapidly what works and what does not.

Enhancing Analyses of Randomized Controlled Trials

Many types of interventions are particularly well suited to RCT evaluations. For example, observational studies of cognitive engagement, social networks, or screening interventions are particularly problematic because of the powerful selection processes at work in such exposures. Although quasi-experimental approaches may help remediate these biases, RCTs are both feasible and particularly valuable in these settings. RCTs of both pharmacologic and nonpharmacologic interventions provide unique information for dementia research because they are already randomized for other purposes. Mediation models of RCT-based data can help inform theoretical understanding of disease progression and mechanisms. Instrumental variables analyses applied to RCTs are typically uncontroversial but have not been widely adopted in health research (Glymour et al., 2017). Such analyses would yield more relevant estimates of the impact of interventions *as received* rather than *as randomized*.

Careful comparisons of RCTs and observational studies can provide bias estimates to support interpretation of nonrandomized results and evaluation of heterogeneity in treatment responses. Precision medicine has popularized the idea that responses to treatment may vary substantially across individuals, but the focus has been on genetic determinants of that heterogeneity, whereas social and contextual factors are likely to be equally relevant. Large heterogeneity in treatment responses undermines the interpretation of RCT results because trial participants generally are not representative of the target population for inference purposes. Formal methods for assessing heterogeneity and the application of the assessment results to RCTs would provide more generalizable interpretations of RCT findings (Mehrotra et al., 2019). This is one form of the evidence integration discussed earlier, and further below.

RCTs are typically expensive and slow in comparison with pragmatic trials and quasi-experimental approaches. However, many existing large RCTs have not been fully leveraged for dementia research. For example, many RCTs of cardiovascular risk factor reduction, chronic disease and substance use treatment interventions, social determinants of health or social support, or pharmacologic interventions were never followed up for impacts on dementia. This is rigorous evidence simply awaiting data collection to determine the impacts of these interventions on dementia risk (see, e.g., Robertson et al., 2021; Dahabreh et al., 2021). When RCTs do show that a behavioral or social intervention does not have the desired outcome, qualitative research may help reveal the mechanistic misunderstanding and guide improvements in future interventions.

Moving from Evidence to Implementation

Rigorous evidence will not improve the lives of people affected by dementia unless there is a pipeline from the scientific results to implementation. Implementation entails a new set of challenges beyond establishing that a proposed intervention or treatment could, in theory, reduce disease incidence or improve quality of life (Glasgow et al., 2012; Green et al., 2009, 2014). Implementation needs to be considered not at the end of the pipeline but from the beginning of the research generation process: Who could use this evidence and how would they use it? Is this study going to provide actionable evidence? Research across the spectrum from theory-building to directly actionable work is essential. Various categorizations of work across this spectrum have been offered, but a consistent theme is the value of intentionality in translating evidence into clinical, behavioral, or policy interventions and supporting widespread adoption.

Incorporating stakeholder perspectives from the outset is critical to delivering actionable work that will be implemented. The stakeholders include individuals living with dementia, their families and social networks, and the individuals who would use the evidence and implement innovations. For example, translation efforts focused on changes in clinical processes require adoption by clinicians or health system administrators. Translation efforts focused on local, state, or federal policy adoption require input from advocates and policy makers who understand the range of possible policy options and the kinds of evidence needed to influence the debate.

A key consideration is whether an innovation is likely to scale well. For example, complex, high-touch, expensive intervention programs may be difficult to implement at a scale that will have substantial population health impact. Considerations of scalability should lead researchers—even people working on theory-building interventions—to focus efforts on particular types of risk factors and exposures amenable to scaling. Interventions that depend on individual adoption of long-term behavior change (e.g., increased exercise) without changing the context and resources that facilitate or create barriers to those behaviors are often ineffective. One approach, developed by the World Health Organization, involves itemizing seven characteristics of scalable interventions (using the acronym CORRECT): Credible and based on sound evidence; Observably effective; Relevant for addressing the problems experienced by stakeholders; Relatively better than other options; Easy and simple to understand and adopt; Compatible with stakeholders' established values, norms, and practices; and Testable so stakeholders can see the results (World Health Organization, 2010). Another approach to addressing the problem, seen in the National Institute of Health's Science of Behavior Change initiative,[7] focuses on the small effect sizes common in individual-level interventions.

Formal training programs related to implementation science, which include teaching about developing theory-guided interventions, evidence dissemination, and intentional consideration of how to account for implementation

---

[7] https://commonfund.nih.gov/behaviorchange

settings, have emerged in recent years. This movement has been valuable but will benefit from formal attention to causal inference and adoption of tools from multiple disciplines, including domains outside the typical sphere of clinical or epidemiologic research: communications, economics, policy analysis, legal scholarship, human factors psychology, and organizational psychology.

Because there is currently no effective treatment for dementia and many individuals will survive for many years after diagnosis, interventions to improve quality of life are particularly important (Karlawish, 2021).[8] Like other interventions, those designed to improve quality of life require rigorous study designs that integrate qualitative and quantitative methods to improve quality and allow for adaptation of programs to accommodate context-specific constraints and modifications based on what is learned.

Conducting Pragmatic Clinical Trials Embedded in Health Systems

Traditional explanatory RCTs are designed to evaluate whether an intervention can improve health outcomes under ideal, highly controlled conditions. In the case of nonpharmacologic interventions, research staff deliver the intervention under strict protocols that are generally more intensive and focused relative to similar services provided by health care personnel in such normal settings as hospitals, nursing homes, and physicians' offices. Efficacy trials of nonpharmacologic interventions are expensive and often underpowered, and they commonly generate findings that are not applicable to normal practice (Scales et al., 2018). In contrast, pragmatic clinical trials are embedded in functioning health care systems and are designed to evaluate the effectiveness of interventions implemented under real-world conditions.[9]

Typically, researchers conducting pragmatic trials randomize and deliver the intervention at the level of the unit of care (e.g., nursing home, physician practice) rather than the individual (Mitchell et al., 2020, p. S2). In addition, the intervention is implemented as part of the delivery of routine clinical care rather than by researchers under artificial circumstances. Instead of enrolling

---

[8] A 2021 National Academies of Sciences, Engineering, and Medicine report, *Meeting the Challenge of Caring for Persons Living with Dementia and Their Care Partners and Caregivers*, notes that the results of the systematic review conducted for that report reflect the high uncertainty about benefits of all interventions other than REACH II and collaborative care models. The report does not imply that the other interventions were found to be ineffective; rather, the high uncertainty on which the review's results were based was due to limitations of the evidence base and the approach used in the review to support conclusions on readiness for implementation and dissemination (National Academies of Sciences, Engineering, and Medicine 2021).

[9] The Pragmatic Explanatory Continuum Indicator Summary (PRECIS)-2 framework describes how pragmatic and efficacy trials differ across nine domains, illustrating that most trial design features lie somewhere along the continuum between pragmatic and explanatory; see https://www.precis-2.org.

highly selected participants, such trials minimize restrictive eligibility criteria and attempt to expand recruitment to all individuals receiving care in a particular setting. Researchers using pragmatic trials also aim to leverage existing administrative or electronic health records to identify participants and ascertain outcomes, avoiding the need for a special research infrastructure to collect data. Intervention delivery, participant follow-up, and adherence are typically more flexible and closely aligned with usual care (Mitchell et al., 2020, p. S2). In many cases, people in settings randomly assigned to the control group need not even know they are part of a research study, as their care processes are not affected in any way (Mitchell et al., 2021).

Relative to researcher-implemented trials, pragmatic trials must be undertaken in close collaboration with the health care system. The clinical care problem being addressed must be salient to the system and to the providers on the front line of care. The saliency of the problem of meeting the needs of persons living with dementia and their caregivers will, of course, vary as a function of their prevalence in the care setting. Thus, any individual primary care practice may have relatively few such patients; caring for them may be more time-consuming than caring for other patients but not enough so to require restructuring of the practice's workflow. On the other hand, emergency departments in urban settings or acute care hospitals may be confronted daily with the inadequacy of current models for caring for persons living with dementia, and so may be motivated to test the effectiveness of various interventions to ameliorate the challenges they face in caring for these individuals.

Interventions in such pragmatic trials need not be restricted to hospitals, nursing homes, or other traditional health care systems. Exercise programs or even caregiver support groups, whether in person or online, can be delivered by community-based organizations and may even be paid for under arrangements in Medicare Advantage plans that now may cover nonmedical services. Many such insurance plans already have discounted membership relationships with health clubs, which could be the perfect vehicle for implementing pragmatic trials designed to deliver exercise and other social support programs to older persons at risk of cognitive impairment. These kinds of efforts are likely to be become more common as the line between medical and nonmedical health services blurs, making it possible to evaluate rigorously the effectiveness of these kinds of services.

The discrepancy between intent-to-treat effect estimates (the effect of randomization) and per-protocol effect estimates (the effect that would have occurred had everyone adhered to the assigned treatment) that is typically observed in any randomized study can be especially large in a pragmatic trial. Since researchers using pragmatic trials hope to apply relatively few exclusion criteria and may need to recruit a large number of providers to be part of the study, many providers may fail to implement the intervention protocol as designed and intended. As a result, statistical power is reduced, and the likelihood of detecting the hypothesized effect is small. Engaging with the health care system at all levels is thus important to improve intervention fidelity. Augmenting intent-to-treat analyses with analyses based on instrumental variables or identifying adherent subgroups based on pre-randomization characteristics can yield additional relevant effect estimates.

Thus, even though sample sizes will be very large, and the population of providers and patients will be much more representative than is the case in researcher-based trials, the challenges of implementing pragmatic trials can be considerable. Implementation science—study of the processes necessary to implement an intervention effectively at scale—is coming into its own, but its application to the field of dementia care is in its infancy. Work in this area will be needed to support the translation of interventions that are efficacious into the real world of health care systems serving the population of persons living with dementia.

Evaluating Complex, Dynamic Interventions

Community-based initiatives are often developed by the communities involved and funded by nonresearch sources. These programs are designed to meet the social service or health needs of a specified population rather than to generate knowledge that can be generalized to other settings. Thus, these programs are highly relevant to the local community, including accommodating diversity and encouraging the widest possible participation. Their evaluation, however, is frequently limited to counts of participants and other descriptive or process measures rather than assessment of impact. The Dementia Friendly America Program mentioned in Chapter 5 is an example of such an initiative (Dementia Friendly America, 2021).

Although some efforts have been made to bridge science and service programs (e.g., community-based participatory research), challenges based on the cultures and regulations of the different approaches and goals remain. For example, most research on effectiveness places additional demands on participants (e.g., responding to surveys) and may require informed consent. Some people interested in participation may be excluded based on entry criteria. Randomization or other assignment methods may be needed to establish appropriate comparison groups, which may further discourage participation.

The location of the program's base is also an important factor. Academic institutions have infrastructure to support research but frequently do not have the community contacts needed to implement programs or the trust of the community. Conversely, community-based programs are usually highly pragmatic, allowing considerable flexibility in implementation instead of requiring adherence to strict protocols that may be needed to draw conclusion about effectiveness. Methods for promoting the implementation and evaluation of these programs with respect to participants' health and well-being while minimizing their burden are needed.

Simulations, Microsimulations, Agent-Based Models, and Complex Systems Models

A host of methods that generally fall under the umbrella of complex systems methods—including agent-based models, dynamic models (also known as mathematical or mechanistic models), and dynamic microsimulation models—may prove valuable for examining the possible consequences of certain interventions. In simple causal structures, these models may be equivalent to conventional regression modeling approaches (see, e.g., Ackley et al., 2017), but dynamic models can sometimes more easily represent known biological constraints on a data-generating structure, allow for feedback processes in which variables influence one another in near-continuous time, and represent emergent processes that would not be manifest when individual units are considered in isolation. Many of these methods have been widely used in infectious disease epidemiology but less frequently in chronic disease research (Murray et al., 2017). One challenge for agent-based models, for example, is that they require inputs for parameter values that are typically drawn from conventional observational studies.

Modeling and simulation techniques have been used to support policy through models of dementia prevalence and costs and how they are affected by innovations and changing population health. Dynamic microsimulation models individual-level actions but can then illustrate how community-level patterns may emerge from individual-level decision rules. Agent-based models may provide additional insight by including interactions among individuals, such as patients and physicians or patients and family caregivers. The full value of these methods for dementia research is as yet unclear, but they certainly hold promise. Researchers will need training in these domains as well as expertise in the substantive problems in dementia research to take advantage of these methods.

Formalizing Study Design Approaches

A formal framework is useful for understanding how study design should guide the selection of acceptable exposure and outcome measures. For example, some exposure–outcome measures (e.g., retirement effects on mild cognitive impairment) may be more vulnerable than others to reverse causation (i.e., if early memory loss leads to early retirement), an issue that could be addressed with different choices of measures (e.g., a statutory retirement age requirement or longitudinal cognitive change). Similarly, measurement invariance (the principle that a measurement instrument is capturing the same construct across different subgroups) is a challenge for both exposure and outcome measures. Large samples are needed to evaluate the assumption of measurement invariance, and qualitative methods can be valuable for understanding whether violations are likely and if so, how to correct them. Issues of mode effects—the possibility that people perform differently on a measurement instrument if it is administered in person versus over the phone or on a computer—emerged very strongly in the context of the COVID-19 pandemic.

Currently, researchers have a very ad hoc strategy for selecting study designs and are driven as much by the convenience of an approach or access to data as by scientific priority based on the available evidence and limitations of prior studies. Figure 8-2 illustrates these trade-offs. For example, if the most important challenge in studying, say, participant experiences or the information to be gleaned from biomarkers is

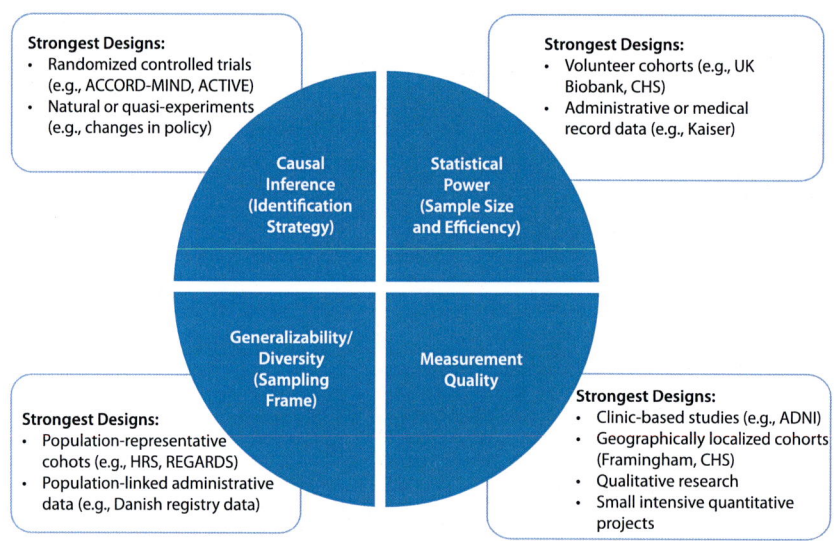

FIGURE 8-2 Desirable features of data sources and examples of alternative study designs most likely to have each feature.
NOTES: The text in the blue wedges refers to the study design issues or priorities (with examples of how these concepts are referred to in different disciplines); the examples in the white boxes refer to the types of data sources that are typically strongest with respect to this dimension of good study design. ACCORD-MIND = Action to Control Cardiovascular Risk in Diabetes Memory in Diabetes study; ACTIVE = Advanced Cognitive Training for Independent and Vital Elderly study; ADNI = Alzheimer's Disease Neuroimaging Initiative; CHS = Cardiovascular Health Study; HRS = Health and Retirement Study; REGARDS = Reasons for Geographic and Racial Differences in Stroke study.

measurement, large population-representative cohorts are unlikely to provide the best approach. The strongest study designs might include qualitative work to yield richer understanding of participant experiences. In the study of technical biomarkers, clinic-based or geographically restricted studies may be best. But it should be recognized that in making such choices, researchers may be compromising on the generalizability of the sample, diversity of inclusion, statistical power, and often causal identification strategies. Likewise, convenience sampling, such as that used in the UK Biobank or All of Us, may increase sample size and therefore statistical power, but at the cost of representativeness. Special attention in such studies (as in All of Us) may help in addressing these issues by aggressively recruiting from underrepresented communities. It is unclear to what extent this recruitment is as good as representative sampling or leads to new types of selection bias—the answer would depend on the setting.

Evidence Integration

Evidence integration, drawing on research triangulation, refers to the idea of combining findings from multiple studies with complementary strengths and weaknesses to develop a better understanding of a problem (Lawlor et al., 2017). Research triangulation is an intentional process of proposing new study designs that address the weaknesses of prior work, for example, by using negative controls, instrumental variables, or study populations with very likely different patterns of confounding. This process is the essence of scientific thinking but is often conducted informally. Recognition of the importance of systematic, principled approaches to evidence integration is growing in part because the sheer volume of research is expanding. Moreover, traditional perspectives on the hierarchy of evidence (with RCTs recognized as providing the highest-quality evidence) are being challenged because excellent, well-conducted RCTs are often not feasible for important research questions. And even with excellent RCTs, findings may not be conclusive because participant samples are small or unrepresentative, follow-up time is relatively short, or there is uncertainty about how variations in the treatment might influence findings. Thus, it is important to supplement even evidence from RCTs with observational evidence. Perfect studies are rare, moreover, and the more similar two studies are, the more likely it is that they share the same limitations. There is often a direct trade-off between desirable study features, such as sample size and quality of measurement. For most important questions, then, it is necessary to patch together evidence from work that uses varied study designs and populations and varies in other research characteristics as well.

Methods for Assessing Heterogeneity and Generalizing Results

Generalizing from study samples to new populations is essential. Major discrepancies between general-population characteristics and the characteristics of people who participate in research studies have been well documented in comparisons of RCTs and clinic-based observational studies, and are also a concern when more or less data-intensive observational studies are compared (Gianattasio et al., 2021). These differences are not well understood, and there has been little effort to date to compare effect estimates formally across highly selected and less-selected samples. This is an area in which machine learning methods may be useful, in that exploratory evaluations across a wide swath of possible modifiers may be enlightening. Although machine learning methods have focused predominantly on prediction questions, recent applications in the context of causal questions have been important (Athey, 2015; Wager and Athey, 2018).

A growing array of quantitative tools can aid in generalizing findings from a study sample to a target population. These tools depend on understanding the drivers of selection, the potential modifiers, and the availability of relevant measures for both study samples and the target population (Bareinboim and Pearl, 2016). Rapid progress on methods for addressing such problems has not yet been widely seen in dementia research (Bareinboim and Pearl, 2016; Westreich et al., 2017, 2019). These methods would help clarify whether what is learned from the often highly selected participants in RCTs is applicable more broadly. They also would indicate whether meaningful heterogeneity exists across populations with respect to predictors of disease incidence or outcomes, and whether this heterogeneity can be accounted for by incorporating sociodemographic, behavioral, or contextual modifiers. For these methods to be successful, however, it will be essential to model and understand the selection process. Unfortunately, the selection mechanisms for convenience samples are opaque and difficult to model well. Just as new data linkages will support novel exposure assessments, new data linkages can also be valuable for investigating heterogeneity and generalizing results beyond the selected samples in some datasets.

Tools for Systematically Combining Evidence

Only a few methods are currently available for systematically combining evidence from multiple sources, and these tools are woefully limited and underused. Meta-analyses emphasize selection of highly parallel studies with similar exposure and outcome definitions and study designs. Meta-analyses are thus of limited utility in evidence integration, which focuses on combining results from varied study designs. Meta-analyses can be especially challenging in dementia research because the studies considered may use quite different methods to address the same question based on the disciplinary background of the researcher, the data available, or particular analytic approaches. Meta-regression methods are used to address a narrow slice of questions related to ways in which easily quantified and routinely reported variables modify the analysis findings. Most meta-analyses give limited attention to evaluating the biases implicit in various study designs and the extent to which different studies address those biases. Better tools are therefore needed for triangulating evidence and quantifying how findings from different study designs fit together.

Needed, for example, are tools with which to establish a crosswalk between studies with different but conceptually related exposure and outcome measures (i.e., to create a mapping between measures that correspond with each other in the two studies and ideally illustrate how transformations can make the measures directly comparable). Modern psychometric methods foster specification of latent variables to allow data pooling but are still underused. Because datasets typically specialize in careful measurement of some but not all domains and/or recruitment of specific populations, ways to analyze heterogeneous datasets jointly are another need.

Still another valuable set of tools facilitates quantification and correction of bias from various sources. For example, "borrowing" of bias estimates across studies so that information on confounding or selection bias from a study with good measures could be used to estimate and correct that bias in a study without such measures could be powerful. Bias quantification might be based on simulations or simple, intuitive calculations (Mayeda et al., 2016; VanderWeele and Ding, 2017). Such statistical tools as reweighting are a standard approach to addressing selection bias. Improvements to basic weighting tools can yield better understanding of the selection process. (Methods building on Robins' g-formula and formalization of counterfactual frameworks can avoid bias or provide simpler ways to quantify bias and extend results from one sample to another; see VanderWeele et al., 2008; Danaei et al., 2016; Dahabreh et al., 2019.) Newer data sources (e.g., social media data; financial transaction data; convenience cohorts, such as those used by UK Biobank or All of Us) have strong selection processes, but the impact of these processes on research results is unclear and likely varies across settings. There is currently no standardized approach to evaluating concerns about selection bias.

Tools for Quantifying Impacts of Policies, Interventions, or Therapies

A disconnect exists between the typical structure of research results (which present, for example, differences in the likelihood of an outcome for different groups, or hazard ratios) and important measures of impact relevant to dementia. In general, outcome measures must be thoughtfully matched to the question at hand. Hazard ratios may be useful for understanding the magnitude of a causal effect but are less useful for personal or policy decision making. Thus, measures that take into account absolute as well as relative risk at both the individual and population levels and account for a broad array of outcomes may be more useful. For example, cost/benefit analyses may provide insight into the broader impact of policy changes in monetary terms, or decision analytic tools may help individuals understand the consequences of behavioral changes in terms of their own personal values or quality of life.

Important diagnostic and therapeutic innovations on the horizon, such as new imaging modalities, fluid biomarkers, and pharmacologic treatments (see Chapter 3), illustrate the importance of tools for quantifying broad impacts. Such innovations may have important clinical consequences, but some will likely have marginal clinical benefit. Thus, diagnostic innovations need to be scrutinized specifically in relation to the potential therapeutic options and the potential impact of those treatments for patients who are identified as at high risk for dementia long before symptoms are evident. Beyond the clinical impacts, technical innovations may alter the social costs of dementia, change the landscape of research, and influence disparities.

It has been noted that diagnosing Alzheimer's disease using only a neuroimaging biomarker exposes people to adverse effects and complications, and, particularly when diagnosis is based solely on biomarker evidence, many people receive completely ineffective treatment (Langa and Burke, 2019). By one estimate, one-half of adults with preclinical Alzheimer's disease are treated with medications priced in the same range as monoclonal antibody drugs to treat cholesterol, which would represent nearly one-third of 2017 total costs for retail prescriptions. Another recent estimate is that if just one-fourth of Medicare beneficiaries currently taking Alzheimer's treatments covered under Part D were prescribed aducanumab, the drug approved by the U.S. Food and Drug Administration just as this report was going to press (see Chapter 9), the cost of drug alone, apart from associated delivery costs, could be $29 billion annually (current total Medicare spending for Part B drugs is $37 billion) (Cubanski and Neuman, 2021). In addition, Medicare beneficiaries would likely face approximately $11,500 in coinsurance costs, or approximately 40 percent of the median annual income of Medicare beneficiaries.

The criteria for the clinical importance of innovations need always to be based on patient- and family-centered outcomes related to quality and length of life. Therefore, tools that can quantify these impacts more easily are needed. It is important to note here that, because of the high costs of some technical innovations, their widespread adoption could result in the displacement of established and effective lower-cost alternatives, such as supportive services. In addition, defining disease in terms of the presence of a biomarker could lead to use of the biomarker as a surrogate outcome in trials of new therapies. Such a change would be troubling. For example, evidence from prior RCTs indicates that it is possible to change biomarker indicators of Alzheimer's without offering clinical benefit (Ackley et al., 2021; Richard et al., 2021). Likewise, the adoption of marginally beneficial diagnostic or therapeutic tools could have a chilling effect on future research to identify effective options or evaluate adverse consequences of medications approved on the basis of minimal evidence (Musiek and Morris, 2021). These problems raise questions of social policy and regulatory design, solidly within the domain of social science research.

It is well established that new technologies in any health domain have the potential to exacerbate inequalities because those individuals who already have resources are best positioned to take advantage of new tools (Phelan and Link, 2005; Phelan et al., 2004, 2010). Anticipating such consequences for equity and proposing policy and systems solutions to ameliorate them are important responsibilities for researchers. Other technical innovations (e.g., low-cost fluid biomarkers) hold promise for improving health equity by promoting access to diagnostic information and improving the inclusivity of biomarker-based research. As discussed in Chapter 3, however, such innovations may bring their own ethical challenges and social consequences. For example, what are the consequences of informing a large fraction of middle-aged adults that they have biomarkers indicating that they could develop Alzheimer's disease when it is not possible to inform them of how likely that outcome is or offer meaningful treatment to delay or prevent symptoms?

Simulation studies may be important tools for helping to anticipate the effects of complex developments in dementia care and treatment and integrate evidence from disparate types of studies. Dynamic microsimulations for cognitive decline and dementia could support the development of both U.S. and international projections of dementia prevalence and costs associated with new diagnostics and treatments, changes in population health, and changes in policies affecting people living with dementia and their caregivers (Zissimopoulos et al., 2014, 2018). Simulations often depend on valid input assumptions from other study designs. Also essential to note is that these tools will not work without data on the "target" population. Thus, a key priority is ensuring that major data sources include sufficient diversity to support well-powered analyses of racial/ethnic groups and intersectionally defined identities. Attention to intersectionality—the multiple identities individuals have that may each interact in shaping health risk or resilience—is essential. For example, it is important to study not only broad racial/ethnic differences in the incidence of and prognosis for dementia but also how they may be different for men versus women, or for gay versus straight men.

Finally, even when interventions are demonstrated to work in the setting of a trial, they may not scale well to new settings. Research is needed to understand what types of interventions scale, and scalable interventions are a research priority. Evaluation of interventions also needs to incorporate potential population impact.

INVESTMENT IN HUMAN CAPITAL AND RESEARCH CAPACITY

None of the above suggestions are feasible without research leaders who have the needed skills, including proficiency with quantitative and qualitative methodologies, applied understanding of the needs of people living with dementia and their networks, insights into biological mechanisms relevant to disease incidence and progression, and skills related to dissemination and implementation. Applicable methods are evolving rapidly, so even recently trained researchers need ways to constantly update and improve their knowledge. Training often occurs in research silos, without clear communication across disciplines. For example, instrumental variables and quasi-experimental methods are not part of the core quantitative methods covered in typical epidemiology training but are central tools for economics. Clinician-scientists are essential to the research workforce but often receive shockingly limited training in statistical methods. On the opposite end of the spectrum, many quantitative methodologists receive almost no exposure to applied or clinical settings where their evidence would be used, which inevitably reduces the impact of their work. Scientific communication and dissemination training is often minimal and may even be considered a problematic distraction from research. Moreover, the lack of racial/ethnic and socioeconomic diversity in the health research workforce has been widely recognized as a major barrier to progress and is equally problematic in dementia research.

Efforts to build researchers' capacity to design and run pragmatic trials, such as the IMbedded Pragmatic Alzheimer's disease and Alzheimer's disease-related dementias Clinical Trials Collaboratory (IMPACT), are promising. IMPACT focuses on developing and disseminating best-practice research methods, including giving due attention to inclusive and representative methods, supporting pilot studies for pragmatic trials, taking account of issues of training and knowledge generation, and catalyzing collaboration. Smaller initiatives have also proven useful but provide fewer direct training activities. Institutional training grants restrict the training period in ways that make truly challenging interdisciplinary experiences less likely. The typical cost of living for students also discourages extended training activities and restricts the pipeline of researchers because of the need for substantial subsidies. Despite these challenges, networks dedicated to interdisciplinary training and combining substantive and technical skills, such as the Training in Advanced Data and Analytics for Behavioral and Social Sciences Research Program, can have powerful influences on the field. Investing in training, across the career spectrum, pays off.

RESEARCH DIRECTIONS

This is a moment of opportunity for investments in strengthening research methods for the study of dementia in four areas: *data sources* that support new, more inclusive, and more rigorous research; *measurement* of factors that influence both dementia risk and progression, of patient- and family-centered outcomes related to dementia, and of outcomes that are appropriate for diverse populations and settings; *study designs* that offer greater rigor and relevance to diverse populations; and *meta-research methods* with which to integrate disparate sources of evidence and guide decision making.

These opportunities are interrelated: better data sources will support the development of more rigorous study designs; innovations in measurement will make previously nonviable data sources potentially useful; and thinking about the weaknesses implicit in any single study will help researchers better integrate the available evidence to provide guidance for the development of systems, policies, and interventions to prevent dementia, improve prognosis and quality of life for people living with dementia, and ameliorate the adverse consequences of the disease for families and society. Advances in these areas will be relevant to and strengthen research in every area discussed in this report. Social and behavioral scientists from numerous specific disciplines are the natural leaders in meeting these methodological challenges.

The committee identified five priority areas for research in the domain of improved methodologies for dementia research. These priorities are summarized in Conclusion 8-1 and detailed in Table 8-1.

CONCLUSION 8-1: Advances in research methodology are needed to support progress in virtually every domain of dementia research. Progress in five areas will support a research agenda to reduce the negative impacts of dementia by strengthening data collection and research methodology:
1. **Expansion of data infrastructure.**
2. **Improved measurement of exposures and outcomes.**
3. **Support for the adoption of more rigorous study designs, particularly in the realm of implementation science, so that research findings can be successfully integrated into clinical and community practices.**

4. Development of systematic approaches for integrating evidence from disparate studies.
5. Improved inclusion and representation among both research participants and researchers.

TABLE 8-1 Detailed Research Needs

1: Expansion of Data Infrastructure	• Fostering of new applications for existing data sources, including those from beyond the health care context (e.g., by improving the extraction of relevant constructs from existing data sources) • Development of new tools for data linkage across health care system, payer, and community-based data systems, including standards for variables and protocols • Funding to support documentation, archiving, and sharing of existing datasets and follow-up of previously abandoned datasets, including RCTs that evaluated relevant treatments but did not originally include dementia-relevant outcomes • Creation of a "reference database" by linking multiple data sources that researchers can use for comparison against localized samples and selection of settings for new studies • Evaluation of biases in who is selected into research studies; how data are collected; and how measurements are made, including algorithmic bias • Increased focus and accountability related to inclusion in research participation and development of a testable scientific framework for conducting inclusive research
2: Improved Measurement	• Evaluation of the correspondence between evolving biomarkers and clinical/functional outcomes of relevance to people living with dementia • Development of standardized definitions/tools for identifying dementia and capturing stages of disease • Development of reliable and valid early markers of subsequent disease—potentially based on novel, nontraditional data sources—to foster research on causes of disease • Research to improve measurement validity across disease stages, outcome domains, and assessment modes • Expanded inclusive measurement strategies to yield valid measures for diverse populations, including heterogeneous cultural settings, racial/ethnic identities, gender/sexual minority groups, and linguistic backgrounds • Tools to support valid crosswalks between assessments from different instruments or modalities • Fostering of exploratory research to evaluate novel exposures that may influence disease risk across the life course • Development of improved measures of consent to participate in research

TABLE 8-1 Continued

3: Support for the Adoption of More Rigorous Study Designs	• Broadening of the repertoire of tools for estimating causal effects in nonrandomized settings • Development of opportunities for quasi-experimental studies, natural experiments, instrumental variables analyses, regression discontinuity methods, difference-in-difference methods, and other approaches that do not depend on the "no-confounding of exposure–outcome association" assumption • Investment in more comprehensive analyses of RCTs to evaluate mediation, bias, and generalizability, particularly in parallel with real-world data • Support for implementation science's focus on scalable interventions and how new discoveries are disseminated and adopted (e.g., via new policies, behavioral interventions, or systems changes) • Development of platforms to facilitate fielding of pragmatic trials embedded in health care systems and analysis of the results of those trials • Investment in qualitative work to identify new questions, improve the cultural validity of measurements, and better understand why past interventions succeeded or failed • Improved strategies for evaluating complex, dynamic interventions, such as community-based initiatives • Development of guidelines for conceptualizing study design trade-offs that could be used to prioritize research investments
4: Development of Systematic Approaches for Evidence Integration	• Fostering of research on heterogeneity in treatment response/exposure effects across populations, and methods to support generalizing from samples in existing studies to other populations • Expansion of meta-analytic and related approaches to integrate findings from heterogeneous study designs more flexibly and correct for bias • Quantifying of the population health and health equity impacts of proposed policies, interventions, or therapies • Facilitation of linkage of data, including data from electronic health records, claims, research studies, and records of community-based organizations (e.g., consenting, nonrandomized control groups; proxy respondents)
5: Improved Inclusion and Representation Among Research Participants and Researchers	• Bolstering of training efforts to accommodate changing standards of living, continue to foster diversity and representation in the research workforce, and emphasize the interdisciplinary skills noted elsewhere

REFERENCES

Ackley, S., Mayeda, E., Worden, L., Enanoria, W., Glymour, M., and Porco, T. (2017). Compartmental model diagrams as causal representations in relation to DAGs. *Epidemiologic Methods*, 6(1), 20160007. https://doi.org/10.1515/em-2016-0007

Ackley, S.F., Zimmerman, S.C., Brenowitz, W.D., Tchetgen, E.J., Gold, A.L., Manly, J.J., Mayeda, E.R., Filshtein, T.J., Power, M.C., Elahi, F.M., and Brickman, A.M. (2021). Effect of reductions in amyloid levels on cognitive change in randomized trials: Instrumental variable meta-analysis. *British Medical Journal*, 372(156). https://doi.org/10.1136/bmj.n156

Athey, S. (2015). Machine learning and causal inference for policy evaluation. *Proceedings of the 21st ACM SIGKDD International Conference on Knowledge Discovery and Data Mining*, 5–6. https://doi.org/10.1145/2783258.2785466

Bareinboim, E., and Pearl, J. (2016). Causal inference and the data-fusion problem. *Proceedings of the National Academy of Sciences*, 113(27), 7345–7352. https://doi.org/10.1073/pnas.1510507113

Bärnighausen, T., Røttingen, J.A., Rockers, P., Shemilt, I., and Tugwell, P. (2017). Quasi-experimental study designs series—Paper 1: Introduction: Two historical lineages. *Journal of Clinical Epidemiology*, 89, 4–11. https://doi.org/10.1016/j.jclinepi.2017.02.020

Beekly, D.L., Ramos, E.M., van Belle, G., Deitrich, W., Clark, A.D., Jacka, M.E., and Kukull, W.A. (2004). The National Alzheimer's Coordinating Center (NACC) database: An Alzheimer disease database. *Alzheimer Disease & Associated Disorders*, 18(4), 270–277.

Berkman, L.F. (1986). The association between educational attainment and mental status examinations: Of etiologic significance for senile dementias or not? *Journal of Chronic Diseases*, 39(3), 171–174.

Besser, L., Kukull, W., Knopman, D., Chui, H., Galasko, D., Weintraub, S., Jicha, G., Carlsson, C., Burns, J., Quinn, J., Sweet, R., Rascovsky, K., Teylan, M., Beekly, D., Thomas, G., Bollenbeck, M., Monsell, S., Mock, C., Zhou, X., Thomas, N., Robichaud, E., Dean, M., Hubbard, J., Jacka, M., Schwabe-Fry, K., Wu, J., Phelps, C., and Morris, J.C. (2018). The neuropsychology work group, directors, and clinical core leaders of the National Institute on Aging-funded US Alzheimer's disease centers version 3 of the National Alzheimer's Coordinating Center's uniform data set. *Alzheimer Disease & Associated Disorders* 32(4), 351–358. https://doi.org/10.1097/WAD.0000000000000279

Bild, D.E., Bluemke, D.A., Burke, G.L., Detrano, R., Diez Roux, A.V., Folsom, A.R., Greenland, P., Jacobs Jr., D.R., Kronmal, R., Liu, K., and Nelson, J.C. (2002). Multi-ethnic study of atherosclerosis: Objectives and design. *American Journal of Epidemiology*, 156(9), 871–881.

Brewster, P., Barnes, L., Haan, M., Johnson, J.K., Manly, J.J., Nápoles, A.M., Whitmer, R.A., Carvajal-Carmona, L., Early, D., Farias, S., and Mayeda, E.R. (2019). Progress and future challenges in aging and diversity research in the United States. *Alzheimer's & Dementia*, 15(7), 995–1003.

Bynum, J.P.W., Dorr, D.A., Lima, J., McCarthy, E.P., McCreedy, E., Platt, R., and Vydiswaran, V.G.V. (2020). Using healthcare data in embedded pragmatic clinical trials among people living with dementia and their caregivers: State of the art. *Journal of the American Geriatrics Society*, 68(Suppl 2), S49–S54. https://doi.org/10.1111/jgs.16617

Caniglia, E.C., Rojas-Saunero, L.P., Hilal, S., Licher, S., Logan, R., Stricker, B., Ikram, M.A., and Swanson, S.A. (2020). Emulating a target trial of statin use and risk of dementia using cohort data. *Neurology*, 95(10):e1322–1332.

Cubanski, J., and Neuman, T. (2021). *FDA's approval of Biogen's new Alzheimer's drug has huge cost implications for Medicare beneficiaries*. Kaiser Family Foundation. https://www.kff.org/medicare/issue-brief/fdas-approval-of-biogens-new-alzheimers-drug-has-huge-cost-implications-for-medicare-and-beneficiaries

Dahabreh, I.J., Robins, J.M., Haneuse, S.J., and Hernán, M.A. (2019). Generalizing causal inferences from randomized trials: Counterfactual and graphical identification. *arXiv*, 1906.10792.

Dahabreh, I.J., Haneuse, S.J.P.A., Robins, J.M., Robertson, S.E., Buchanan, A.L., Stuart, E.A., and Hernán, M.A. (2021). Study designs for extending causal inferences from a randomized trial to a target population. *American Journal of Epidemiology*, 190(8), 1632–1642. https://doi.org/10.1093/aje/kwaa270

Dahl, A., Berg, S., and Nilsson, S.E. (2007). Identification of dementia in epidemiological research: A study on the usefulness of various data sources. *Aging Clinical and Experimental Research*, 19(5), 381–389.

Danaei, G., Robins, J.M., Young, J., Hu, F.B., Manson, J.E., and Hernán, M.A. (2016). Estimated effect of weight loss on risk of coronary heart disease and mortality in middle-aged or older women: Sensitivity analysis for unmeasured confounding by undiagnosed disease. *Epidemiology*, 27(2), 302.

Dankwa-Mullan, I., Pérez-Stable, E., Gardner, K., Zhang, X., and Rosario, A. (Eds.). (2021). *The Science of Health Disparities Research*. Hoboken, NJ: John Wiley and Sons.

Dementia Friendly America. (2021). *What is DFA?* https://www.dfamerica.org/what-is-dfa

Fried, L.P., Borhani, N.O., Enright, P., Furberg, C.D., Gardin, J.M., Kronmal, R.A., Kuller, L.H., Manolio, T.A., Mittelmark, M.B., Newman, A., and O'Leary, D.H. (1991). The cardiovascular health study: Design and rationale. *Annals of Epidemiology*, 1(3), 263–276.

Fry, A., Littlejohns, T.J., Sudlow, C., Doherty, N., Adamska, L., Sprosen, T., Collins, R., and Allen, N.E. (2017). Comparison of sociodemographic and health-related characteristics of UK Biobank participants with those of the general population. *American Journal of Epidemiology*, 186(9), 1026–1034.

Gershon, R., Nowinski, C., Peipert, J.D., Bedjeti, K., Ustsinovich, V., Hook, J., Fox, R., and Weintraub, S. (2020). Use of the NIH Toolbox for assessment of mild cognitive impairment and Alzheimer's disease in general population, African American and Spanish speaking samples of older adults: Neuropsychology: Cognitive and functional assessment in diverse populations. *Alzheimer's & Dementia*, 16(S6), e043372. https://doi.org/10.1002/alz.043372

Gianattasio, K.Z., Wu, Q., Glymour, M.M., and Power, M.C. (2019). Comparison of methods for algorithmic classification of dementia status in the Health and Retirement Study. *Epidemiology*, 30(2), 291.

Gianattasio, K.Z., Ciarleglio, A., and Power, M.C. (2020). Development of algorithmic dementia ascertainment for racial/ethnic disparities research in the US Health and Retirement Study. *Epidemiology*, 31(1), 126–133.

Gianattasio, K.Z., Bennett, E.E., Wei, J., Mehrotra, M.L., Mosley, T., Gottesman, R.F., Wong, D.F., Stuart, E.A., Griswold, M.E., Couper, D., and Glymour, M.M. (2021). Generalizability of findings from a clinical sample to a community-based sample: A comparison of ADNI and ARIC. *Alzheimer's & Dementia*. https://doi.org/10.1002/alz.12293

Gilmore-Bykovskyi, A., Jackson, J.D., and Wilkins, C.H. (2021). The urgency of justice in research: Beyond COVID-19. *Trends in Molecular Medicine*, 27(2), 97–100. https://doi.org/10.1016/j.molmed.2020.11.004

Glasgow, R.E., Vinson, C., Chambers, D., Khoury, M.J., Kaplan, R.M., and Hunter, C. (2012). National Institutes of Health approaches to dissemination and implementation science: Current and future directions. *American Journal of Public Health*, 102(7), 1274–1281.

Glymour, M.M., Walter, S., and Tchetgen Tchetgen, E.J. (2017). Natural experiments and instrumental variables analyses in social epidemiology. In J. Oakes and J. Kaufman (Eds.), *Methods in Social Epidemiology* (pp. 493–537). Hoboken, NJ: John Wiley & Sons.

Glymour, M.M., Brickman, A.M., Kivimaki, M., Mayeda, E.R., Chêne, G., Dufouil, C., and Manly, J.J. (2018). Will biomarker-based diagnosis of Alzheimer's disease maximize scientific progress? Evaluating proposed diagnostic criteria. *European Journal of Epidemiology*, 33(7), 607–612.

Green, L.W., Ottoson, J.M., Garcia, C., and Hiatt, R.A. (2009). Diffusion theory and knowledge dissemination, utilization, and integration in public health. *Annual Review of Public Health*, 30, 151–174. https://doi.org/10.1146/annurev.publhealth.031308.100049

Green, L.W., Ottoson, J.M., García, C., Hiatt, R.A., and Roditis, M.L. (2014). Diffusion theory and knowledge dissemination, utilization and integration. *Frontiers in Public Health Services & Systems Research*, 3(1), 3.

Gross, A.L., Khobragade, P.Y., Meijer, E., and Saxton, J.A. (2020). Measurement and structure of cognition in the Longitudinal Aging Study in India–Diagnostic Assessment of Dementia. *Journal of the American Geriatrics Society*, 68(S3), S11–S19. https://doi.org/10.1111/jgs.16738

Handley, M.A., Lyles, C.R., McCulloch, C., and Cattamanchi, A. (2018). Selecting and improving quasi-experimental designs in effectiveness and implementation research. *Annual Review of Public Health*, 39, 5–25. https://doi.org/10.1146/annurev-publhealth-040617-014128

Haneuse, S., and Daniels, M. (2016). A general framework for considering selection bias in EHR-Based studies: What data are observed and why? *Journal of Electronic Health Data and Methods*, 4(1), 1203. https://doi.org/10.13063/2327-9214.1203

Hernán, M., Brumback, B., and Robins, J. (2000). Marginal structural models to estimate the causal effect of zidovudine on the survival of HIV-positive men. *Epidemiology*, 11(5), 561–570. https://doi.org/10.1097/00001648-200009000-00012

Hernán, M., Hernández-Díaz, S., and Robins, J. (2004). A structural approach to selection bias. *Epidemiology*, 15(5), 615–625. https://doi.org/10.1097/01.ede.0000135174.63482.43

Hernán, M.A., Alonso, A., Logan, R., Grodstein, F., Michels, K.B., Stampfer, M.J., Willett, W.C., Manson, J.E., and Robins, J.M. (2008). Observational studies analyzed like randomized experiments: An application to postmenopausal hormone therapy and coronary heart disease. *Epidemiology*, 19(6), 766.

Hernán, M.A., Robins, J.M. (2016). Using big data to emulate a target trial when a randomized trial Is not available, *American Journal of Epidemiology*,183(8), 758–764, https://doi.org/10.1093/aje/kwv254

Jack Jr., C.R., Bennett, D.A., Blennow, K., Carrillo, M.C., Dunn, B., Haeberlein, S.B., Holtzman, D.M., Jagust, W., Jessen, F., Karlawish, J., and Liu, E. (2018). NIA-AA research framework: Toward a biological definition of Alzheimer's disease. *Alzheimer's & Dementia*, 14(4), 535–562.

James, B.D., Boyle, P.A., Buchman, A.S., Barnes, L.L., and Bennett, D.A. (2011). Life space and risk of Alzheimer disease, mild cognitive impairment, and cognitive decline in old age. *American Journal of Geriatric Psychiatry*, 19(11), 961–969.

Jutkowitz, E., Bynum, J.P.W., Mitchell, S.L., Cocoros, N.M., Shapira, O., Haynes, K., Nair, V.P., McMahill-Walraven, C.N., Platt, R., and McCarthy, E.P. (2020). Diagnosed prevalence of Alzheimer's disease and related dementias in Medicare Advantage plans. *Alzheimer's & Dementia: Diagnosis, Assessment & Disease Monitoring*, 12(1), e12048. https://doi.org/10.1002/dad2.12048

Karlawish, J. (2021). *The Problem of Alzheimer's: How Science, Culture, and Politics Turned a Rare Disease into a Crisis and What We Can Do About It*. New York: St. Martin's Press. https://us.macmillan.com/books/9781250218742

Kobayashi, L.C., Gross, A.L., Gibbons, L.E., Tommet, D., Sanders, R.E., Choi, S.E., Mukherjee, S., Glymour, M., Manly, J.J., Berkman, L.F., and Crane, P.K. (2020). You say tomato, I say radish: Can brief cognitive assessments in the US Health Retirement Study be harmonized with its International Partner Studies? *Journals of Gerontology, Series B*. https://doi.org/10.1093/geronb/gbaa205

Krysinska, K., Sachdev, P., Breitner, J., Kivipelto, M., Kukull, W., and Brodaty, H. (2017). Dementia registries around the globe and their applications: A systematic review. *Alzheimer's & Dementia*, *13*(9), 1031–1047. https://doi.org/10.1016/j.jalz.2017.04.005

Labrecque, J.A., and Swanson, S.A. (2017). Target trial emulation: Teaching epidemiology and beyond. *European Journal of Epidemiology*, *32*(6), 473–475. https://doi.org/10.1093/aje/kwv254

Langa, K.M., and Burke, J.F. (2019). Preclinical Alzheimer disease—Early diagnosis or overdiagnosis? *JAMA Internal Medicine*, *179*(9), 1161–1162. https://doi.org/10.1001/jamainternmed.2019.2629

Langa, K.M., Plassman, B.L., Wallace, R.B., Herzog, A.R., Heeringa, S.G., Ofstedal, M.B., Burke, J.R., Fisher, G.G., Fultz, N.H., Hurd, M.D., and Potter, G.G. (2005). The aging, demographics, and memory study: Study design and methods. *Neuroepidemiology*, *25*(4), 181–191

Lawlor, D., Tilling, K., and Davey Smith, G. (2017). Triangulation in aetiological epidemiology. *International Journal of Epidemiology*, *45*(6), 1866–1886. https://doi.org/10.1093/ije/dyw314

Matthay, E.C., Hagan, E., Gottlieb, L.M., Tan, M.L., Vlahov, D., Adler, N.E., and Glymour, M.M. (2020). Alternative causal inference methods in population health research: Evaluating tradeoffs and triangulating evidence. *SSM-Population Health*, *10*, 100526. 10.1016/j.ssmph.2019.100526

Mayeda, E.R., Tchetgen Tchetgen, E.J., Power, M.C., Weuve, J., Jacqmin-Gadda, H., Marden, J.R., Vittinghoff, E., Keiding, N., and Glymour, M.M. (2016). A simulation platform for quantifying survival bias: An application to research on determinants of cognitive decline. *American Journal of Epidemiology*, *184*(5), 378–387.

McCleery, J., Flicker, L., Richard, E., and Quinn, T. (2019). When is Alzheimer's not dementia—Cochrane commentary on The National Institute on Ageing and Alzheimer's Association Research Framework for Alzheimer's Disease. *Age and Ageing*, *48*(2), 174–177. https://doi.org/10.1093/ageing/afy167

McDonald, S., Hultsch, D., and Dixon, R. (2003). Performance variability is related to change in cognition: Evidence from the Victoria Longitudinal Study. *Psychology and Aging*, *18*(3), 510–523. https://doi.org/10.1037/0882-7974.18.3.510

Mehrotra, M.L., Petersen, M.L., and Geng, E.H. (2019). Understanding HIV program effects: A structural approach to context using the transportability framework. *Journal of Acquired Immune Deficiency Syndromes*, *82*, S199–S205.

Mitchell, S.L., Mor, V., Harrison, J., and McCarthy, E.P. (2020). Embedded pragmatic trials in dementia care: Realizing the vision of the NIA IMPACT Collaboratory. *Journal of the American Geriatrics Society*, *68*(Suppl 2), S1–S7. https://doi.org/10.1111/jgs.16621

Mitchell, S., Volandes, A., Gutman, R., Gozalo, P., Ogarek, J., Loomer, L., McCreedy, E., Zhai, R., and Mor, V. (2021). Advance care planning video intervention among long-stay nursing home residents: A pragmatic cluster randomized clinical trial. *JAMA Internal Medicine*, *180*(8), 1070–1078. https://doi.org/jamainternmed.2020.2366

Mukherjee, S., Mez, J., Trittschuh, E.H., Saykin, A.J., Gibbons, L.E., Fardo, D.W., Wessels, M., Bauman, J., Moore, M., Choi, S.E., and Gross, A.L. (2020). Genetic data and cognitively defined late-onset Alzheimer's disease subgroups. *Molecular Psychiatry*, *25*(11), 2942–2951.

Murray, E.J., Robins, J.M., Seage, G.R., Freedberg, K.A., and Hernán, M.A. (2017). A comparison of agent-based models and the parametric g-formula for causal inference. *American Journal of Epidemiology*, *186*(2), 131–142.

Musiek, E.S., and Morris, J.C. (2021). Possible Consequences of the approval of a disease-modifying therapy for Alzheimer disease. *JAMA Neurology*, *78*(2), 141–142. https://doi.org/10.1001/jamaneurol.2020.4478

National Academies of Sciences, Engineering, and Medicine (2021). *Meeting the Challenge of Caring for Persons Living with Dementia and Their Care Partners and Caregivers: A Way Forward.* Washington, DC: The National Academies Press. https://doi.org/10.17226/26026

NACC (National Alzheimer's Coordinating Center). (2021). *UDS Subject Demographics by Cognitive Status.* https://naccdata.org/requesting-data/data-summary/uds

National Institutes of Health. (2021). *All of Us Research Hub: The Basics Survey.* https://databrowser.researchallofus.org/survey/the-basics

Nicholas, L.H., Langa, K.M., Bynum, J.P., and Hsu, J.W. (2021). Financial presentation of Alzheimer disease and related dementias. *JAMA Internal Medicine, 181*(2), 220–227.

Obermeyer, Z., Powers, B., Vogeli, C., and Mullainathan, S. (2019, October 25). Dissecting racial bias in an algorithm used to manage the health of populations. *Science, 366*(6464), 447–453. https://doi.org/10.1126/science.aax2342

Oldenburg, C.E., Moscoe, E., and Bärnighausen, T. (2016). Regression discontinuity for causal effect estimation in epidemiology. *Current Epidemiology Reports, 3*(3), 233–241.

Pearl, J. (2009). *Causality: Models, Reasoning, and Inference.* Cambridge: Cambridge University Press. http://bayes.cs.ucla.edu/BOOK-2K

Phelan, J.C., and Link, B.G. (2005). Controlling disease and creating disparities: A fundamental cause perspective. *Journals of Gerontology, Series B, 60*(Special_Issue_2), S27–S33.

Phelan, J.C., Link, B.G., Diez-Roux, A., Kawachi, I., and Levin B. (2004). "Fundamental causes" of social inequalities in mortality: A test of the theory. *Journal of Health and Social Behavior, 45*(3), 265–285.

Phelan, J.C., Link, B.G., and Tehranifar, P. (2010). Social conditions as fundamental causes of health inequalities: Theory, evidence, and policy implications. *Journal of Health and Social Behavior, 51*(Suppl 1), S28–S40.

Plassman, B., Langa, K., Fisher, G., Heeringa, S., Weir, D., Ofstedal, M.B., Burke, J., Hurd, M., Potter, G., Rodgers, W., Steffens, D., McArdle, J., Willis, R., and Wallace, R. (2008). Prevalence of cognitive impairment without dementia in the United States. *Annals of Internal Medicine.* https://doi.org/10.7326/0003-4819-148-6-200803180-00005

Power, M.C., Gianattasio, K.Z., and Ciarleglio, A. (2020). Implications of the use of algorithmic diagnoses or Medicare claims to ascertain dementia. *Neuroepidemiology, 54*(6), 462–471.

Richard, E., den Brok, M.G., and van Gool, W.A. (2021). Bayes analysis supports null hypothesis of anti amyloid beta therapy in Alzheimer's disease. *Alzheimer's & Dementia, 17*(6), 1051–1055. https://doi.org/10.1002/alz.12379

Robertson, S.E., Leith, A., Schmid, C.H., and Dahabreh, I.J. (2021). Assessing heterogeneity of treatment effects in observational studies. *American Journal of Epidemiology, 190*(6), 1088–1100. https://doi.org/10.1093/aje/kwaa235

Robins, J.M., Hernán, M., and Brumback, B. (2000). Marginal structural models and causal inference in epidemiology. *Epidemiology, 11*(5), 550–560. https://doi.org/10.1097/00001648-200009000-00011

Rojas-Saunero, L.P., Hilal, S., Murray, E.J., Logan, R.W., Ikram, M.A., and Swanson, S.A. (2021). Hypothetical blood-pressure-lowering interventions and risk of stroke and dementia. *European Journal of Epidemiology, 36*(1), 69–79.

Salganik, M. (2019). *Bit by Bit: Social Research in the Digital Age.* New Jersey: Princeton University Press.

Scales, K., Zimmerman, S., and Miller, S.J. (2018). Evidence-based nonpharmacological practices to address behavioral and psychological symptoms of dementia. *Gerontologist, 58*(1), S88–S102. https://doi.org/10.1093/geront/gnx167

Thorogood, A., Mäki-Petäjä-Leinonen, A., Brodaty, H., Dalpé, G., Gastmans, C., Gauthier, S., Gove, D., Harding, R., Knoppers, B., Rossor, M., and Bobrow, M. (2018). Consent recommendations for research and international data sharing involving persons with dementia. *Alzheimer's & Dementia, 14*(10), 1334–1343. https://doi.org/10.1016/j.jalz.2018.05.011

VanderWeele, T.J., and Ding, P. (2017). Sensitivity analysis in observational research: Introducing the E-value. *Annals of Internal Medicine, 167*(4), 268–274.

VanderWeele, T.J., Hernán, M.A., and Robins, J.M. (2008). Causal directed acyclic graphs and the direction of unmeasured confounding bias. *Epidemiology, 19*(5), 720.

Wager, S., and Athey, S. (2018). Estimation and inference of heterogeneous treatment effects using random forests. *Journal of the American Statistical Association, 113*(523), 1228–1242.

Walter, S., Dufouil, C., Gross, A.L., Jones, R.N., Mungas, D., Filshtein, T.J., Manly, J.J., Arpawong, T.E., and Glymour, M.M. (2019). Neuropsychological test performance and MRI markers of dementia risk. *Alzheimer Disease & Associated Disorders, 33*(3), 179–185.

Weintraub, S., Salmon, D., Mercaldo, N., Ferris, S., Graff-Radford, N., Chui, H., Cummings, J., DeCarli, C., Foster, N., Galasko, D., Peskind, E., Dietrich, W., Beekly, D., Kukull, W., and Morris, J. (2009). The Alzheimer's Disease Centers' Uniform Data Set (UDS). *Alzheimer Disease and Associated Disorders, 23*(2), 91–101. https://doi.org/10.1097/WAD.0b013e318191c7dd

Weintraub, S., Besser, L., Dodge, H.H., Teylan, M., Ferris, S., Goldstein, F.C., Giordani, B., Kramer, J., Loewenstein, D., Marson, D., Mungas, D., Salmon, D., Welsh-Bohmer, K., Zhou, X.H., Shirk, S.D., Atri, A., Kukull, W.A., Phelps, C., and Morris, J.C. (2018). Version 3 of the Alzheimer Disease Centers' neuropsychological test battery in the Uniform Data Set (UDS). *Alzheimer Disease and Associated Disorders, 32*(1), 10–17. https://doi.org/10.1097/WAD.0000000000000223

Westreich, D., Edwards, J.K., Lesko, C.R., Stuart, E., and Cole, S.R. (2017). Transportability of trial results using inverse odds of sampling weights. *American Journal of Epidemiology, 186*(8), 1010–1014.

Westreich, D., Edwards, J.K., Lesko, C.R., Cole, S.R., and Stuart, E.A. (2019). Target validity and the hierarchy of study designs. *American Journal of Epidemiology, 188*(2), 438–443.

Weuve, J., Proust-Lima, C., Power, M.C., Gross, A.L., Hofer, S.M., Thiébaut, R., Chêne, G., Glymour, M.M., Dufouil, C., and MELODEM Initiative. (2015). Guidelines for reporting methodological challenges and evaluating potential bias in dementia research. *Alzheimer's & Dementia, 11*(9), 1098–1109.

White, A.D., Folsom, A.R., Chambless, L.E., Sharret, A.R., Yang, K., Conwill, D., Higgins, M., Williams, O.D., Tyroler, H.A., and ARIC Investigators. (1996). Community surveillance of coronary heart disease in the Atherosclerosis Risk in Communities (ARIC) Study: Methods and initial two years' experience. *Journal of Clinical Epidemiology, 49*(2), 223–233.

Wilkinson, T., Ly, A., Schnier, C., Rannikmäe, K., Bush, K., Brayne, C., Quinn, T.J., Sudlow, C.L., UK Biobank Neurodegenerative Outcomes Group, and Dementias Platform. (2018). Identifying dementia cases with routinely collected health data: A systematic review. *Alzheimer's & Dementia, 14*(8), 1038–1051. https://doi.org/10.1016/j.jalz.2018.02/016

World Health Organization (2010). *Nine Steps for Developing a Scaling-Up Strategy.* https://apps.who.int/iris/bitstream/handle/10665/44432/9789241500319_eng.pdf

Zissimopoulos, J., Crimmins, E., and St. Clair, P. (2014). The value of delaying Alzheimer's disease onset. *Forum for Health Economics and Policy, 18*(1), 25–39. https://doi.org/10.1515/fhep-2014-0013

Zissimopoulos, J., Tysinger, B., St. Clair, P., and Crimmins, E. (2018). The impact of changes in population health and mortality on future prevalence of Alzheimer's disease and other dementias in the United States. *Journals of Gerontology, Series B*, *73*(Suppl_1), S38S47. https://doi.org/10.1093/geronb/gbx147

9

Ten-Year Research Priorities

Ten years from now, dementia will still be affecting millions of people and their families—by one estimate, more than 130 million new diagnoses are expected worldwide by that time.[1] Even if therapies are developed that can modify the course of disease, individuals who are now approaching the age when these diseases are most common have already been exposed to both risk and protective factors. It is not yet possible to circumvent the dementias that will affect this population, but it will be possible to apply research to alter the repercussions of these diseases and improve the experience of living with dementia for individuals and family members.

The committee was charged with developing a 10-year research agenda for the social and behavioral sciences to meet the goal of reducing the overall negative impact of dementia. To develop this agenda, we examined the landscape of dementia and dementia care from multiple perspectives and considered diverse types of impacts. We looked across the life span to understand the factors that affect the development and course of dementia and how people experience its symptoms. We asked those living with dementia and caregivers what would make their lives better—not just in terms of medical care but in multiple domains. We looked across many entities and features of the environment that shape the experience of dementia in the United States, from the characteristics of neighborhoods and health care systems to objectives for dementia care. We examined evidence about the

---

[1]Alzheimer's Association. (2021). *2021 Alzheimer's Disease Facts and Figures.* https://alz-journals.onlinelibrary.wiley.com/doi/10.1002/alz.12328

reasons for the stark disparities in the prevalence of dementia—and the way it is experienced—across neighborhoods and population groups. Chapters 2 through 8 describe what we learned about the impacts of dementia from multiple perspectives. We explored the state of the research about each of these aspects of the landscape of dementia and identified the highest-priority areas for further research that could help reduce its negative impacts. As noted in Chapter 1, in so doing we looked for

- challenges that are both common and serious for people living with dementia and their caregivers that can be addressed through research in the social and behavioral sciences;
- gaps in the research available to support meaningful developments in interventions or policies; and
- reason to believe that those gaps could be filled within a decade using data and methods that are currently or could become available.

The conclusions in Chapters 2 through 8 summarize the research directions we identified; Appendix D provides a complete list of the conclusions and detailed research directions with which each of those chapters concludes. Collectively, these conclusions and detailed research needs constitute a substantial body of work that can provide the basis for powerful benefits to people living with dementia, their families and communities, and society. The committee envisioned a world that better supports people living with dementia because of research conducted over the coming decade, and in which the development of interventions and policies is based on improved understanding and corresponds to what matters to those living with dementia. We identified research opportunities, outlined below, that are ripe for development in each of these areas.

Understanding of modifiable factors that can prevent Alzheimer's disease and related dementias or reduce or delay their symptoms (Conclusion 2-1):
- The causal effects of social factors.
- The effects of health-related behaviors and their management over the life course.
- Modifiable drivers of racial/ethnic inequality in dementia incidence.
- The mechanisms through which socioeconomic factors influence brain health.
- Modifiable risk factors that can be the basis for precise recommendations to individuals about decision making and for population-level policies to promote brain health.

- Effective means of communicating the magnitude and degree of potential risk and protective factors to support informed decision making.

Ways to substantively improve the experience of individuals living with dementia by supporting their dignity and well-being, including balancing safety and autonomy (Conclusions 3-1 and 3-2):

- Improved screening and diagnosis, including guidance for clinicians that also addresses issues related to disclosure.
- Guidance to support ethical and responsible decision making by and for people living with dementia.
- Outcome measures that reflect the perspectives and values of people living with dementia, their family caregivers, and communities.
- Improved design and evaluation of nonpharmacologic interventions to slow or prevent cognitive and functional decline, reduce or ameliorate behavioral and psychological symptoms, improve comfort and well-being, and adequately and equitably serve diverse populations.

Ways to substantively improve the experience of family caregivers (Conclusion 4-1):

- Identification of the highest-priority needs for resources and support for family caregivers, particularly assessment of how they vary across race, ethnicity, and community.
- Means of identifying the assets that family caregivers bring to their work, as well as their needs for supplemental skills and training.
- Innovations to support and enhance family caregiving and address practical and logistical challenges in multiple domains, including appropriate use of technology to coordinate caregiving, extend independence, and promote comfort.
- Continued progress in data collection and research methods.

Ways to facilitate the development of communities that support people living with dementia and caregivers, allow those with dementia to live independently for as long as possible, maintain social connections, and mitigate the negative effects of past and current socioeconomic and environmental stressors (Conclusion 5-1):

- Systematic analysis of the characteristics of communities that influence the risk of developing dementia and the experience of living

with the disease, with particular attention to the sources of disparities in dementia incidence and disease trajectory.
- Collection of data to document the opportunities and resources available in communities and evaluation of their impact, with particular attention to disparities in population groups' access to resources.
- Analysis of the community characteristics needed to foster dementia friendly environments, including assessment of alternative community models and ways to serve diverse populations.
- Evaluation of innovative approaches to adapting housing, services, and supports so that persons with dementia can remain in the community and out of institutional care.

Ways to substantially strengthen the quality and structure of health care and long-term care (Conclusions 6-1 and 6-2):

- Documentation of the diagnosis and care management received by persons living with dementia from their primary care providers.
- Clarification of disease trajectories to help health systems plan care for persons living with dementia.
- Identification of effective methods for providing dementia-related services throughout the disease trajectory.
- Development and evaluation of standardized systems of coordinated care for comprehensively managing multiple comorbidities for persons with dementia.
- Identification of effective approaches for integrating and coordinating care services across health care delivery and community-based organizations.
- Identification of future long-term and end-of-life needs and available care for persons living with dementia.
- Description and monitoring of factors that contribute to problems with nursing home quality.
- Development and evaluation of alternatives to traditional nursing home facilities.
- Improved understanding of how and when patients use palliative and hospice care and variations in available end-of-life care across regions and populations.

Ways to substantially strengthen the arrangements through which most dementia care is funded—traditional Medicare, Medicare Advantage, alternative payment models, and Medicaid (Conclusion 6-3):

- Comparison of the effects of different financing structures on the quality of care and clinical outcomes.

- Examination of ways to modify incentives in reimbursement models to optimize care and reduce unnecessary hospitalizations.
- Development and testing of approaches to integrated financing of medical and social services.

Ways to improve understanding of the economic impact of dementia and identify high value, cost-effective interventions (Conclusion 7-1):

- Assessment and quantification of the total economic impact of dementia for individuals and families, including current and future national costs.
- Improved understanding of drivers of dementia-related costs.
- Estimation of the value to individuals, families, and society of innovations in prevention; diagnostics; and treatment, including pharmacologic treatments.

Taking advantage of all of these research opportunities will depend on advances in research methodology; the committee identified goals for moving forward in this area as well.

Key methodological objectives to support needed research (Conclusion 8-1):

- Expansion of data infrastructure and improved data collection.
- Improved measurement of exposures and outcomes.
- Support for the adoption of more rigorous study designs, particularly in the realm of implementation science so that research findings can be successfully integrated into clinical and community practices.
- Development of systematic approaches for integrating evidence from disparate studies.
- Improved inclusion and representation among both research participants and researchers.

RESEARCH AGENDA

These conclusions are the foundation for a research agenda that establishes clear priorities for the coming decade. Recognizing that resources are finite, the committee focused on critical areas of study to ensure that research undertaken in the next 10 years will contribute more than the sum of its parts. These priorities emerged from themes laid out throughout this report and can be used to structure funding for a research agenda that addresses the full range of negative impacts of dementia, and to guide decisions about the research likely to have the greatest impact in the coming decade.

> CONCLUSION 9-1: A 10-year research agenda for the behavioral and social sciences will have maximal impact in reducing the negative impacts of dementia and improving quality of life if it distributes attention and resources across five priorities:
> 1. Improvements in the lives of people affected by dementia, including those who develop it and their families and caregivers, as well as in the social and clinical networks that surround them, through research on factors that affect the development of disease and its outcomes, promising innovative practices and new models of care, and policies that can facilitate the dissemination of interventions found to be effective.
> 2. Rectifying of disparities across groups and geographic regions that affect who develops dementia, how the disease progresses, outcomes and quality of life, and access to health care and supportive services.
> 3. Development of innovations with the potential to improve the quality of care and social supports for individuals and communities and to support improved quality of life (e.g., reducing financial abuse and stressors, finding relevant affordable housing and care facilities, gaining access to important services).
> 4. Easing of the financial and economic costs of dementia to individuals, families, and society and balancing of long-term costs with long-term outcomes across the life span.
> 5. Pursuit of advances in research capability, including study design, measurement, analysis, and evidence integration, as well as the development of data infrastructure needed to study key dementia-related topics.

Table 9-1 shows how specific research priorities identified in Chapters 2 through 8 correspond to these five broad priorities.

In addition to these broad priorities, we offer guidelines for the design of an effective portfolio of research.

TABLE 9-1 Priorities for a 10-Year Research Agenda

Research Priority	Research Conclusions
1: Improving the Lives of People Touched by Dementia	2-1
	3-1
	3-2
	4-1
	5-1
	6-1
	6-2
	6-3
2: Rectifying Inequities and Disparities	2-1
	3-2
	4-1
	5-1
	6-1
	7-1
3: Developing Innovations	3-1
	3-2
	4-1
	5-1
	6-1
	6-2
	6-3
4: Easing and Balancing Costs	6-3
	7-1
5: Pursuing Advances in Research Capability	2-1
	3-2
	4-1
	8-1

CONCLUSION 9-2: A 10-year research agenda will be optimally effective if it

- is coordinated to ensure that the various research topics identified in this report are addressed sufficiently without redundancy and competing initiatives;
- consistently takes into account fundamental socioeconomic factors that influence who develops dementia, access to high-quality care, and outcomes;
- includes pragmatic, implementation, and dissemination research needed to ensure that findings can be implemented effectively in clinical and community settings; and
- addresses potential policy implications that are articulated beginning in the planning stages and assessed during the course of the investigations.

CALL TO ACTION

A 10-year research agenda that meets these objectives will require sustained leadership; integration of effort across multiple, sometimes competing domains; and the capacity to deliver research findings to individuals, communities, and health systems that bring meaningful change in the lives of people with dementia and their caregivers. Sustained funding, creativity, and collaboration are essential to the success of a project of this scope and difficulty. Alzheimer's disease and related dementias are common, fatal illnesses. Millions of Americans face the consequences of the disease either for themselves or their loved ones. The illness itself creates suffering, but there are also significant negative impacts from modifiable factors, many of which are socially determined. Much more can be done within the social and behavioral sciences to identify and mitigate those factors. This research agenda defines goals and priorities for the vital task of supporting better lives for people with dementia and caregivers, but its existence alone will not be sufficient: action is needed to ensure that the United States benefits from the potential in this body of research. To this end, the committee makes the following recommendation:

RECOMMENDATION 9-1: Funders of dementia-related research, including federal agencies, such as the National Institutes of Health and the Agency for Healthcare Research and Quality, along with relevant philanthropic and other organizations, such as the Patient-Centered Outcomes Research Institute, should use guidelines for the awarding of research grants to establish incentives for

- coordination of research objectives with the research agenda priorities identified in this report to ensure that key areas are funded without undue overlap and to foster links across research efforts;
- interdisciplinary research and inclusion of stakeholders in research partnerships;
- attention to topics that have not typically been part of standard medical research but are important to those living with dementia, including isolation, financial security, and housing options;
- rigorous evaluation and implementation research needed to translate findings into programs with impact on a broad scale; and
- dissemination of research findings to policy makers.

This report has documented the multifold challenges dementia is expected to bring in the coming decades. It was written as the COVID-19 pandemic was both exposing and exacerbating long-standing deficiencies in the support system for people living with dementia. That reality has highlighted not only the vulnerability of these individuals but also the critical importance of research and policy in shaping the contexts and circumstances in which they and their caregivers live.

Just as this report was going to press, the U.S. Food and Drug Administration (FDA) made the controversial decision to approve aducanumab for the treatment of dementia. Many people living with dementia and advocates greeted the decision with joy, hoping that the drug will meet a desperate need. Many others, especially in the scientific community, objected to the agency's choice to disregard the near-unanimous advice of its advisory panel, which found that the data analysis was flawed and did not demonstrate that the benefits of the drug outweigh its risks. Advocates for aducanumab argue that it showed modest benefit for a subgroup of trial participants. While trial participants were limited to those with mild cognitive impairment (MCI) and early-stage Alzheimer's disease (and included less than one-fourth minority participants), the FDA has labeled the drug for "treatment of Alzheimer's disease." In addition to the concern that any benefit to mildly impaired individuals such as those included in the trials is likely to be modest, it appears unlikely that the millions of people in the United States today who are living with moderate to severe Alzheimer's disease and other forms of dementia can expect any benefit from aducanumab.

The consequences of the FDA's decision are difficult to predict, but it will immediately present clinicians, patients, insurers, policy makers, and others with challenging decisions. Many members of the public might assume that a new drug for Alzheimer's disease will sweep away the problems of people living with dementia. On the contrary, this new treatment will not diminish the pressing need for the research described in this report. Indeed, the FDA's action illustrates many of the research challenges and needs facing the field of dementia research discussed in this report, and could affect responses to the research agenda we have laid out.

Moreover, complex policy issues are raised by the high cost of aducanumab. As discussed in Chapter 7, the cost of the drug itself, approximately $56,000 per year per patient, could reach as much as $112 billion per year and additional costs for delivery of the drug—including infusion services, scans, specialists, and equipment—could add tens of thousands more per eligible patient.[2] The desire to receive this drug will likely create increased demand for early diagnosis and associated testing, which may have additional benefits but will also increase costs overall. The bulk of

---

[2]Robbins, R., and Belluck, P. (2021, June 10). Alzheimer's drug is bonanza for Biogen, most likely at taxpayer expense. *New York Times.* https://www.nytimes.com/2021/06/08/business/aducanumab-alzheimers-cost.html

these costs will be borne by Medicare, depending on insurance-coverage decisions and how widely aducanumab is prescribed.[3]

While the costs of aducanumab may affect all Medicare enrollees, any benefits of the medication would likely accrue only to those with MCI or mild dementia. The rapidly growing and diverse population living with dementia will continue to require support across the broad range of domains covered in this report. What effect will the demand for this level of expenditure have on resources—already stretched thin—available to support the broader group of individuals and communities and to develop and implement interventions to reduce dementia risk across the life span? How will states, health plans, and health care systems balance investments in care programs known to be effective for many while also responding to high demand for a costly drug intended to benefit a smaller group?

The approval process for this drug raises additional policy questions, highlighting the need for a sound and ethical drug approval process that evaluates the appropriate role of scientific evidence, advocacy, economic interests, and politics. Social and behavioral science research can help improve safeguards to provide Americans with access to effective and safe medications.

Roll-out of this drug also will highlight the inequities in access to medical care, insurance coverage, and other supports discussed in this report. Demand for aducanumab will further emphasize inequities in access for people living in rural areas, in socioeconomically disadvantaged circumstances, and in racial/ethnic minority communities, even as relatively few members of these populations participated in the clinical trials assessing the drug's risks and benefits. Out-of-pocket costs are likely to be significant because of high deductible amounts and uncovered services, further disadvantaging lower-income populations. Regardless of the fundamental questions about the drug's efficacy, selective access to such an expensive drug will underscore the harsh inequities in the current system of care.

Although the approval of aducanumab has complicated the dementia landscape, it has not changed the need for a broad research roadmap for the behavioral and social sciences over the next decade to support those living with dementia and caregivers. This report notes promising intervention programs that require additional confirmatory evidence. It describes social and behavioral research that can provide the foundation for the development of programs and policies, as well as ethical safeguards, that would serve the needs of all Americans affected by dementia. And it must

---

[3] Cubanski, J., and Neuman, T. (2021, June 10). FDA's approval of Biogen's new Alzheimer's drug has huge cost implications for Medicare and beneficiaries. Kaiser Family Foundation. https://www.kff.org/medicare/issue-brief/fdas-approval-of-biogens-new-alzheimers-drug-has-huge-cost-implications-for-medicare-and-beneficiaries

be understood that funding for the research agenda proposed in this report may require difficult choices within the federal agencies and others to whom the committee's recommendations are directed.

The committee's objective was to set priorities for research aimed at reducing the negative impacts of dementia, taking into account broad societal and community-level impacts on risk and prevention and on access to care and resources, as well as developments that can improve the quality and delivery of care and improve the lives of persons with dementia and their caregivers. Scrupulous reliance on evidence is the foundation on which society can protect and improve the public health of the nation. It is our hope that by identifying these priorities for social and behavioral science research and making recommendations for how they can be pursued in a coordinated fashion, this report will help produce research that improves the lives of everyone affected by dementia. By 2030, an estimated 8.5 million Americans will have Alzheimer's disease, and many more will have other forms of dementia. If the nation is to ensure that their lives are better than those of people living with dementia in 2021, the time to act is now.

Appendix A

Biographical Sketches of Committee and Advisory Panel Members

COMMITTEE MEMBERS

Tia Powell (*Chair*) is director of the Montefiore Einstein Center for Bioethics, holds the Shoshannah Trachtenberg Frackman chair in medical ethics, and is professor of epidemiology and psychiatry at the Albert Einstein College of Medicine. Powell focuses on bioethics issues related to public policy, dementia, consultation, end-of-life care, the LGBT population, and public health disasters. She served 4 years as executive director of the New York State Task Force on Life and the Law, which functions as New York State's bioethics commission. Powell has worked with the National Academies of Sciences, Engineering, and Medicine on many projects and has also worked with the Centers for Disease Control, New York state and city, and professional organizations on issues related to public health ethics and disasters. She is a member of the American Psychiatric Association ethics committee, and a fellow of the New York Academy of Medicine and the Hastings Center. She is the author of *Dementia Reimagined: Building a Life of Joy and Dignity from Beginning to End*, published by Penguin Random House. Powell received a B.A. from Harvard College and an M.D. from Yale Medical School.

Karen S. Cook (*Vice Chair*) is Ray Lyman Wilbur professor of sociology, director of the Institute for Research in the Social Sciences, and former vice provost for faculty development and diversity at Stanford University. She conducts research on social interaction, social networks, social exchange, and trust. She has served on a number of National Academy of Sciences

(NAS) consensus study committees including on risk, voting, adult education, science communication, and security. She has also served on the NAS Council and is currently chair of Class V. She is also a trustee of the Russell Sage Foundation in New York. Cook was elected to the American Academy of Arts and Sciences in 1996 and to NAS in 2007. In 2004, she received the American Sociological Association Social Psychology Section's Cooley Mead Award for Career Contributions to Social Psychology. Cook received a Ph.D. in sociology from Stanford University.

Margarita Alegría is chief of the Disparities Research Unit at Massachusetts General Hospital and a professor in the departments of medicine and psychiatry at Harvard Medical School. Her research is focused on the improvement of health care services delivery for diverse racial and ethnic populations, conceptual and methodological issues with multicultural populations, and ways to bring the community's perspective into the design and implementation of health services. Alegría is currently the principal investigator of four National Institutes of Health–funded research studies: The Impact of Medicaid Plans on Access to and Quality of Substance Use Disorder (SUD) Treatment, Building Community Capacity for Disability Prevention for Minority Elders, Building Infrastructure for Community Capacity in Accelerating Integrated Care, and Latino Youths Coping with Discrimination: A Multi-Level Investigation in Micro- and Macro-Time. In 2011, she was elected as a member of the National Academy of Medicine in acknowledgment of her scientific contributions to her field. Alegría has also received notable awards, including most recently the 2020 Rema Lapouse Award for Achievement in Epidemiology, Mental Health, and Applied Public Health Statistics by the American Public Health Association. She obtained a B.A. in psychology from Georgetown University in 1978 and a Ph.D. from Temple University in 1989.

Deborah Blacker is a professor of psychiatry at Harvard Medical School and deputy chair and professor in the Department of Epidemiology at the Harvard T.H. Chan School of Public Health (HSPH). She is a geriatric psychiatrist and epidemiologist based at Massachusetts General Hospital, where she directs the Gerontology Research Unit and serves as associate chief for research in the Department of Psychiatry. Blacker's work is focused on the epidemiology, genetics, assessment, and early recognition of Alzheimer's disease. She serves as leader of the Research Education Component and coleader of the Clinical Core for the Massachusetts Alzheimer's Disease Research Center, and as leader of the Analytic Core for the Harvard Aging Brain Study. Blacker is involved in multiple local and national studies regarding Alzheimer's disease genetics and epidemiology, and leads the

AlzRisk project to develop a curated online catalog of studies on the risk factors for Alzheimer's disease. She is also actively involved in teaching and methodological research at HSPH, where she codirects a training program in psychiatric genetics and translational research, and teaches a course on assessment methods in psychiatric research. Blacker served on the Neurocognitive Disorders Workgroup for the *Diagnostic and Statistical Manual of Mental Disorders (DSM-5)* and the American Psychiatric Association's Workgroup to Revise the Practice Guideline for Dementia. She received an M.D. from Harvard Medical School and an Sc.D. in epidemiology from HSPH.

M. Maria Glymour is a professor in the University of California, San Francisco (UCSF) Department of Epidemiology and Biostatistics and currently serves as director for the UCSF Ph.D. program in epidemiology and translational science. She coleads a National Institutes of Health–sponsored training grant on aging and chronic disease, and coleads the Methods for Longitudinal Studies in Dementia initiative to improve research methods related to cognitive aging, Alzheimer's, and dementia. Glymour's research is focused on how social factors experienced across the life course (from infancy to adulthood) influence cognitive function, Alzheimer's disease and related dementias, stroke, and other health outcomes in late life. She is especially interested in how exposures amenable to policy interventions shape health. Another line of her work is focused on strengthening quantitative methods for research on cognitive aging and ADRD. Specific topics have included the geographic patterning of stroke and dementia, the socioeconomic inequalities in healthy aging, the causal effects of education on later-life health, the influence of selection and survival biases in models of cognitive aging, life-course timing of dementia risk factors, and longitudinal modeling of cognitive change and dementia. Prior to joining UCSF, Glymour was an assistant professor at the Harvard School of Public Health. She completed an Sc.D. at the Harvard School of Public Health and postdoctoral training at Columbia University.

Roee Gutman is an associate professor of biostatistics at Brown University. His areas of research interest are Bayesian data analysis, missing data, file linkage, causal inference, matching, and bioinformatics. Gutman has been and continues to be involved in many comparative effectiveness studies, in which he contributes in terms of both statistical theory and its implementation. He brings vast experience in analyzing many types of secondary datasets from various sources (e.g., Medicare claims data, registries, Veteran's Affairs health data), as well as data collected through large pragmatic cluster randomized trials. Gutman received a Ph.D. in statistics from Harvard University.

Mark D. Hayward is a professor of sociology, Centennial Commission professor in the liberal arts, and a faculty research associate of the Population Research Center at the University of Texas at Austin. Recently, he began a collaborative National Institute on Aging–supported project with Eileen Crimmins, examining trends and disparities in the dementia experience of the older U.S. population. At its core, this study is designed to inform our understanding of how education—a crucial Alzheimer's disease risk factor—influences the cognitive health of older Americans. Hayward has served with the National Academies of Sciences, Engineering, and Medicine's Committee on Population. He was chair of The Future Directions for the Demography of Aging: A Workshop and also was a member of the Committee on Accounting for Socioeconomic Status in Medicare Payment Programs. He received a Ph.D. in sociology from Indiana University.

Ruth Katz is senior vice president for public policy at LeadingAge, the nation's largest association representing not-for-profit providers of aging services. She joined LeadingAge in January 2018, after a 27-year career in the Office of the Secretary of the U.S. Department of Health and Human Services (HHS). For the past 20 years, Katz served as the senior career official in the Office of the Assistant Secretary for Planning and Evaluation (ASPE). She is a trusted leader, coalition builder, research translator, and policy influencer, known for leading teams that work on—and seek to be a nexus between—policy analysis and research. At ASPE, Katz led the founding and operation of the National Alzheimer's Project Act Advisory Council, and she led the creation of the first national plan and updates that followed. She also led the convening of the ASPE/National Institutes of Health Research Summit on social science research on Alzheimer's disease and related dementias. Katz was the staff leader for the HHS early implementation work on the Community Living Assistance Services and Supports (CLASS) Act program and led the drafting of the report to repeal CLASS. She oversaw numerous policy research projects on aging, disability, long-term care, and mental health topics, and served on secretarial work groups, including those responding to the opioid crisis. She received an M.Ed. from The George Washington University.

Spero M. Manson (Pembina Chippewa) is a distinguished professor of public health and psychiatry, occupies the Colorado Trust Chair in American Indian Health, and directs the Centers for American Indian & Alaska Native Health in the Colorado School of Public Health at the University of Colorado Anschutz Medical Campus. His programs include 10 national centers, which pursue research, program development, training, and collaboration with 250 Native communities, spanning rural, reservation, urban, and village settings across the country. Manson has acquired $250 million in sponsored research to support this work and published more than 250 articles on the assessment, epidemiology, treatment, and prevention of physical, alcohol, drug, and mental health problems over the developmental life span of Native people. He was elected to the National Academy of Medicine in 2002, and he is widely acknowledged as one of the nation's leading authorities in regard to Indian and Native health. Manson received a Ph.D. in anthropology at the University of Minnesota.

Terrie E. Moffitt is the Nannerl O. Keohane university professor of psychology and neuroscience at Duke University and a professor of social development at King's College London. She studies how genetic and environmental risks together shape the developmental course of problem behaviors. While her initial interest was in antisocial, violent, and criminal behavior, Moffitt now also studies mental health and substance abuse, including how mental health and brain function affect the body's physical health and aging. She is working on testing whether chronic psychiatric disorders and lifelong poor cognitive abilities accelerate the pace of aging. Moffitt codirects the Dunedin Longitudinal Study, which has followed 1,000 people born in 1972 in New Zealand from birth to age 45. She also codirects the Environmental Risk Longitudinal Twin Study, which has followed 1,100 British families with twins born in 1994–1995 from birth to age 24. Moffitt is a trustee of the Nuffield Foundation and a fellow of the Academy of Medical Sciences, the American Society of Criminology, the British Academy, the American Psychopathological Association, Academia Europaea, the American Academy of Political & Social Science, the Association for Psychological Science, and King's College London. She has served with investigative panels for such institutions as the Nuffield Council on Bioethics and the National Academy of Sciences. Moffitt received a Ph.D. in clinical psychology at the University of Southern California.

Vincent Mor is Florence Price Grant professor of community health in the Brown University School of Public Health and a research health scientist at the Providence Veterans Affairs Medical Center. He was on the faculty of the Department of Community Health in the Brown Medical School from 1981 until it became the Department of Health Services, Policy, and Practice in the School of Public Health. Mor was tenured in 1987 and promoted to professor in 1990. He helped found the department's graduate program in 1986 and directed the Center for Gerontology and Health Care Research for 10 years. He served as chair of the Department of Community Health from 1996 to 2010. As chair, he instituted an expansion of the department's graduate programs, growing the doctoral programs in epidemiology and biostatistics, and adding a Ph.D. program in health services research. His work has been continuously funded by the National Institutes of Health since 1984. He has held a MERIT award from the National Institute on Aging (NIA), has been a Robert Wood Johnson health policy investigator, and was awarded the Distinguished Investigator award from AcademyHealth. He currently directs an NIA-funded program project on long-term care services and supports in America. He received a Ph.D. at the Florence Heller School for Advanced Studies in social welfare at Brandeis University.

David B. Reuben is director of the Multicampus Program in Geriatric Medicine and Gerontology and chief of the Division of Geriatrics at the University of California, Los Angeles (UCLA) Center for Health Sciences. He is chair of the Archstone Foundation, professor at the David Geffen School of Medicine at UCLA, and director of the UCLA Alzheimer's and Dementia Care Program. Reuben is past president of the American Geriatrics Society and former board chair of the American Board of Internal Medicine. In 2012, he received one of the first Innovation Challenge awards from the Center for Medicare & Medicaid Innovation to develop a model program for providing comprehensive, coordinated care for patients with Alzheimer's disease and other dementias. In 2014, Reuben was one of three principal investigators to be awarded a grant for a multicenter clinical trial (the STRIDE study) by the Patient-Centered Outcomes Research Institute (PCORI) and the National Institute on Aging (NIA) to reduce serious fall-related injuries; it is the largest grant that PCORI has awarded. In 2018, he was awarded a multisite PCORI- and NIA-funded pragmatic trial to compare the effectiveness of health system–based versus community-based versus usual dementia care. Reuben continues to provide primary care for frail older persons, including making house calls. He received an M.D. from the Emory University School of Medicine.

Roland J. Thorpe Jr. is an associate professor in the Department of Health, Behavior and Society at the John Hopkins University Bloomberg School of Public Health; founding director of the Program for Research in Men's Health in the Hopkins Center for Health Disparities Solutions (HCHDS); deputy director of the HCHDS; and director of the Johns Hopkins Alzheimer's Disease Resource Center for Minority Aging Research. He holds joint appointments in the divisions of geriatric medicine and gerontology and in neurology at the Johns Hopkins University School of Medicine and in the undergraduate program in public health in the Krieger School of Arts & Sciences. Thorpe's research is focused on functional and health status disparities related to race, place, and socioeconomic status across the life course of community-dwelling adults with a focus on African American men. Most of his work has been funded by the National Institute on Aging and the National Institute on Minority Health and Health Disparities. Thorpe has published in various outlets including the *Journal of*

Gerontology: Medical Sciences, *Social Science & Medicine*, the *American Journal of Public Health*, and *Biodemography and Social Biology*. He is a member of the National Committee on Vital and Health Statistics and recently completed a 4-year term on the Advisory Committee on Minority Health at the U.S. Department of Health and Human Services. Thorpe earned an M.S. and a Ph.D. from Purdue University.

Rachel M. Werner is Robert D. Eilers professor, health care management and economics, and is executive director of the Leonard Davis Institute of Health Economics, both at the University of Pennsylvania. She is an internationally recognized expert in health economics and health policy, particularly how provider payment and financial incentives affect the care of older adults. Werner's research has been published in high-impact, peer-reviewed journals, including *Journal of the American Medical Association*, the *New England Journal of Medicine*, and *Health Affairs*. Beyond publication, she has influenced policy as a member of numerous national committees and as an advisor to the federal government on quality measurement and quality improvement incentives. In a particularly policy-relevant study, she found that a five-star rating system has a much greater effect on consumer choice of nursing home than more complicated measures of quality. She is a core investigator with the Veterans Health Administration (VHA) Center for Health Equity Research and Promotion and directed one of four national centers to evaluate the effectiveness of VHA's medical home model. She has received numerous awards for her work, including the Presidential Early Career Award for Scientists and Engineers and Outstanding Investigator Award from the American Federation for Medical Research. She was elected to the National Academy of Medicine in 2018. She received an M.D. and a Ph.D. in health economics from the University of Pennsylvania.

Kristine Yaffe is a professor of psychiatry, neurology, and epidemiology; the Roy and Marie Scola endowed chair and vice chair of research in psychiatry; and the director of the Center for Population Brain Health at the University of California, San Francisco (UCSF). She is an internationally recognized expert in the field of cognitive aging and dementia. As principal investigator of multiple grants from the National Institutes of Health, the U.S. Department of Defense, and several foundations, Yaffe is particularly interested in identifying novel risk factors for cognitive impairment that may lead to strategies for preventing cognitive decline. She has published more than 500 peer-reviewed articles in numerous prestigious journals including *The Lancet*, *The British Medical Journal*, the *Journal of the American Medical Association*, and *The New England Journal of Medicine*. Yaffe served as cochair of the Institute of Medicine's Committee on Cognitive Aging, which released a report in 2015 entitled *Cognitive Aging:*

Progress in Understanding and Opportunities for Action. She is currently a member of the Beeson Scientific Advisory Board and the Global Council on Brain Health and has received several awards for her distinguished scholarly work, including the American Association for Geriatric Psychiatry's Distinguished Scientist Award and the American Academy of Neurology's Potamkin Prize for Alzheimer's Research. Yaffe completed postdoctoral training in epidemiology and geriatric psychiatry at UCSF. She received a B.S. in biology-psychology from Yale University and an M.D. from the University of Pennsylvania.

Julie M. Zissimopoulos is an associate professor in the Sol Price School of Public Policy at the University of Southern California (USC). In addition to her faculty appointment, she serves as director of the Aging and Cognition Research Program and Research Training at the Schaeffer Center for Health Policy and Economics. She is director of USC's Resource Center for Minority Aging Research, and Center for Advancing Sociodemographic and Economic Study of Alzheimer's Disease and Related Dementias, both focused on reducing the burden of Alzheimer's disease and funded by the National Institute on Aging (NIA). Her research applies insights and methods from economics to several health policy areas, such as racial and ethnic disparities in dementia risk and health care and costs of Alzheimer's disease, medical expenditures, caregiving, and financial support between generations of family members. Zissimopoulos currently leads an NIA-funded research project on the use of and response to drug therapies for non-Alzheimer's disease conditions that influence risk of Alzheimer's disease, and racial and ethnic disparities in health care treatment for Alzheimer's disease. Her recently published research appears in numerous publications, including *JAMA Neurology*, the *Journal of Gerontology: Social Sciences*, *Daedalus—Journal of the American Academy of Arts & Science*, and the *Journal of Health Economics*. She received a B.A., summa cum laude, from Boston College; an M.A. from Columbia University; and a Ph.D. in economics from the University of California, Los Angeles.

ADVISORY PANEL TO THE COMMITTEE

Cynthia Huling Hummel recently completed a term of service as a member of the National Advisory Council on Alzheimer's Research, Care, and Services. She has served as a national early-stage advisor for the Alzheimer's Association. She presented at the 2017 and 2019 National Institutes of Health Alzheimer's Research Summits and has given many other talks in her role as an advocate. Huling Hummel is also active on a local level, co-leading a respite care group called "Faithful Friends" and serving on a local committee that plans social programs for those with Alzheimer's disease and related dementias. She is especially interested in Alzheimer's research and enrolled in the Alzheimer's Disease Neuroimaging Initiative study in 2010. A retired pastor, Huling Hummel speaks to faith communities about offering dementia friendly programs and services. She received a B.S. from Rutgers College, an M.Div. from New Brunswick Theological Seminary, and a D.Min. from McCormick Theological Seminary.

Marie Martinez Israelite serves as director of victim services at the Human Trafficking Institute. She previously served as chief of the Victim Assistance Program at Homeland Security Investigations, where she directed policy efforts; program development; and victim services for all federal crime victims, including survivors of human trafficking and child exploitation. Israelite has held several positions within the U.S. Department of Homeland Security and the U.S. Department of Justice related to human trafficking, sexual assault, and domestic violence prevention and services. Most recently, she served as a senior program manager with ICF, where she facilitated the work of the U.S. Advisory Council on Human Trafficking. Her mother, a retired pediatrician, was diagnosed with Alzheimer's disease in 2017, and Israelite shares caregiving responsibilities with her mother's younger sister and her brothers. She received a B.A. from Bucknell University and an M.S.W. from the University of Pennsylvania.

John-Richard (JR) Pagan is a disabled veteran with a background in marriage and family therapy. In 2012, he began a doctorate degree in clinical psychology; 1 year into the program, at age 47, he began to suffer cognitive challenges that interfered with his studies. Although Pagan received a diagnosis that included mild cognitive impairment and sudden-onset adult attention deficit disorder, he was dismissed from the program. At this time, Veterans Affairs medical doctors have only been able to definitively diagnose his condition as a progressive neurodegenerative disease with moderate cognitive impairments in processing, language, and attention, thus meeting the requirements for early-stage dementia with additional symptoms relating to mobility and autonomic dysfunction. Pagan continues to advocate for his own health and the health of others who live with Lewy body dementia and other dementias. He is active in his spiritual and social community, and often describes his immediate family as the most vital part of his ongoing support team.

Edward Patterson was diagnosed with Alzheimer's disease in 2018 at the age of 71. Patterson, who formerly worked in the financial sales industry, states that it was his husband who first started noticing changes in his cognition. The first warning signs were difficulty completing stressful tasks, such as making airline reservations, and episodes of repetition. His husband also noticed that his mood was affected—he seemed to have a short fuse and quick mood swings. Patterson brought up the issue with his doctor, and after receiving an Alzheimer's diagnosis, stayed home and did not talk much to others about what was going on. Eventually, he started looking for information and resources related to Alzheimer's and came across individuals living with the disease speaking publicly about their experience. "Their messages woke me up, and got me going," Patterson says. He "went public" with his diagnosis on Facebook and joined the Florida Gulf Coast chapter of the Alzheimer's Association, where he is involved in advocacy, fundraising, and programming.

Brian Van Buren is an Alzheimer's advocate and public speaker, a board member of the Western Carolina Chapter of the Alzheimer's Association, and an advisory council member for the Dementia Action Alliance. He was diagnosed in 2015 with early-onset Alzheimer's, and he was a caretaker for his mother, who died in January from Alzheimer's. After losing his job as an international flight attendant, Van Buren reimagined himself as an advocate, giving his voice to Alzheimer's. As an African American man, he felt he needed to give a face to the disease, and he seeks to address marginalized and LGBTQ communities. He was featured in a video for AARP's announcement presenting $60 million to fund dementia research.

Geraldine Woolfolk, a retired teacher, has had decades of experience as a caregiver for her father, her mother, and then her husband, who developed early-onset Alzheimer's disease. As an adult education teacher for almost 25 years, she held leadership roles in the development and delivery of programs specifically designed for people with Alzheimer's disease and related dementias (ADRD), as well as for their families. Woolfolk continues to be active with ADRD support groups, forums, and conferences. She provides information, referrals, and presentations for individuals, families, and groups dealing with Alzheimer's disease and she advocates at all levels of government. Woolfolk has lobbied legislators and policy makers for increased funding for ADRD research and caregiver support projects that will enable families to keep their loved ones in the home environment and out of institutional settings for as long as possible. In 2011, Woolfolk was appointed to the first National Alzheimer's Project Act Advisory Council, on which she served for 6 years. She has a B.A. in music and an MPA.

Appendix B

The Paid Health Care Workforce

A detailed examination of issues related to the paid workforce that supports people living with dementia and their families was beyond the scope of this report, but these individuals are critical to the future of dementia care (see Chapter 1). The health care system and the entities that provide direct care to people living with dementia (both in their homes and in residential facilities) employ millions of people, who range from highly trained medical specialists and other clinicians to the individuals who provide assistance with bathing and toileting. Some work exclusively with people living with dementia, but the majority work with other geriatric or disabled patients and clients, and serve the general public as well. Today, the United States is facing moderate to severe shortages of most categories of workers needed to care for people living with dementia, and these shortages are growing.

Over the past two decades, the National Academies of Sciences, Engineering, and Medicine (and, previously, the Institute of Medicine [IOM]) have conducted a series of studies addressing workforce issues, but none have focused specifically on dementia care, and none have directly addressed the direct care force. This appendix draws on several of these reports to highlight recent developments related to dementia care, and provides the research recommendations offered by the 2017 National Research Summit on Dementia Care.

THE PROFESSIONAL WORKFORCE

A 2008 IOM report proposes a three-pronged approach to preparing a workforce to support an aging U.S. population: increasing the recruitment and retention of geriatric specialists and caregivers, enhancing the competence of all individuals in the delivery of health care, and redesigning models of care and broadening provider and patient roles to achieve greater flexibility (IOM, 2008).

The needed dementia experts identified in the first of these prongs include physicians trained and board-certified in neurology, psychiatry, or geriatric medicine who devote a substantial proportion of patient contact time to the evaluation and care of adults with acquired cognitive impairment or dementia (Johnson et al., 2013). At present, there are few of these experts, and their numbers do not even meet current demand. For example, the number of geriatricians in the United States has declined from more than 7,100 in 2008, when the IOM released the above report, to approximately 6,800 currently, including fewer than 1,600 geriatric psychiatrists (American Geriatrics Society; American Board of Medical Specialists, 2020). This shortfall of dementia experts is expected to grow.

Predicted shortages of generalist health care providers needed for the second prong of the IOM approach (enhancing the competence of all individuals in the delivery of health care) are also likely to affect people living with dementia. The Association of American Medical Colleges (2020) predicts that the nation will have between 21,000 and 22,000 fewer primary care physicians than it needs by 2032. Shortages of nurses are already a serious problem across health care settings (National Academies of Sciences, Engineering, and Medicine [NASEM] 2021a). Since 2012, 60,000 registered nurses have left the health care workforce each year (Buerhaus et al., 2017). Nevertheless, the number of nurse practitioners is growing, and there is substantial evidence supporting the effectiveness of their care of persons living with dementia (Auerbach, Buerhaus, and Staiger, 2020; Poghosyan et al., 2021). Moreover, a recent National Academies study of dementia care identified collaborative care, including nurse practitioners, as one of the few evidence-based interventions for dementia care (NASEM, 2021b).

Rural communities are often particularly hard hit by shortages of professional, licensed care providers, leaving older adults with limited access to vital services (IOM, 2008). In 2010, for example, 90 percent of the geriatric workforce was serving urban areas (Lester et al., 2020; Hintenach et al., 2019). Compounding these shortages is the fact that older adults living in rural areas are at higher risk for developing dementia (Weise et al., 2014).

Substantial efforts have been made to increase the expertise of all health care providers. In 2015, the Health Resources and Services Administration's (HRSA's) Geriatrics Workforce Enhancement Program (GWEP) provided $35.7 million to 44 academic medical centers in the United States with the goal of transforming geriatric education and training. The central focus of the program is on integrating geriatrics into primary care through education and training. Special emphasis has been placed on collaborating with community partners to address gaps in health care for older adults and to promote individual-, system-, and population-level changes. Thirty-eight of the first 44 awardees created training programs in Alzheimer's disease and related dementias to educate families; caregivers; direct care workers; and health professions students, faculty, and providers. In 2019, HRSA funded its second cohort of 48 GWEP programs across 35 states and 2 territories (Guam and Puerto Rico), and provided extension grants to 15 former GWEP awardees. All GWEP awardees are educating and training the workforce on how to care for persons living with dementia. Of the $35.7 million GWEP budget, $8.7 million was for dementia education and training activities. In academic year 2018–2019 (latest available data), GWEP grants provided 445 courses and trainings in Alzheimer's disease and related dementias for 73,115 health care providers and 24,434 caregivers (Office of the Assistant Secretary for Planning and Evaluation, 2020).

The effectiveness of such training on the care received by persons with dementia remains unknown. Similarly, the supply of specialists in hospice and palliative medicine is already insufficient to provide treatment for everyone with an advanced illness, and limited knowledge of basic palliative care among nonspecialists has led to deficiencies with respect to end-of-life care (IOM, 2015). The 2015 IOM report *Dying in America: Improving Quality and Honoring Individual Preferences Near the End of Life* suggests enhancing the curricula for medical schools, increasing interprofessional collaboration, and building communications skills in graduate and undergraduate education to better prepare physicians, nurses, and other professional health care workers to meet patients' basic palliative care needs, suggestions that mirror similar findings regarding health care delivery for older adults described below (IOM, 2015). The 2015 National Academies' report *Improving Diagnosis in Health Care* also recommends that greater emphasis on teamwork and education be an essential component of education and training around the diagnostic process (NASEM, 2015).

Finally, there has been substantial progress on the third prong of the IOM approach, redesigning models of care and broadening provider and patient roles to achieve greater flexibility. These models hold the potential for more efficient and effective use of the limited workforce. Examples of such models of care are provided in Chapter 6. Yet to date, these models have seen limited spread, largely because of the lack of payment structures that adequately cover the costs of providing services (Lees et al., 2020).

THE DIRECT CARE WORKFORCE

The direct care dementia workforce, comprising certified nursing assistants (CNAs), home health aides, and personal care aides, provides care primarily in nursing homes, home care, and community settings. They represent the most numerous paid dementia providers and make up nearly one-third of the overall U.S. health care workforce (Warshaw and Bragg, 2014; Osterman, 2017). More than 4 million CNAs, home health aides, and personal care aides provided long-term services and supports in 2017, and by 2024 this workforce will grow to 5.2 million (Espinoza, 2017). These workers "hold in their hands the quality of care and quality of life of individuals with dementia" (Gilster et al., 2018).

The jobs performed by direct care workers may entail high levels of physical and emotional stress—for example, requiring workers to lift and clean persons who may resist assistance or respond with fear and aggression. Because people living with dementia often need 24-hour care, many of these workers have demanding schedules. Yet their salaries are typically low, and many such jobs come with limited or no benefits. Indeed, direct care providers were exempt from federal minimum wage and overtime standards for many years, until that ruling was set aside in 2017. Now, they are generally entitled to minimum wage and other protections long enjoyed by fast food workers, but many still lack health benefits and paid time off, a problem highlighted during the COVID-19 pandemic. Many work full time yet still must rely on food stamps and other government programs to support their families (PHI, 2018).

Direct care workers are disproportionately women and members of minority groups, and approximately one-quarter to one-third are recent immigrants (PHI, 2018; IOM, 2008). Immigrants who serve as health care workers may not be fluent English speakers and may lack knowledge of U.S. work culture and laws. Those who are undocumented face additional challenges, and race and gender discrimination have affected many workers in this field (Espinoza, 2017; Hartmann and Hayes, 2017). Studies of this population indicate that foreign-born home care workers face the worst gender pay gaps, are disproportionately poor, and are often subject to abuse and exploitation (Gould et al., 2016; Zallman et al., 2019; Green and Ayalon, 2018). Recent immigrants frequently need training to qualify for jobs, as well as support in navigating legal frameworks for entry, work, and long-term legal status (Hartmann and Hayes, 2017). The diversity of the direct care workforce also presents challenges to providing culturally sensitive care, as the person living with dementia and the direct care worker frequently do not share the same cultural background.

Pay for this workforce varies by location and the tightness of the job market, but in 2019, the median annual income for home health aides was $25,280 ($12.10 per hour) and for CNAs was $29,640 ($14.25 per hour) (BLS, 2020). Two in five home care workers report working part time (less than 35 hours per week) (PHI, 2018). Many direct care workers are employed by multiple companies and/or are paid under the table

(Campbell, 2018). Turnover rates among direct care workers range from 40 percent to more than 100 percent (Glister et al., 2018).

States have two routes for regulating the quality of the direct care workforce—through regulations imposed on facilities that employ the workers and through the certification of categories of workers (Burke and Orlowski, 2015). However, many workers are employed in settings other than residential facilities, especially private homes, or have not obtained the certifications that require training in dementia care. Moreover, states vary significantly in what they require for job categories related to dementia care. For example, there are three states that require training for administering medication, providing assistance with feeding, and providing respite care, respectively, but there is no overlap among these three states (Burke and Orlowski, 2015). One reason for the variation may be lack of consensus on definitions of the elements of quality caregiving and competencies that care providers need to have (Weiss et al., 2017).

RECOMMENDATIONS OF THE 2017 NATIONAL RESEARCH SUMMIT ON DEMENTIA CARE

The task force established after the 2017 National Research Summit on Dementia Care to address the goals of improving the quality of care and services for persons living with dementia has offered recommendations for research to address gaps in education and training in four areas (Weiss et al., 2020):

1. recruitment and retention of a dementia-capable workforce,
2. financing and cost of workforce education and training,
3. interprofessional education and training for care coordination and management of dementia care, and
4. translation and implementation of effective dementia care.

For each of these areas, the task force offers more detailed research objectives.

The 2020 National Research Summit on Care, Services, and Supports for Persons with Dementia and Their Caregivers also addressed workforce issues and identified several specific gaps and opportunities for further research, including the following (National Institute on Aging, 2020):

2.4 Develop and evaluate training for direct care workers to identify specific competencies and modalities that best contribute to improved health, quality of life, and financial and social outcomes for PLWD [persons living with dementia], their care partners, and the direct care workers themselves.

2.5 Analyze the impact of heterogeneity among PLWD and the direct care worker and clinician workforce (paid and unpaid) and develop and test approaches that promote cultural awareness and respect, cultural competence, and communication skills.

2.6 Determine the relative effectiveness and efficiency of interprofessional workforce models in providing high-quality care to PLWD, and how to support workforce collaboration across home, community, and residential settings.

2.7 Analyze the interactions between care partners, direct care workers, and clinicians, in relation to technologies designed for the care of PLWD; determine how technological change will affect future workforce needs, and design and evaluate effective education and training for care partners, direct care workers, and clinicians to use new technologies effectively.

3.2 Determine the core competencies, domains, and quality metrics needed to ensure that medical care for PLWD is consistent with evidence-based clinical standards.

REFERENCES

American Board of Medical Specialists. (2020). *AMBS Board Certification Report*. https://www.abms.org/wp-content/uploads/2020/11/ABMS-Board-Certification-Report-2019-2020.pdf

American Geriatrics Society. (n.d.). *Geriatrics Workforce by the Numbers*. https://www.americangeriatrics.org/geriatrics-profession/about-geriatrics/geriatrics-workforce-numbers

Association of American Medical Colleges. (2020). *The Complexities of Physician Supply and Demand: Projections from 2018 to 2033*. https://www.aamc.org/media/45976/download

Auerbach, D.I., Buerhaus, P.I., and Staiger, D.O. (2020). Implications of the rapid growth of the nurse practitioner workforce in the US. *Health Affairs*, 39(2). https://doi.org/10.1377/hlthaff.2019.00686

Buerhaus, P., Auerbach, D., and Staiger, D. (2017). How should we prepare for the wave of retiring baby boomer nurses? *Health Affairs Blog*. https://doi.org/10.1377/hblog20170503.059894

Bureau of Labor Statistics, U.S. Department of Labor, Occupational Outlook Handbook, Nursing Assistants and Orderlies. https://www.bls.gov/ooh/healthcare/nursing-assistants.htm

Burke, G., and Orlowski, G. (2015). Paper 3: A review of dementia training standards across professional licensure. In *Training to Serve People with Dementia: Is our Health Care System Ready?* Justice in Aging. https://www.justiceinaging.org/wp-content/uploads/2015/08/Training-to-serve-people-with-dementia-Alz3_FINAL.pdf

Campbell, S. (2018). *U.S. Home Care Workers: Key Facts*. PHI. https://phinational.org/resource/u-s-home-care-workers-key-facts-2018

Espinoza, R. (2017). *Immigrants and the Direct Care Workforce*. PHI. https://phinational.org/wp-content/uploads/2017/06/immigrants_and_the_direct_care_workforce_-_phi_-_june_2017.pdf

Gilster, S., Boltz, M., and Dalessandro, J. (2018). Long-term care workforce issues: Practice principles for quality dementia care. *Gerontologist*, 58(Suppl_1), S103–S113. https://doi.org/10.1093/geront/gnx174

Gould, E., Schieder, J., and Geier, K. (2016). *What is the Gender Pay Gap and Is It Real?* Economic Policy Institute. https://www.epi.org/publication/what-is-the-gender-pay-gap-and-is-it-real

Green, O., and Ayalon, L. (2018). Violations of workers' rights and exposure to work-related abuse of live-in migrant and live-out local home care workers—A preliminary study: Implications for health policy and practice. *Israel Journal of Health Policy Research*, 7(1). 10.1186/s13584-018-0224-1

Hartmann, H., and Hayes, J. (2017). The growing need for home care workers: Improving a low-paid, female-dominated occupation and the conditions of its immigrant workers. *Public Policy and Aging Report*, 27(3), 88–95. https://doi.org/10.1093/ppar/prx017

Hintenach, A., Raphael, O., and Hung, W. (2019). Training programs on geriatrics in rural areas: A review. *Current Geriatrics Reports*, 8, 117–122. https://doi.org/10.1007/s13670-019-0283-3

Howes, C. (2004). Upgrading California's health care workforce: The impact of political action and unionization. In *The State of California Labor* (pp. 71–105). University of California. https://escholarship.org/uc/item/1h28v106

IOM (Institute of Medicine). (2008). *Retooling for an Aging America: Building the Health Care Workforce*. Washington, DC: The National Academies Press. https://doi.org/10.17226/12089

———. (2015). *Dying in America: Improving Quality and Honoring Individual Preferences Near the End of Life*. Washington, DC: The National Academies Press. https://doi.org/10.17226/18748

Johnson, K.A., Minoshima, S., Bohnen, N.I., Donohoe, K.J., Foster, N.L., Herscovitch, P., Karlawish, J.H., Rowe, C.C., Hedrick, S., Pappas, V., Carrillo, M.C., Hartley, D.M., and Amyloid Imaging Task Force of the Alzheimer's Association and Society for Nuclear Medicine and Molecular Imaging. (2013). Update on appropriate use criteria for amyloid PET imaging: Dementia experts, mild cognitive impairment, and education. Amyloid Imaging Task Force of the Alzheimer's Association and Society for Nuclear Medicine and Molecular Imaging. *Alzheimer's & Dementia*, 9(4), e106-9. https://doi.org/10.1016/j.jalz.2013.06.001

Lees Haggerty, K., Epstein-Lubow, G., Spragens, L.H., Stoeckle, R.J., Evertson, L.C., Jennings, L.A., and Reuben, D.B. (2020). Recommendations to improve payment policies for comprehensive dementia care. *Journal of the American Geriatrics Society*, 68(11), 2478–2485. https://doi.org/10.1111/jgs.16807

Lester, P., Dharmarajan, T.S., and Weinstein, E. (2020). The looming geriatrician shortage: Ramifications and solutions. *Journal of Aging and Health*, 32(9), 1052–1062. https://doi.org/10.1177/0898264319879325

NASEM (National Academies of Sciences, Engineering, and Medicine). (2015). *Improving Diagnosis in Health Care*. Washington, DC: The National Academies Press. https://doi.org/10.17226/21794

———. (2021a). *The Future of Nursing 2020-2030: Charting a Path to Achieve Health Equity*. Washington, DC: The National Academies Press. https://doi.org/10.17226/25982

———. (2021b). *Living with Dementia and Their Care Partners and Caregivers: A Way Forward*. Washington, DC: The National Academies Press. https://doi.org/10.17226/26026

National Institute on Aging. (2020). *National Research Summit on Care, Services, and Supports for Persons Living with Dementia and Their Caregivers*. National Institutes of Health. https://www.nia.nih.gov/sites/default/files/2021-01/DementiaCareSummitReport.pdf

Office of the Assistant Secretary for Planning and Evaluation. (2020). *National Plan to Address Alzheimer's Disease: 2020 Update. Strategy 2.A: Build a Workforce with the Skills to Provide High-Quality Care.* https://aspe.hhs.gov/report/national-plan-address-alzheimers-disease-2020-update/strategy-2a-build-workforce-skills-provide-high-quality-care

Osterman, P. (2017). *Who Will Care for Us? Long-Term Care and the Long-Term Workforce.* New York: Russell Sage Foundation. https://doi.org/10.7758/9781610448673

PHI (2018). U.S. home care workers: Key facts. https://phinational.org/wp-content/uploads/2018/08/U.S.-Home-Care-Workers-2018-PHI.pdf

Poghosyan, L., Brooks, J., Hovsepian, V., Pollifrone, M., Schlak, A., and Sadak, T. (2021). The growing primary care nurse practitioner workforce: A solution for the aging population living with dementia. *American Journal of Geriatric Psychiatry, 29*(6), 517–526. https://doi.org/10.1016/j.jagp.2021.01.135

Warshaw, G., and Bragg, E. (2014). Preparing the health care workforce to care for adults with Alzheimer's disease and related dementias. *Health Affairs, 33*(4). https://doi.org/10.1377/hlthaff.2013.1232

Wiese, L.K., Williams, C.L., Tappen, R.M. (2014). Analysis of barriers to cognitive screening in rural populations in the United States, advances in nursing science, *37(4)*, 327-339 doi: 10.1097/ANS.0000000000000049

Weiss, J., Tumosa, N., Perweiler, E., Bailey, D., Blackwell, E., Forceia, M.A., Miles, T., Tebb, S., Trudeau, S., and Worstell, M. (2017). *Workforce Gaps in Dementia Education and Training: Stakeholder Group Paper.* Research Summit on Dementia Care. https://aspe.hhs.gov/system/files/pdf/257826/WorkforceGaps.pdf

Weiss, J., Tumosa, N., Perweiler, E., Forciea, M.A., Miles, T., Blackwell, E., Tebb, S., Bailey, D., Trudeau, S., and Worstell. (2020). Critical workforce gaps in dementia education and training. *Journal of the American Geriatrics Society, 68*(3), 625–629. 10.1111/jgs.16341

Zallman, L., Finnegan, K., Himmelstein, D., Touw, S., and Woolhandler, S. (2019). Care for America's elderly and disabled people relies on immigrant labor. *Health Affairs, 38*(6). https://doi.org/10.1377/hlthaff.2018.05514

Appendix C

Synthesis of Reviews of Nonpharmacologic Interventions

Author	Method	Dates of Studies Reviewed	Population	No. of Studies Included	Included Study Designs
Cotelli et al., 2019	Systematic review	2005–2016	Persons living with mild cognitive impairment, Alzheimer's disease, or frontotemporal dementia	5	Randomized controlled trial
Tay et al., 2019	Systematic review	1998–2017	Persons living with dementia	11	• Quasi-experimental • Randomized controlled trial
Lim et al., 2019	Systematic review	2009–2017	Persons in the early stages of dementia or mild cognitive impairment	9	• Nonrandomized controlled trial • Nonrandomized prospective study • Randomized controlled trial
Bahar-Fuchs et al., 2019	Systematic review and meta-analysis	1988–2018	Persons living with mild to moderate dementia	33 (32 included in meta-analysis)	Randomized controlled trial

Types of Interventions	Outcomes Examined for Persons Living with Dementia	Key Findings
Cognitive telerehabilitation	Cognitive ability	• Overall, studies were of low quality. • Telerehabilitation may be comparable to face-to-face cognitive rehabilitation.
Cognitive-behavioral therapy	• Anxiety • Depression	• Preliminary evidence indicates cognitive-behavioral therapy is effective at reducing anxiety and depressive symptoms among persons with dementia. • More rigorous trials are need.
Tai chi	• Short-term cognitive function • Global cognitive functions • Working memory and executive function • Verbal learning and memory • Self-perception of memory • Attention and concentration • Semantic memory • Visuospatial skills	Tai chi has the potential to improve short-term cognitive function in the early stages of dementia.
Cognitive training	• Global cognition • Clinical disease severity • Delayed memory ability • Capacity to perform activities of daily living • Mood and well-being of participant • Mood and well-being of informant/caregiver • Participant/treatment burden (retention rates)	• Moderate-quality evidence indicates cognitive training relative to control, but not alternative treatment, is associated with small to moderate effects on global cognition and verbal semantic fluency. • Medium- to long-term follow-up evidence of cognitive training is low.

Continued

Author	Method	Dates of Studies Reviewed	Population	No. of Studies Included	Included Study Designs
Yen and Lin, 2018	Systematic review	2004–2010	Older adults living with and without dementia	16	• Nonexperimental studies • Qualitative studies • Randomized controlled trial
van der Steen et al., 2018	Systematic review and meta-analysis	1993–2016	Persons living with dementia	22 (21 included in meta-analysis)	Randomized controlled trial
van den Berg et al., 2018	Systematic review	1991–2017	Persons living with dementia	17	• Case reports • Chart review • Prospective cohort
Spencer et al., 2018	Systematic review	2009	Persons living with dementia	1	Cluster randomized controlled study
Russell-Williams et al., 2018	Review	2010–2016	Persons living with dementia, mild cognitive impairment, or subjective cognitive decline	10	• Randomized controlled trial • Quasi-experimental

APPENDIX C

Types of Interventions	Outcomes Examined for Persons Living with Dementia	Key Findings
Reminiscence therapy	• Daily functioning • Cognition • Depression • Mood status • Self-esteem • Life satisfaction	• Findings were not separated for populations with and without dementia. • Reminiscence therapy is associated with improved quality of life and depressive symptoms among older adults.
Music therapy	• Emotional well-being (quality of life and positive affect) • Mood and affect • Behaviors • Cognition	• Low-quality evidence indicates music-based interventions may improve emotional well-being and quality of life and reduce anxiety. • Moderate-quality evidence indicates music-based interventions reduce depressive symptoms and overall behaviors, but there is no effect on agitation/aggression. • Low-quality evidence indicates music-based interventions have no effect on cognition. • Conclusions could not be drawn regarding the effect of music-based interventions on social behavior or outcomes at long-term follow-up.
Electroconvulsive therapy	Agitation and aggression	Clinical improvements were observed in most of the studies, but the lack of randomized controlled trials limits inference.
De-escalation techniques for managing aggression	• Aggression • Behaviors	A single study with high risk of bias found no difference in change in overall behavior.
Meditation: – Mindfulness – Kirtan kriya meditation – Mindfulness-based Alzheimer's stimulation	• Stress • Cognition • Quality of life	• Medication may result in improvements in stress, cognition, and quality of life. • More rigorous studies are needed.

Continued

Author	Method	Dates of Studies Reviewed	Population	No. of Studies Included	Included Study Designs
Peluso et al., 2018	Review	1995–2016	Persons living with dementia and/or psychiatric disorders	16	• Nonrandomized clinical trial • Randomized controlled trial
Oltra-Cucarella et al., 2018	Systematic review and meta-analysis	1993–2016	Persons living with Alzheimer's disease or mixed dementias	33	• Nonrandomized clinical trial • Randomized controlled trial
Mohler et al., 2018	Systematic review and meta-analysis	2000–2015	Persons living with dementia	8 (7 included in meta-analysis)	• Controlled clinical trial • Randomized controlled trial
Lorusso and Bosch, 2018	Systematic review	2001–2014	Persons living with dementia	12	• Quasi-experimental • Randomized controlled trial
Liang et al., 2018	Systematic review and network meta-analysis	2004–2016	Persons living with Alzheimer's disease or mild cognitive impairment	17	Randomized controlled trial
Hu et al., 2018	Systematic review and meta-analysis	1999–2016	Persons living with cognitive impairment, including dementia and mild cognitive impairment	10	• Quasi-experimental • Randomized controlled trial

APPENDIX C

Types of Interventions	Outcomes Examined for Persons Living with Dementia	Key Findings
Animal-assisted therapy	• Cognition • Behavior • Depression • Physical function • Quality of life • Social function	Preliminary evidence from studies of low quality indicates that in persons with dementia, animal-assisted therapy may decrease problem behaviors and improve quality of life and social skills.
Cognition-focused interventions: – Cognitive rehabilitation – Cognitive training – Cognitive stimulation	• Cognition • Attention • Memory • Naming • Executive functioning • Physical functioning	Cognition-focused interventions have limited effects on cognition or function compared with non–cognition focused interventions.
Tailored activities	• Behavior • Quality of life • Affect • Mood • Cost	• For persons with dementia living in long-term care facilities, low-quality evidence indicates tailored activities may marginally improve behaviors. • Evidence was inconclusive for quality of life, affect, and mood-related outcomes.
Multisensory environments	• Behavior • Mood	• Multisensory interventions may reduce behaviors and have a positive impact on mood. • Long-term effects are mixed, and rigorous studies are needed.
• Physical exercise • Music therapy • Computerized cognitive training • Nutrition therapy	• Cognitive functioning • Behavior	• For persons with mild to moderate dementia, physical exercise may improve cognition. • For persons with mild to moderate dementia, computerized cognitive training may improve behavior.
Animal-assisted intervention	• Behaviors • Daily living activities • Cognition • Quality of life	• For persons with cognitive impairment, animal-assisted interventions may reduce problem behaviors. • For persons with cognitive impairment, animal-assisted interventions may have no effect on daily activities, cognition, or quality of life.

Continued

Author	Method	Dates of Studies Reviewed	Population	No. of Studies Included	Included Study Designs
Herke et al., 2018	Systematic review	1986–2015	Persons living with dementia	9	Randomized controlled trial
Fusar-Poli et al., 2018	Systematic review and meta-analysis	2009–2014	Persons living with dementia	6	Randomized controlled trial
Frederiksen et al., 2018	Systematic review	2006–2017	Persons living with no cognitive impairment (6 studies) Individuals with subjective memory complaints, mild cognitive impairment, or Alzheimer's disease (2 studies)	8	Randomized controlled trial
Duan et al., 2018	Systematic review and network meta-analysis	2006–2016	Persons living with dementia	10	Randomized controlled trial

APPENDIX C

Types of Interventions	Outcomes Examined for Persons Living with Dementia	Key Findings
Environmental or behavior modifications for food and fluid intake	• Food and fluid intake • Nutritional status • Secondary outcomes: mealtime behavior, global and specific cognitive function, daily function, quality of life	Conclusions could not be made due to heterogeneity in interventions and poor study design.
Music therapy	• Cognition • Attention • Executive function • Learning and memory • Language • Motor skills	• Overall music therapy had no effect on all outcomes. • A secondary analysis found that active music therapy had a positive effect on global cognition.
Physical exercise	• Hippocampal volume • Biomarkers: cerebrospinal fluid, amyloid-B, tau	For persons with dementia, two small studies found physical exercise had no effect on biomarker outcomes.
• Home-based exercise • Group exercise • Walking program • Reminiscence therapy • Art therapy • Psychosocial interventions + acetylcholinesterase inhibitor • Cognitive stimulation + acetylcholinesterase inhibitor (continued)	• Cognition • Compliance	• Psychosocial interventions including walking, home/group exercise, reminiscence therapy, and art therapy are more effective than usual care on measures of cognition. • Nonpharmacologic intervention + acetylcholinesterase inhibitor is more effective than acetylcholinesterase inhibitor alone on measures of cognition. • Compliance was greater for persons in walking and home-based exercise interventions compared with those in group exercise and art therapy interventions.

Continued

Author	Method	Dates of Studies Reviewed	Population	No. of Studies Included	Included Study Designs
Duan et al., 2018 (continued)					
Deshmukh et al., 2018	Systematic review	2006–2011	Persons living with dementia	2	Randomized controlled trial
Theleritis et al., 2018	Systematic review	1998–2016	Persons living with dementia	43	• Quasi-experimental study • Randomized controlled trial
Wu et al., 2017	Systematic review and meta-analysis	2005–2015	Persons living with dementia	11	• Quasi-experimental studies • Randomized controlled trial
Wood et al., 2017	Systematic mapping review	2001–2015	Persons living with dementia	10	• Quasi-experimental studies • Randomized controlled trial

APPENDIX C 303

Types of Interventions	Outcomes Examined for Persons Living with Dementia	Key Findings
• Mindfulness-based Alzheimer's stimulation + acetylcholinesterase inhibitor • Progressive muscle relaxation + acetylcholinesterase inhibitor • Cognitive training + acetylcholinesterase inhibitor		
Art therapy	• Cognition • Depression • Quality of life	Evidence is insufficient to draw conclusions regarding the effect of art therapy on outcomes.
Nonpharmacologic: – Staff training – Multisensory – Walking – Emotion-oriented care – Individualized activity – Reminiscence therapy – Music – Art therapy – Cognitive therapy	Apathy	• Most studies do not include apathy as a primary outcome measure. • Nonpharmacologic treatment for apathy is safe and may be effective, but overall, more rigorous studies are needed.
• Massage • Touch therapy	Behaviors	Low-quality evidence is insufficient to draw conclusions.
Animal-assisted therapies incorporating dogs	Quality of life	• For persons with dementia residing in long-term care facilities, animal-assisted therapy may improve quality of life. • More rigorous studies are needed.

Continued

Author	Method	Dates of Studies Reviewed	Population	No. of Studies Included	Included Study Designs
Theleritis et al., 2017	Systematic review and meta-analysis	2004–2016	Persons living with Alzheimer's disease	22	• Quasi-experimental studies • Randomized controlled trial
Streater et al., 2017	Systematic and scoping review	1982–2013	Persons living with dementia	7	• Quasi-experimental studies • Randomized controlled trial

Types of Interventions	Outcomes Examined for Persons Living with Dementia	Key Findings
Nonpharmacologic: – Cognitive training (group sessions) – Reminiscence therapy (group sessions) – Individualized cognitive rehabilitation program (individual sessions) – Biography-orientated mobilization – Music and art therapy – Nursing home staff education program – Multisensory – Cognitive stimulation, physical activity, and socialization – Activities	Apathy	• Most studies do not include apathy as a primary outcome measure. • Heterogeneity of studies and poor study designs limit inferences, but several nonpharmacologic interventions are effective in reducing apathy.
Crisis management: – Psychiatry service – Outreach support – Crisis resolution home treatment team – Mental and behavioral health – Individualized care plan	• Hospitalizations • Institutionalization • Quality of life • Cognition • Activities of daily living • Mortality • Use of medication • Patient/caregiver satisfaction	• The overall effectiveness of crisis management on key outcomes is inconclusive. • More rigorous studies are needed.

Continued

Author	Method	Dates of Studies Reviewed	Population	No. of Studies Included	Included Study Designs
Smallfield and Heckenlaible, 2017	Systematic review	2006–2014	Persons living with Alzheimer's disease and related neurocognitive disorders	52	• Quasi-experimental studies • Randomized controlled trial
Lewis et al., 2017	Systematic review	2008–2015	Persons living with cognitive impairment	7 (6 included in meta-analysis)	Randomized controlled trial
Karssemeijer et al., 2017	Systematic review and meta-analysis	2008–2017	Persons living with mild cognitive impairment or dementia	10	Randomized controlled trial
Karkou and Meekums, 2017	Systematic review	N/A	Persons living with dementia	0	Randomized controlled trial

Types of Interventions	Outcomes Examined for Persons Living with Dementia	Key Findings
Interventions to maintain self-care and leisure: – Occupation-based – Sleep – Cognitive – Physical exercise – Multicomponent interventions	• Physical functioning • Sleep • Leisure • Social engagement	• For persons with dementia, evidence is strong for the effect of occupation-based interventions and cognitive interventions on maintaining functional performance. • Evidence is strong for physical exercise for improving sleep and physical function.
Supervised home- or community-based exercise programs longer than 3 months	• Function (basic and instrumental activities of daily living) • Falls • Hospital readmission	• For older adults with cognitive impairment, long-term exercise programs improved functional independence compared with usual care. • Two randomized trials suggest long-term exercise programs may reduce falls.
Combined cognitive–physical interventions	• Cognitive function • Activities of daily living • Mood	• For persons with dementia, there is a small to medium positive effect of combined cognitive–physical interventions on global cognitive function compared with usual care. • There is a moderate to large positive effect of combined cognitive–physical interventions on activities of daily living. • There is a small to medium positive effect of combined cognitive–physical interventions on mood.
Dance movement therapy	• Behavior • Social interaction	No studies met the inclusion criteria.

Continued

Author	Method	Dates of Studies Reviewed	Population	No. of Studies Included	Included Study Designs
Ijaopo, 2017	Systematic review	2008–2017	Persons living with dementia	10	• Randomized controlled trial (7) • Reviews (3)
Garrido et al., 2017	Critical synthesis	2006–2016	Persons living with dementia	28	• Nonrandomized clinical trial • Randomized controlled trial
Dimitriou and Tsolaki, 2017	Systematic review	1998–2013	Persons living with dementia	11	Randomized controlled trial
Anderson et al., 2017	Systematic review	2008–2015	Persons living with dementia	7	Randomized controlled trial
Abraha et al., 2017	Systematic review	1997–2007	Persons living with dementia	3	• Quasi-randomized controlled trial • Randomized controlled trial
Charry-Sanchez et al., 2018	Systematic review	2000–2017	Persons living with dementia, depression, and other conditions	23 (8 on dementia)	• Quasi-experimental • Randomized controlled trial

APPENDIX C

Types of Interventions	Outcomes Examined for Persons Living with Dementia	Key Findings
• Therapeutic touch • Tailored activity program • Lavender oil • Music therapy • Electroconvulsive therapy • Acupressure • Reviews of various nonpharmacologic strategies	• Agitation • Behavior	Evidence is limited on the effect of nonpharmacologic interventions on reducing severe agitation.
Prerecorded music alone or in combination with other musical activities	Behaviors	For persons with dementia, prerecorded music can be effective in reducing behavioral symptoms, including agitation.
Sensory stimulation interventions: – Massage – Acupuncture – Bright light	Sleep disturbances	Bright light therapy may help reduce sleeping problems compared with usual care.
Complementary and alternative medicine: – Reflexology – Aromatherapy – Therapeutic touch – Foot massage – Aromatherapy and hand massage – Aromatherapy with donepezil	• Behavior • Pain	Complementary and alternative medicine may reduce behavioral symptoms compared with control conditions.
Simulated presence therapy (audio or video recording)	• Behaviors • Quality of life	Low quality evidence indicates the effects of simulated presence on behavioral outcomes is uncertain.
Animal-assisted therapies	• Cognition • Behavior • Mood • Physical function	For persons living with dementia, animal–assisted therapy shows promise in short-term management of behaviors, but study designs limit inferences.

Continued

Author	Method	Dates of Studies Reviewed	Population	No. of Studies Included	Included Study Designs
Chiu et al., 2018	Systematic review and meta-analysis	1981–2016	Persons living with dementia	11	Randomized controlled trial
Creighton et al., 2013	Systematic review	1989–2012	Persons living with dementia	34	• Quasi-experimental • Randomized controlled trial
Fakhoury et al., 2017	Literature review	2000–2015	Persons living with dementia	6	Randomized controlled trial
Fleiner et al., 2017	Systematic review	1994–2009	Persons living with dementia	5	• Quasi-experiential • Randomized controlled trial
Folkerts et al., 2017	Systematic review and meta-analysis	1981–2016	Persons living with dementia	27 (15 included in meta-analysis)	• Quasi-experiential • Randomized controlled trial
Garcia-Casal et al., 2017	Systematic review and meta-analysis	2003–2014	Persons living with dementia	12	• Quasi-experiential • Randomized controlled trial

Types of Interventions	Outcomes Examined for Persons Living with Dementia	Key Findings
Reality orientation therapy alone or combined with reminiscence therapy or cognitive training	• Cognition • Behavior • Depressive symptoms	• Reality orientation is associated with a moderate effect on cognitive function. • Intervention has no effect on behavior or depressive symptoms.
Spaced retrieval: – Name–face associations – Object–name associations – Cue–behavior associations – Mixed goals/ other	• Recall • Behavior	Spaced-retrieval interventions are viable and may be effective in improving recall and reducing problem behaviors, but more rigorous study designs are needed.
Music therapy	Behavior	Findings across studies are mixed.
Short-term structured exercise	Behavior	Structured exercise may reduce problem behaviors. Larger and more rigorous study designs are needed.
Cognitive intervention: – Reminiscence therapy – Cognitive training – Cognitive rehabilitation – Cognitive stimulation – Multimodal interventions	• Cognition • Global scales for dementia symptoms • Quality of life • Behavior • Mood • Physical function	• Cognitive interventions moderately improve global cognition, autobiographical memory, and behaviors. • Cognitive interventions are associated with small improvements in quality of life.
Computer-based cognitive training: – Cognitive recreation – Cognitive rehabilitation – Cognitive stimulation – Cognitive training	Cognition	• Computer-based cognitive training is associated with moderate improvements in cognition and anxiety. • Computer-based cognitive training is associated with a small reduction in depression. • Computer-based cognitive training is associated with no effect on activities of daily living.

Continued

Author	Method	Dates of Studies Reviewed	Population	No. of Studies Included	Included Study Designs
Jutkowitz et al., 2016	Systematic review and meta-analysis	1999–2014	Persons living with dementia	19	Randomized controlled trial
Klimova et al., 2017	Literature review	2010–2014	Persons living with dementia	6	• Quasi-experiential • Randomized controlled trial
Woods et al., 2018	Systematic review and meta-analysis	1987–2016	Persons with dementia	22 (16 included in meta-analysis)	Randomized controlled trial
Levy et al., 2017	Systematic review	1995–2015	Older adults	40 (39 on dementia)	• Quasi-experiential • Randomized controlled trial

Types of Interventions	Outcomes Examined for Persons Living with Dementia	Key Findings
Care-delivery interventions: – Dementia care mapping – Person centered care – Clinical protocols – Emotion-oriented care – Staff education	• Agitation • Aggression • Behaviors • Psychotropic use • Depression	Evidence was insufficient to draw conclusions on the effect of care-delivery interventions on agitation/aggression or problem behaviors.
Dancing therapy	Any outcomes	Limited data suggest dancing therapy may positively impact cognition, physical function, and mood.
Reminiscence therapy	• Quality of life • Communication • Depression • Cognition	Heterogeneity of study designs makes inferences challenging, but overall, effects are small and inconsistent.
Complementary and alternative medicine: – Acupressure – Aromatherapy – Massage – Therapeutic touch – Reflexology – Natural products – Japanese medicine – Osteopathy – Healing touch	• Agitation • Delirium	• Complementary and alternative medicine had a small effect on reducing agitation. • Conclusions could not be drawn regarding the effect of complementary and alternative medicine on delirium.

Continued

Author	Method	Dates of Studies Reviewed	Population	No. of Studies Included	Included Study Designs
Morrin et al., 2018	Systematic review	1995–2017	Persons living with Lewy body dementia	15	Quasi-experiential
Nyman et al., 2018	Systematic review	2003–2015	Persons living with dementia	9 (reported in 19 articles)	Randomized controlled trial
O'Caoimh et al., 2019	Systematic review and meta-analysis	1992–2018	Persons living with mild cognitive impairment or dementia	48	• Quasi-experiential • Randomized controlled trial
Zhang et al., 2017	Systematic review and meta-analysis	1987–2016	Persons living with dementia	34	• Controlled clinical trial • Randomized controlled trial

SOURCE: Adapted from Gaugler et al., 2020. [commissioned paper]

Types of Interventions	Outcomes Examined for Persons Living with Dementia	Key Findings
Nonpharmacologic interventions: – Deep brain stimulation – Transcranial direct current stimulation – Exercise – Electro-convulsive therapy – Repetitive transcranial magnetic stimulation	• Cognition • Physical function • Quality of life • Behavior • Mood	• Evidence for the effect of nonpharmacologic interventions for persons with Lewy body dementia is inconclusive. • More rigorous study designs are needed.
Behavior change (e.g., goal setting, social support, credible source) to promote physical activity	• Participation in physical activity • Physical activity • Adherence	• Some behavior change strategies are associated with increased participation in physical activity. • More rigorous study designs are needed.
Nonpharmacologic interventions: – Light therapy – Multimodal – Transcutaneous electrical nerve stimulation – Exercise – Acupressure/acupuncture – Cognitive-behavioral therapy	• Sleep • Cognition • Mood • Behavior • Quality of life	• Nonpharmacologic interventions may significantly improve sleep efficiency outcomes compared with control conditions, but overall, evidence is insufficient. • More rigorous study designs are needed.
Music therapy	• Behavior • Cognitive function • Depression • Anxiety • Quality of life	• Music therapy compared with inactive control condition associated with reductions in behaviors and anxiety. • The effect of music therapy on cognitive function, depression, and quality of life is unclear.

REFERENCES

Abraha, I., Rimland, J.M., Lozano-Montoya, I., Dell'Aquila, G., Velez-Diaz-Pallares, M., Trotta, F.M., Cruz-Jentoft, A.J., and Cherubini, A. (2017). Simulated presence therapy for dementia. *Cochrane Database of Systematic Reviews*, 4, Cd011882. https://doi.org/10.1002/14651858.CD011882.pub2

Anderson, A.R., Deng, J., Anthony, R.S., Atalla, S.A., and Monroe, T.B. (2017). Using complementary and alternative medicine to treat pain and agitation in dementia: A review of randomized controlled trials from long-term care with potential use in critical care. *Critical Care Nursing Clinics of North America*, 29(4), 519–537. https://doi.org/10.1016/j.cnc.2017.08.010

Bahar-Fuchs, A., Martyr, A., Goh, A.M., Sabates, J., and Clare, L. (2019). Cognitive training for people with mild to moderate dementia. *Cochrane Database of Systematic Reviews*, 3, CD013069. https://doi.org/10.1002/14651858.CD013069.pub2

Charry-Sanchez, J.D., Pradilla, I., and Talero-Gutierrez, C. (2018). Animal-assisted therapy in adults: A systematic review. *Complementary Therapies in Clinical Practice*, 32, 169–180. https://doi.org/10.1016/j.ctcp.2018.06.011

Chiu, H.Y., Chen, P.Y., Chen, Y.T., and Huang, H.C. (2018). Reality orientation therapy benefits cognition in older people with dementia: A meta-analysis. *International Journal of Nursing Studies*, 86, 20–28. https://doi.org/10.1016/j.ijnurstu.2018.06.008

Cotelli, M., Manenti, R., Brambilla, M., Gobbi, E., Ferrari, C., Binetti, G., and Cappa, S.F. (2019). Cognitive telerehabilitation in mild cognitive impairment, Alzheimer's disease and frontotemporal dementia: A systematic review. *Journal of Telemedicine and Telecare*, 25(2), 67–79. https://doi.org/10.1177/1357633x17740390

Creighton, A.S., van der Ploeg, E.S., and O'Connor, D.W. (2013). A literature review of spaced retrieval interventions: A direct memory intervention for people with dementia. *International Psychogeriatrics*, 25(11), 1743–1763. https://doi.org/10.1017/s1041610213001233

Deshmukh, S.R., Holmes, J., and Cardno, A. (2018). Art therapy for people with dementia. *Cochrane Database of Systematic Reviews*, 9, Cd011073. https://doi.org/10.1002/14651858.CD011073.pub2

Dimitriou, T.D., and Tsolaki, M. (2017). Evaluation of the efficacy of randomized controlled trials of sensory stimulation interventions for sleeping disturbances in patients with dementia: A systematic review. *Clinical Interventions in Aging*, 12, 543–548. https://doi.org/10.2147/cia.s115397

Duan, Y., Lu, L., Chen, J., Wu, C., Liang, J., Zheng, Y., Wu, J., Rong, P., and Tang, C. (2018). Psychosocial interventions for Alzheimer's disease cognitive symptoms: A Bayesian network meta-analysis. *BMC Geriatrics*, 18(1), 175. https://doi.org/10.1186/s12877-018-0864-6

Fakhoury, N., Wilhelm, N., Sobota, K. F., and Kroustos, K. R. (2017). Impact of music therapy on dementia behaviors: A literature review. *The Consultant Pharmacist*, 32(10), 623–628. https://doi.org/10.4140/TCP.n.2017.623

Fleiner, T., Leucht, S., Forstl, H., Zijlstra, W., and Haussermann, P. (2017). Effects of short-term exercise interventions on behavioral and psychological symptoms in patients with dementia: A systematic review. *Journal of Alzheimers Disease*, 55(4), 1583–1594. https://doi.org/10.3233/jad-160683

Folkerts, A.K., Roheger, M., Franklin, J., Middelstadt, J., and Kalbe, E. (2017). Cognitive interventions in patients with dementia living in long-term care facilities: Systematic review and meta-analysis. *Archives of Gerontology and Geriatrics*, 73, 204–221. https://doi.org/10.1016/j.archger.2017.07.017

Frederiksen, K.S., Gjerum, L., Waldemar, G., and Hasselbalch, S.G. (2018). Effects of physical exercise on Alzheimer's disease biomarkers: A systematic review of intervention studies. *Journal of Alzheimer's Disease*, 61(1), 359–372. https://doi.org/10.3233/jad-170567

Fusar-Poli, L., Bieleninik, L., Brondino, N., Chen, X.J., and Gold, C. (2018). The effect of music therapy on cognitive functions in patients with dementia: A systematic review and meta-analysis. *Aging & Mental Health*, 22(9), 1097–1106. https://doi.org/10.1080/13607863.2017.1348474

Garcia-Casal, J.A., Loizeau, A., Csipke, E., Franco-Martin, M., Perea-Bartolome, M.V., and Orrell, M. (2017). Computer-based cognitive interventions for people living with dementia: A systematic literature review and meta-analysis. *Aging & Mental Health*, 21(5), 454-467. https://doi.org/10.1080/13607863.2015.1132677

Garrido, S., Dunne, L., Chang, E., Perez, J., Stevens, C.J., and Haertsch, M. (2017). The use of music playlists for people with dementia: A critical synthesis. *Journal of Alzheimers Disease*, 60(3), 1129–1142. https://doi.org/10.3233/jad-170612

Gaugler, J., Jutkowitz, E., and Gitlin, L.N. (2020). *Non-Pharmacological Interventions for Persons Living with Alzheimer's Disease: Decadal Review and Recommendations.* Paper prepared for the National Academies of Sciences, Engineering, and Medicine's Committee on Decadal Survey of Behavioral and Social Science Research on Alzheimer's Disease and Alzheimer's Disease-Related Dementias. https://www.nationalacademies.org/event/10-17-2019/meeting-2-decadal-survey-of-behavioral-and-social-science-research-on-alzheimers-disease-and-alzheimers-disease-related-dementias

Herke, M., Fink, A., Langer, G., Wustmann, T., Watzke, S., Hanff, A. M., and Burckhardt, M. (2018). Environmental and behavioural modifications for improving food and fluid intake in people with dementia. *Cochrane Database of Systematic Reviews*, 7, Cd011542. https://doi.org/10.1002/14651858.CD011542.pub2

Hu, M., Zhang, P., Leng, M., Li, C., and Chen, L. (2018). Animal-assisted intervention for individuals with cognitive impairment: A meta-analysis of randomized controlled trials and quasi-randomized controlled trials. *Psychiatry Research*, 260, 418–427. https://doi.org/10.1016/j.psychres.2017.12.016

Ijaopo, E.O. (2017). Dementia-related agitation: A review of non-pharmacological interventions and analysis of risks and benefits of pharmacotherapy. *Translational Psychiatry*, 7(10), e1250. https://doi.org/10.1038/tp.2017.199

Jutkowitz, E., Brasure, M., Fuchs, E., Shippee, T., Kane, R.A., Fink, H.A., Butler, M., Sylvanus, T., and Kane, R.L. (2016). Care-delivery interventions to manage agitation and aggression in dementia nursing home and assisted living residents: A systematic review and meta-analysis. *Journal of the American Geriatrics Society*, 64(3), 477–488. https://doi.org/10.1111/jgs.13936

Karkou, V., and Meekums, B. (2017). Dance movement therapy for dementia. *Cochrane Database of Systematic Reviews*, 2, Cd011022. https://doi.org/10.1002/14651858.CD011022.pub2

Karssemeijer, E.G.A., Aaronson, J.A., Bossers, W.J., Smits, T., Olde Rikkert, M.G.M., and Kessels, R.P.C. (2017). Positive effects of combined cognitive and physical exercise training on cognitive function in older adults with mild cognitive impairment or dementia: A meta-analysis. *Ageing Research and Reviews*, 40, 75–83. https://doi.org/10.1016/j.arr.2017.09.003

Klimova, B., Valis, M., and Kuca, K. (2017). Dancing as an intervention tool for people with dementia: A mini-review dancing and dementia. *Current Alzheimer Research*, 14(12), 1264–1269. https://doi.org/10.2174/1567205014666170713161422

Levy, I., Attias, S., Ben-Arye, E., Bloch, B., and Schiff, E. (2017). Complementary medicine for treatment of agitation and delirium in older persons: A systematic review and narrative synthesis. *International Journal of Geriatric Psychiatry*, 32(5), 492–508. https://doi.org/10.1002/gps.4685

Lewis, M., Peiris, C.L., and Shields, N. (2017). Long-term home and community-based exercise programs improve function in community-dwelling older people with cognitive impairment: A systematic review. *Journal of Physiotherapy*, 63(1), 23–29. https://doi.org/10.1016/j.jphys.2016.11.005

Liang, J.H., Xu, Y., Lin, L., Jia, R.X., Zhang, H.B., and Hang, L. (2018). Comparison of multiple interventions for older adults with Alzheimer disease or mild cognitive impairment: A PRISMA-compliant network meta-analysis. *Medicine*, 97(20), e10744. https://doi.org/10.1097/md.0000000000010744

Lim, K.H., Pysklywec, A., Plante, M., and Demers, L. (2019). The effectiveness of Tai Chi for short-term cognitive function improvement in the early stages of dementia in the elderly: A systematic literature review. *Clinical Interventions in Aging*, 14, 827–839. https://doi.org/10.2147/cia.s202055

Lorusso, L.N., and Bosch, S.J. (2018). Impact of multisensory environments on behavior for people with dementia: A systematic literature review. *The Gerontologist*, 58(3), e168–e179. https://doi.org/10.1093/geront/gnw168

Mohler, R., Renom, A., Renom, H., and Meyer, G. (2018). Personally tailored activities for improving psychosocial outcomes for people with dementia in long-term care. *Cochrane Database of Systematic Reviews*, 2, Cd009812. https://doi.org/10.1002/14651858.CD009812.pub2

Morrin, H., Fang, T., Servant, D., Aarsland, D., and Rajkumar, A.P. (2018). Systematic review of the efficacy of non-pharmacological interventions in people with Lewy body dementia. *International Psychogeriatrics*, 30(3), 395–407. https://doi.org/10.1017/s1041610217002010

Nyman, S.R., Adamczewska, N., and Howlett, N. (2018). Systematic review of behaviour change techniques to promote participation in physical activity among people with dementia. *British Journal of Health Psychology*, 23(1), 148–170. https://doi.org/10.1111/bjhp.12279

O'Caoimh, R., Mannion, H., Sezgin, D., O'Donovan, M.R., Liew, A., and Molloy, D.W. (2019). Non-pharmacological treatments for sleep disturbance in mild cognitive impairment and dementia: A systematic review and meta-analysis. *Maturitas*, 127, 82–94. https://doi.org/10.1016/j.maturitas.2019.06.007

Oltra-Cucarella, J., Ferrer-Cascales, R., Clare, L., Morris, S.B., Espert, R., Tirapu, J., and Sanchez-SanSegundo, M. (2018). Differential effects of cognition-focused interventions for people with Alzheimer's disease: A meta-analysis. *Neuropsychology*, 32(6), 664–679. https://doi.org/10.1037/neu0000449

Peluso, S., De Rosa, A., De Lucia, N., Antenora, A., Illario, M., Esposito, M., and De Michele, G. (2018). Animal-Assisted therapy in elderly patients: Evidence and controversies in dementia and psychiatric disorders and future perspectives in other neurological diseases. *Journal of Geriatric Psychiatry and Neurology*, 31(3), 149–157. https://doi.org/10.1177/0891988718774634

Russell-Williams, J., Jaroudi, W., Perich, T., Hoscheidt, S., El Haj, M., and Moustafa, A.A. (2018). Mindfulness and meditation: Treating cognitive impairment and reducing stress in dementia. *Reviews in the Neurosciences*, 29(7), 791–804. https://doi.org/10.1515/revneuro-2017-0066

Smallfield, S., and Heckenlaible, C. (2017). Effectiveness of occupational therapy interventions to enhance occupational performance for adults with Alzheimer's disease and related major neurocognitive disorders: A systematic review. *American Journal of Occupational Therapy*, *71*(5), 7105180010p–7105180010p. https://doi.org/10.5014/ajot.2017.024752

Spencer, S., Johnson, P., and Smith, I.C. (2018). De-escalation techniques for managing non-psychosis induced aggression in adults. *Cochrane Database of Systematic Reviews*, *7*, Cd012034. https://doi.org/10.1002/14651858.CD012034.pub2

Streater, A., Coleston-Shields, D.M., Yates, J., Stanyon, M., and Orrell, M. (2017). A scoping review of crisis teams managing dementia in older people. *Clinical Interventions in Aging*, *12*, 1589–1603. https://doi.org/10.2147/cia.s142341

Tay, K.W., Subramaniam, P., and Oei, T.P. (2019). Cognitive behavioural therapy can be effective in treating anxiety and depression in persons with dementia: A systematic review. *Psychogeriatrics*, *19*(3), 264–275. https://doi.org/10.1111/psyg.12391

Theleritis, C., Siarkos, K., Katirtzoglou, E., and Politis, A. (2017). Pharmacological and non-pharmacological treatment for apathy in Alzheimer disease: A systematic review across modalities. *Journal of Geriatric Psychiatry and Neurology*, *30*(1), 26–49. https://doi.org/10.1177/0891988716678684

Theleritis, C., Siarkos, K., Politis, A.A., Katirtzoglou, E., and Politis, A. (2018). A systematic review of non-pharmacological treatments for apathy in dementia. *International Journal of Geriatric Psychiatry*, *33*(2), e177–e192. https://doi.org/10.1002/gps.4783

van den Berg, J.F., Kruithof, H.C., Kok, R.M., Verwijk, E., and Spaans, H.P. (2018). Electroconvulsive therapy for agitation and aggression in dementia: A systematic review. *American Journal of Geriatric Psychiatry*, *26*(4), 419–434. https://doi.org/10.1016/j.jagp.2017.09.023

van der Steen, J.T., Smaling, H.J., van der Wouden, J.C., Bruinsma, M.S., Scholten, R.J., and Vink, A.C. (2018). Music-based therapeutic interventions for people with dementia. *Cochrane Database of Systematic Reviews*, *7*, Cd003477. https://doi.org/10.1002/14651858.CD003477.pub4

Wood, W., Fields, B., Rose, M., and McLure, M. (2017). Animal-assisted therapies and dementia: A systematic mapping review using the Lived Environment Life Quality (LELQ) Model. *American Journal of Occupational Therapy*, *71*(5), 7105190030p–7105190030p. https://doi.org/10.5014/ajot.2017.027219

Woods, B., O'Philbin, L., Farrell, E., Spector, A., and Orrell, M. (2018). Reminiscence therapy for dementia. *Cochrane Database Systematic Review*, *3*(3), CD001120. https://doi.org/10.1002/14651858.CD001120.pub3

Wu, J., Wang, Y., and Wang, Z. (2017). The effectiveness of massage and touch on behavioural and psychological symptoms of dementia: A quantitative systematic review and meta-analysis. *Journal of Advanced Nursing*, *73*(10), 2283–2295. https://doi.org/10.1111/jan.13311

Yen, H.Y., and Lin, L.J. (2018). A systematic review of reminiscence therapy for older adults in Taiwan. *Journal of Nursing Research*, *26*(2), 138–150. https://doi.org/10.1097/jnr.0000000000000233

Zhang, Y., Cai, J., An, L., Hui, F., Ren, T., Ma, H., and Zhao, Q. (2017). Does music therapy enhance behavioral and cognitive function in elderly dementia patients? A systematic review and meta-analysis. *Ageing Research Reviews*, *35*, 1–11. https://doi.org/10.1016/j.arr.2016.12.003

Appendix D

Complete Research Agenda

This appendix contains the complete text of the committee's conclusions, research directions, and recommendation, by chapter.

CHAPTER 2: PREVENTION AND PROTECTIVE FACTORS

CONCLUSION 2-1: For health care and public health professionals to take advantage of modifiable factors to prevent Alzheimer's disease and related dementias or reduce or delay their symptoms, research is needed in six broad areas:
1. The causal effects of social factors on the incidence and rate of progression of dementia, including factors from multiple domains (socioeconomic resources, social network, structural drivers of exposure); at multiple levels (individual, family, and community); and at multiple life-course periods (e.g., childhood, early to mid-adulthood, old age).
2. The effects of health-related behaviors and their management over the life course.
3. Modifiable drivers of racial/ethnic inequality in dementia incidence, as well as other dimensions of inequality (e.g., geography).
4. The mechanisms through which socioeconomic factors influence brain health, including physiologic changes, behavioral mechanisms, and medical care pathways.
5. Detailed understanding of identified risk factors to support more precise recommendations to individuals about decision making and inform population-level policies for altering social contexts,

modifying the environment, or changing social policies/systems to promote brain health.
6. Effective means of communicating the magnitude and degree of potential risk and protective factors to support informed decision making.

TABLE 2-1 Detailed Research Needs

1 and 2: Causal Effects of Social Factors and Health-Related Behaviors Over the Life Course	• Identification of causal social and behavioral risk factors versus those that are attributable to noncausal structures; understanding of the influence of confounding reverse causation and selection bias on apparent associations between established risk factors and dementia
• Identification of specific dimensions of complex social exposures or behaviors that are relevant to dementia risk, such as aspects of education (e.g., attainment, quality, context), social support (instrumental, emotional, informational), or physical activity (aerobic vs. strength, duration, intensity), as well as of when in the life span they must be modified to have an effect
• Studies of the extent to which the influence of socioeconomic resources or behaviors is dependent on context and capacity to utilize a resource
• Research to improve understanding of how dementia develops across the life span and at what age the first behavioral or other manifestations emerge
• Identification of study designs that can be used to evaluate alternative possible explanations for observational associations
• Identification of the mediators/mechanisms linking social factors and dementia risk, in particular, mechanisms that might be modified
• Where feasible, use of randomized controlled trial (RCT) methodology in the study of behavior change and follow-up for dementia and related outcomes, ensuring that the methodology is sufficiently powered such that it involves large sample sizes, longitudinal interventions, and extended follow-up periods necessary to examine cognitive decline
3: Inequality in Dementia	• Research on how interlocking systems of structural racism create disparities in dementia risk
• Study of how the risk factors evaluated in typical research samples operate differentially in underrepresented groups
• Examination of sources of resilience that reduce risk in individuals exposed to disproportionate, racially stratified risk factors

TABLE 2-1 Continued

3: Inequality in Dementia (continued)	• Exploration of the effects of individual, interpersonal discrimination on dementia risk and the mechanisms through which those effects may occur • Assessment of how promising interventions to delay or prevent dementia may affect disparities • Monitoring trends and progress in reducing disparities in dementia incidence, care, and outcomes
4: Mechanisms Through Which Socioeconomic Factors Operate	• Study of the physiologic changes, behavioral patterns, social resources, and medical care mechanisms underlying connections between socioeconomic factors and dementia risk
5: Interventions Involving Changes in Policies, Systems, or Individual Behaviors	• Development and improvement of interventions to modify identified risk factors and reduce both the overall population incidence of dementia and disparities in its incidence and outcomes • Identification of critical elements of preventive factors that can be translated into policy interventions • Exploration of ways to redesign structural and environmental elements that shape the behavioral patterns of individuals (e.g., to improve access to exercise and healthy food) • Identification of the opportunity costs of proposed interventions
6: Effective Means of Communicating About Risk and Protective Factors	• Research on the tailoring of communication about the quality of evidence regarding suspected risk factors to different communities to help individuals make informed decisions

CHAPTER 3: IMPROVING OUTCOMES FOR INDIVIDUALS LIVING WITH DEMENTIA

CONCLUSION 3-1: Research in the following areas related to diagnosis and decision-making support has the potential to substantively improve the experience of individuals living with dementia by supporting their dignity and well-being:
- Improved screening and diagnosis to identify persons living with dementia, including guidance for clinicians that also addresses issues related to disclosure.
- Development of guidance to support ethical and responsible decision making by and for people living with dementia.

TABLE 3-3 Detailed Research Needs: Diagnosis and Decision-Making Support

1: Improved Screening and Diagnosis	• Social science research addressing the use of biomarkers, including accuracy in unselected populations, clinical utility, and the positive and negative implications of disclosure to patients and families. • Studies of screening, including the comparative effectiveness of different approaches; evidence-based guidance on whom and when to screen; and improved accuracy of screening approaches, particularly for minority and less-educated populations. • Improved coordination of resources for patients once diagnosed, including medical care, information, social supports, and community resources. • Public education strategies to heighten awareness of impaired cognition and the need for diagnostic evaluation. • Evaluation of dementia education programs for health care providers.
2: Support for Ethical and Responsible Decision Making	• Development and evaluation of approaches to including persons with dementia in conversations about their preferences and care, and guidance for adapting communication as the severity of disease increases. • Improved guidance on balancing the goals of autonomy and safety for the person living with dementia and others who could be harmed, as well as training for clinicians and others in applying this guidance. • Improved education for families about the types of decisions affected by dementia. • Improved methods (e.g., shorter, less expensive, more accurate) for assessing capacity for various types of decision making. • Improved guidance for advance care planning for health care, financial management, housing, and other nonmedical choices. • Improved methods for predicting disease progression and survival, including digital markers.

CONCLUSION 3-2: Research in the following areas has the potential to advance the development of interventions to support the well-being and quality of life of people living with dementia:
- Development and validation of outcome measures that reflect the perspectives of people living with dementia, their family caregivers, and communities.
- Improved design and evaluation of nonpharmacologic interventions to slow or prevent cognitive and functional decline, reduce or ameliorate behavioral and psychological symptoms, improve comfort and well-being, and adequately and equitably serve diverse populations.

TABLE 3-4 Detailed Research Needs: Support for Well-Being and Quality of Life

1: Development and Validation of Outcome Measures	• Identification of outcomes of interest that apply across contexts (e.g., health care system, community, residential care) to support alignment of research. • Development and validation of person-centered and caregiver-centered outcome measures and outcomes that reflect positive aspects of dementia and dementia care. • Leveraging of existing data sources, such as claims data. • Identification and development of outcomes that effectively capture well-being and health-related quality of life across all stages of disease and symptomatology. • Development of outcome measures that can be communicated by persons living with dementia when they have capacity and by family caregivers or other proxies when they no longer have capacity.
2: Improved Design and Evaluation of Nonpharmacologic Interventions	• Clinical and pragmatic trials to test the efficacy and effectiveness of promising but unproven nonpharmacologic interventions. • Research on methods of dissemination and adaptation of interventions to varied contexts and populations.

CHAPTER 4: CAREGIVERS: DIVERSITY IN DEMOGRAPHICS, CAPACITIES, AND NEEDS

CONCLUSION 4-1: Research in the following four areas has the potential to substantially improve the experience of family caregivers:
1. Identification of the highest-priority needs for resources and support for family caregivers, particularly assessment of how caregivers' needs vary across race, ethnicity, and community.
2. Means of identifying the assets that family caregivers bring to their work, as well as their needs for supplemental skills and training and other resources to enhance their capacity to provide care while maintaining the safety and well-being of both the recipients of their care and themselves.
3. Continued development and evaluation of innovations to support and enhance family caregiving and address the practical and logistical challenges involved.
4. Continued progress in data collection and research methods.

TABLE 4-2 Detailed Research Needs

1: Meeting Highest-Priority Needs	• Improved description of family caregivers, with attention to the heterogeneity and disparities within the group, including such caregiver characteristics as age, ethnicity, education, skills, wealth, social capital, and geographic location, as well as to future projections of available caregivers, long-distance caregivers, and culturally diverse caregivers. • Improved understanding of the number and distribution of people living with dementia who do not have family caregivers, and ways to identify their unmet needs and design appropriate interventions. • Improved understanding of the changing needs of caregivers throughout the stages of dementia and the life course of caregivers. • Assessment of caregivers who balance multiple caring roles and the effects of the stress they experience. • Ways to identify the caregivers in greatest need and provide them with adequate support. • Expansion of the concept and measurement of caregiver needs to incorporate stresses associated with medical and nursing tasks and navigation of a complex landscape of long-term care supports and services. • Training for physicians, nurses, direct care providers, and other team members in identifying caregiver stresses and providing information about relevant resources to assist them. • Examination of systemic barriers to communication between providers and caregivers and navigation of the health care system. • Assessment of practices and experiences related to dementia diagnosis and care, including questions about caregiver access to the electronic health record and provider responsibility for identifying needs and impairments.
2: Caregiver Screening and Assessment	• Identification of caregiver strengths and deficits across different populations and development of supports that are culturally relevant. • Examination of the connections between caregiver education and training and access to resources and outcomes for patients. • Design of an evaluation of effective, accessible educational materials for caregivers. • Research into technological approaches to assessment and training, including web-based education, use of smartphones, etc. Improved access to Internet-based resources is essential to address the "digital divide." • Improved understanding of family dynamics and networks, family functioning and well-being, division of labor, and role definitions and their links to better outcomes.

TABLE 4-2 Continued

3: Intervention Development and Evaluation	• Assessment of the efficacy of interventions for caregivers who vary by age, ethnicity, education, skills, wealth, social capital, and geography, as well as ways to integrate them routinely into care plans. • Study of the alignment of interventions with identified unmet needs of people living with dementia and caregivers, including housing options, transportation, social connection/isolation, money management, and protection from financial abuse. • Improved understanding of care coordination, reduction of poorly managed care transitions, and identification of appropriate placements. • Development and evaluation of strategies for fostering supportive contact between family caregivers and nursing home residents. • Development and improvement of technological interventions to support people living with dementia and their caregivers in ways that limit privacy intrusions while enhancing freedom and safety, including computer and smartphone applications, as well as physical devices that assist with such high-stress caring activities as toileting and bathing. • Development and evaluation of interventions for persons with dementia living alone and/or without family or friend caregivers.
4: Data Collection and Research Methods	• Development of methods for collecting actionable and relevant context- and setting-specific data on the challenges faced by caregivers and the related stresses. • Improved study designs to facilitate adaptation beyond the research setting. • Implementation studies for improved understanding of how to scale up effective interventions from research settings to the real world. • Improved measurement of objective (physiological) outcomes and their relationship to subjective measures.

CHAPTER 5: THE ROLE OF THE COMMUNITY

CONCLUSION 5-1: Research in four areas is needed to facilitate the development of communities that are well equipped to support people living with dementia and their caregivers and families, allowing those with dementia to live independently for as long as possible and mitigating the negative effects of past and current socioeconomic and environmental stressors:

1. **Systematic analysis of the characteristics of communities that influence the risk of developing dementia and the experience of living**

with the disease, with particular attention to the sources of disparities in dementia incidence and disease trajectory.
2. Collection of data to document the opportunities and resources available in communities both historically and currently and evaluation of their impact, with particular attention to disparities in population groups' access to resources and including development of the infrastructure needed for data collection.
3. Analysis of the community characteristics needed to foster dementia friendly environments, including assessment of alternative community models that foster dementia friendly environments in communities that have different constellations of resources and serve diverse populations.
4. Evaluation of innovative approaches to adapting housing, services, and supports so that persons with dementia can remain in the community and out of institutional care.

TABLE 5-1 Detailed Research Needs

1: Community Characteristics That Affect Dementia Risk	• How race/ethnicity, gender, socioeconomic status, urban/rural residence, structural racism, and segregated neighborhoods may influence the development and trajectory of dementia throughout the life span • The impact of exposure to neighborhood-level social and environmental stressors on the health and quality of life of individuals living with dementia • Evidence-based evaluations of structural interventions and policies designed to improve care and quality of life for people with dementia and caregivers, that is, interventions focused not on changing the behaviors of individuals but on the structures that shape behavioral change
2: Opportunities and Resources	• Development of systematic means of assessing local needs and challenges and identifying gaps that are not well addressed by existing services and supports • Development of a community needs assessment to identify the effects of resources available in the community, such as religious institutions, adult day centers, or residential care facilities, on addressing the needs of individuals living with dementia and their caregivers • Identification of policies that can coordinate federal and state funding efforts to develop effective community supports • Identification of strategies for mobilizing community health and social welfare networks to address dementia disparities for traditionally underserved groups • Development of refined evaluation methods and indicators of effectiveness for interventions aimed at improving accessibility, availability, acceptability, affordability, adequacy, and awareness of services

TABLE 5-1 Continued

2: Opportunities and Resources (continued)	• Interventions to reduce exposure to such community stressors as environmental pollution, crime, and neighborhood disorder • Development/refinement of means of monitoring the accessibility and quality of services and supports for accountability purposes • Identification of models and infrastructures for testing hypotheses about the relationships among interconnected community organizations addressing the needs of individuals living with dementia and their caregivers
3: Characteristics of Dementia Friendly Communities	• Identification of community and cultural values that affect how individuals perceive dementia and of best practices among cultural groups for providing educational materials about dementia and community-based dementia care services • Analysis of emerging data to understand community agencies and analyze utilization of services on the local and national levels, focusing in particular on disparities • Refinement of reliable means of measuring the outcomes that community-level policies are designed to foster • Development of improved means of supporting collaboration among and facilitating the development of local organizations and resources • Analysis of structures and approaches for fostering collaboration among and the development of local organizations and resources
4: Innovative Approaches	• Evaluation of innovative housing arrangements • Pilot testing to determine how effective programs can be taken to large scale • Development of new types of modeling approaches for understanding how community factors operate as part of a system to influence dementia risk and the lived experience of dementia

CHAPTER 6: HEALTH CARE, LONG-TERM CARE, AND END-OF-LIFE CARE

CONCLUSION 6-1: Research in the following areas has the potential to substantially strengthen the quality and structure of the health care provided to people living with dementia:
- **Documentation of the diagnosis and care management received by persons living with dementia from their primary care providers.**
- **Clarification of disease trajectories to help health systems plan care for persons living with dementia.**
- **Identification of effective methods for providing dementia-related services (e.g., screening and detection, diagnosis, care management and planning, transition management) for individuals living with dementia throughout the disease trajectory.**

- Development and evaluation of standardized systems of coordinated care for comprehensively managing multiple comorbidities for persons with dementia.
- Identification of effective approaches for integrating care services across health care delivery and community-based organizations.

TABLE 6-1 Detailed Research Needs

1: Documentation of Care Received from Primary Care Providers	• Documentation of existing practices and experiences of diagnosis and subsequent care management; how those practices and experiences are associated with stages of disease and symptom progression, and how they vary across type of dementia as well as racial, ethnic, and socioeconomic groups and geography • Assessment of the effectiveness of patient and caregiver support and management systems embedded in health care systems, and system capacity for mounting comprehensive, multifaceted interventions • Assessment of the effectiveness of population health management systems designed to identify and care for persons living with dementia and their caregivers as implemented by health plans and accountable care organizations • Identification of care gaps and unmet needs of persons living with dementia and caregiver support • Identification of gaps in current standardized systems of coordinated care, including management of multiple comorbidities • Identification of effective care practices that can be disseminated
2: Clarification of Disease Trajectories	• Observational studies examining how persons with dementia progress clinically and in their use of services, including behavioral health care, long-term care, and end-of life care, and how these trajectories vary across type of dementia; racial, ethnic, and socioeconomic groups; and geography, as well as among those with comorbidities
3: Identification of Effective Methods for Providing Dementia Care Services	• Studies that optimize how screening is conducted and results are communicated • Studies of the impact of strategies for integrating dementia-focused interventions into the workflow of primary care practices • Clinical trials to test the effectiveness of promising strategies for providing persons living with dementia with diagnostic and longitudinal care for all their health care needs, including care for behavioral problems and comorbid conditions, in various settings

TABLE 6-1 Continued

3: Identification of Effective Methods for Providing Dementia Care Services (continued)	• Studies of the impact of advance care planning at all stages of dementia and assessment of preferences, including patients' preferences regarding palliative, hospice, and end-of-life care • Development and evaluation of systems for comprehensive care at the population level, including study of the use of existing and emerging models
4 and 5: Standardized Systems of Coordinated Care and Integrated Care Services	• Studies of the application of principles of design, implementation, and diffusion that integrate science and engineering (e.g., agile management) to promote dissemination of care innovations for people living with dementia • Studies of the application of network science tools and processes in the dissemination of innovations • Investigation of strategies for disseminating evidence-based models of dementia care in rural areas and demographically diverse populations • Development and evaluation of comprehensive care models that span health care and community-based organizations • Studies of the use of electronic health record systems for integration across platforms and providers, including caregivers, to promote more efficient transactions between care facilities and community-based partners and track the effects of interventions • Creation and evaluation of innovative financing structures that support persons with dementia and caregivers receiving both health care and social services

CONCLUSION 6-2: Research in the following areas has the potential to substantially strengthen the quality and structure of long-term and end-of-life care provided to people living with dementia:
- Identification of future long-term and end-of-life needs and available care for persons living with dementia.
- Description and monitoring of factors that contribute to problems with nursing home quality, particularly in light of the acceleration of those problems caused by the COVID-19 pandemic, to provide evidence for ongoing changes to the long-term care system.
- Development and evaluation of alternatives to traditional nursing home facilities, including home care options and innovative facility designs.
- Improved understanding of how and when patients use palliative and hospice care options and variation in the end-of-life care available across regions and populations.

TABLE 6-2 Detailed Research Needs

1: Long-Term and End-of-Life Patient Needs and Available Care	• Studies that produce demographic projections, including dementia-specific microsimulation models, based on the anticipated family structure of households in the United States and the availability of family caregivers able and willing to undertake the task of providing care for persons living with late-stage dementia • Studies of how patients and families are informed about their options and how decisions are made, including use of advance directives
2: Improved Nursing Home Quality	• Effects of changes (or differences) in Medicaid payment models on the quality of nursing home and community-based services
3: Development and Evaluation of Alternative Long-Term Care Options	• Studies of the implications for patients and families of greater reliance on home care • Analysis of how innovative alternatives may function in varied settings (e.g., low-income, urban, rural) • Analysis of how alternative staffing models function with patients at different stages of impairment • Comparison of effects of alternative sites and modes of care (e.g., home, assisted living facilities, small residential facilities) on caregivers and clinical outcomes for persons with dementia, as well as on utilization of facilities and services and costs
4: Use of and Variation in End-of-Life Care	• Effects of different types of dementia care programs and payment structures on the timing of hospice referrals • Evaluation of the feasibility of a palliative/home care benefit for patients and families willing to forgo aggressive, life-prolonging services and treatments

CONCLUSION 6-3: Research in the following areas has the potential to substantially strengthen the arrangements through which most dementia care is funded—traditional Medicare, Medicare Advantage, alternative payment models, and Medicaid:
- Comparison of the effects of different financing structures on the quality of care and clinical outcomes for persons living with dementia, as well as effects on their caregivers.
- Examination of ways to modify incentives in reimbursement models to optimize care and reduce unnecessary hospitalizations and other negative outcomes for people living with dementia.
- Development and testing of approaches to integrated financing of medical and social services.

TABLE 6-3 Detailed Research Needs

1: Comparative Effectiveness of Financing Structures	• Comparison of the quality of care, clinical and quality-of-life outcomes, and costs experienced by Medicare beneficiaries living with dementia versus those in managed care plans • Comparison of the outcomes of persons living with advanced dementia being cared for and managed under various specialized managed care programs and alternative payment models, such as special needs plans, accountable care organizations, and Program of All-Inclusive Care for the Elderly programs
2: Ways to Modify Incentives	• Studies of how Medicare Advantage plans and alternative payment models best provide incentives to implement active care management for people living with dementia
3: Evaluation of Approaches to Integrated Financing	• Identification of optimal means of financing and paying for individual services across health care delivery and community-based organizations provided to individual persons with dementia and their caregivers

CHAPTER 7: ECONOMIC COSTS OF DEMENTIA

CONCLUSION 7-1: Research in the following areas is needed to improve understanding of the economic impact of dementia and identify ways to reduce those costs:
- Assessment and quantification of the total economic impact of dementia for individuals and families, including current and future national costs.
- Improved understanding of drivers of dementia-related costs.
- Estimation of the value to individuals, families, and society of innovations in prevention; diagnostics; and treatment, including pharmacologic treatments.

TABLE 7-1 Detailed Research Needs

1: Total Economic Impact	• Quantifying of dementia-related costs not currently measured, including but not limited to caregivers' physical and mental health care use, current and future wages, employability, financial exploitation, harms related to dementia, and impacts across generations of family members • Quantifying and analysis of long-term financial impacts of dementia on a spouse and family members and the intergenerational transfer of inequality related to dementia care costs • Assessment of distribution of costs: how costs and types of costs vary across racial/ethnic populations and other vulnerable groups, etiological type of dementia, age at dementia onset, life course of disease, and type of health care system serving persons living with dementia • Assessment of how costs are distributed across payers • Analysis of innovations in long-term care financing • Assessment of factors, including methods utilized, that drive differences in cost estimates • Improved means of estimating the impacts of new treatments, including new drugs, on Medicare, on patients and families, and on relevant policies
2: Drivers of Costs	• Identification of the multiple individual, familial, community, and societal drivers of costs, using rigorous methods for quantifying the costs attributable to dementia • Analysis of how health care institutions and organizations affect costs through policies and practices
3: Value of Innovations	• Analysis of the value of innovations in dementia prevention, diagnosis, treatment, and care models, considering both direct and indirect costs and the value of extended life-years and quality of years (social value) • Use of rigorous tools, including but not limited to dynamic microsimulation models, for analyzing and quantifying the cost and health implications of innovations in diagnostics and treatments for dementia • Application of the tools of behavioral economics to identify opportunities to reduce the economic impact of dementia

CHAPTER 8: STRENGTHENING DATA COLLECTION AND RESEARCH METHODOLOGY

CONCLUSION 8-1: Advances in research methodology are needed to support progress in virtually every domain of dementia research. Progress in five areas will support a research agenda to reduce the negative impacts of dementia by strengthening data collection and research methodology:
1. Expansion of data infrastructure.
2. Improved measurement of exposures and outcomes.
3. Support for the adoption of more rigorous study designs, particularly in the realm of implementation science, so that research findings can be successfully integrated into clinical and community practices.
4. Development of systematic approaches for integrating evidence from disparate studies.
5. Improved inclusion and representation among both research participants and researchers.

TABLE 8-1 Detailed Research Needs

1: Expansion of Data Infrastructure	• Fostering of new applications for existing data sources, including those from beyond the health care context (e.g., by improving the extraction of relevant constructs from existing data sources)
	• Development of new tools for data linkage across health care system, payer, and community-based data systems, including standards for variables and protocols
	• Funding to support documentation, archiving, and sharing of existing datasets and follow-up of previously abandoned datasets, including RCTs that evaluated relevant treatments but did not originally include dementia-relevant outcomes
	• Creation of a "reference database" by linking multiple data sources that researchers can use for comparison against localized samples and selection of settings for new studies
	• Evaluation of biases in who is selected into research studies; how data are collected; and how measurements are made, including algorithmic bias
	• Increased focus and accountability related to inclusion in research participation and development of a testable scientific framework for conducting inclusive research

Continued

TABLE 8-1 Continued

2: Improved Measurement	• Evaluation of the correspondence between evolving biomarkers and clinical/functional outcomes of relevance to people living with dementia • Development of standardized definitions/tools for identifying dementia and capturing stages of disease • Development of reliable and valid early markers of subsequent disease—potentially based on novel, nontraditional data sources—to foster research on causes of disease • Research to improve measurement validity across disease stages, outcome domains, and assessment modes • Expanded inclusive measurement strategies to yield valid measures for diverse populations, including heterogeneous cultural settings, racial/ethnic identities, gender/sexual minority groups, and linguistic backgrounds • Tools to support valid crosswalks between assessments from different instruments or modalities • Fostering of exploratory research to evaluate novel exposures that may influence disease risk across the life course • Development of improved measures of consent to participate in research
3: Support for the Adoption of More Rigorous Study Designs	• Broadening of the repertoire of tools for estimating causal effects in nonrandomized settings • Development of opportunities for quasi-experimental studies, natural experiments, instrumental variables analyses, regression discontinuity methods, difference-in-difference methods, and other approaches that do not depend on the "no-confounding of exposure–outcome association" assumption • Investment in more comprehensive analyses of RCTs to evaluate mediation, bias, and generalizability, particularly in parallel with real-world data • Support for implementation science's focus on scalable interventions and how new discoveries are disseminated and adopted (e.g., via new policies, behavioral interventions, or systems changes) • Development of platforms to facilitate fielding of pragmatic trials embedded in health care systems and analysis of the results of those trials • Investment in qualitative work to identify new questions, improve the cultural validity of measurements, and better understand why past interventions succeeded or failed • Improved strategies for evaluating complex, dynamic interventions, such as community-based initiatives • Development of guidelines for conceptualizing study design trade-offs that could be used to prioritize research investments

TABLE 8-1 Continued

4: Development of Systematic Approaches for Evidence Integration	• Fostering of research on heterogeneity in treatment response/exposure effects across populations, and methods to support generalizing from samples in existing studies to other populations • Expansion of meta-analytic and related approaches to integrate findings from heterogeneous study designs more flexibly and correct for bias • Quantifying of the population health and health equity impacts of proposed policies, interventions, or therapies • Facilitation of linkage of data, including data from electronic health records, claims, research studies, and records of community-based organizations (e.g., consenting, nonrandomized control groups; proxy respondents)
5: Improved Inclusion and Representation Among Research Participants and Researchers	• Bolstering of training efforts to accommodate changing standards of living, continue to foster diversity and representation in the research workforce, and emphasize the interdisciplinary skills noted elsewhere

CHAPTER 9: TEN-YEAR RESEARCH PRIORITIES

CONCLUSION 9-1: A 10-year research agenda for the behavioral and social sciences will have maximal impact in reducing the negative impacts of dementia and improving quality of life if it distributes attention and resources across five priorities:

1. Improvements in the lives of people affected by dementia, including those who develop it and their families and caregivers, as well as in the social and clinical networks that surround them, through research on factors that affect the development of disease and its outcomes, promising innovative practices and new models of care, and policies that can facilitate the dissemination of interventions found to be effective.
2. Rectifying of disparities across groups and geographic regions that affect who develops dementia, how the disease progresses, outcomes and quality of life, and access to health care and supportive services.
3. Development of innovations with the potential to improve the quality of care and social supports for individuals and communities and to support improved quality of life (e.g., reducing financial abuse and stressors, finding relevant affordable housing and care facilities, gaining access to important services).
4. Easing of the financial and economic costs of dementia to individuals, families, and society and balancing of long-term costs with long-term outcomes across the life span.

5. Pursuit of advances in research capability, including study design, measurement, analysis, and evidence integration, as well as the development of data infrastructure needed to study key dementia-related topics.

TABLE 9-1 Priorities for a 10-Year Research Agenda

Research Priority	Research Conclusions
1: Improving the Lives of People Touched by Dementia	2-1
	3-1
	3-2
	4-1
	5-1
	6-1
	6-2
	6-3
2: Rectifying Inequities and Disparities	2-1
	3-2
	4-1
	5-1
	6-1
	7-1
3: Developing Innovations	3-1
	3-2
	4-1
	5-1
	6-1
	6-2
	6-3
4: Easing and Balancing Costs	6-3
	7-1
5: Pursuing Advances in Research Capability	2-1
	3-2
	4-1
	8-1

CONCLUSION 9-2: A 10-year research agenda will be optimally effective if it
- is coordinated to ensure that the breadth of topics identified in this report is addressed sufficiently without redundancy and competing initiatives;
- consistently takes into account fundamental socioeconomic factors that influence who develops dementia, access to high-quality care, and outcomes;

- includes pragmatic, implementation, and dissemination research needed to ensure that findings can be implemented effectively in clinical and community settings; and
- addresses potential policy implications that are articulated beginning in the planning stages and assessed during the course of the investigations.

RECOMMENDATION 9-1: Funders of dementia-related research, including federal agencies, such as the National Institutes of Health and the Agency for Healthcare Research and Quality, along with relevant philanthropic and other organizations, such as the Patient-Centered Outcomes Research Institute, should use guidelines for the awarding of research grants to establish incentives for

- coordination of research objectives with the research agenda priorities identified in this report to ensure that key areas are funded without undue overlap and to foster links across research efforts;
- interdisciplinary research and inclusion of stakeholders in research partnerships;
- attention to topics that have not typically been part of standard medical research but are important to those living with dementia, including isolation, financial security, and housing options;
- rigorous evaluation and implementation research needed to translate findings into programs with impact on a broad scale; and
- dissemination of research findings to policy makers.